Monographs on Pathology of Laboratory Animals

Sponsored by the International Life Sciences Institute

The following volumes have appeared so far

Endocrine System
1983. 346 figures. XV, 366 pages. ISBN 3-540-11677-X

Respiratory System
1985. 279 figures. XV, 240 pages. ISBN 3-540-13521-9

Digestive System
1985. 352 figures. XVIII, 386 pages. ISBN 3-540-15815-4

Urinary System
1986. 362 figures. XVIII, 405 pages. ISBN 3-540-16591-6

Genital System
1987. 340 figures. XVII, 304 pages. ISBN 3-540-17604-7

Nervous System
1988. 242 figures. XVI, 233 pages. ISBN 3-540-19416-9

Integument and Mammary Glands
1989. 468 figures. XI, 347 pages. ISBN 3-540-51025-7

Hemopoietic System
1990. 351 figures. XVIII, 336 pages. ISBN 3-540-52212-3

Cardiovascular and Musculoskeletal Systems
1991. 390 figures. XVII, 312 pages. ISBN 3-540-53876-3

The following volumes are in preparation

Non-human Primates I
Non-human Primates II

T. C. Jones U. Mohr R. D. Hunt (Eds.)

Eye and Ear

With 141 Figures and 14 Tables

Springer-Verlag
Berlin Heidelberg New York
London Paris Tokyo
Hong Kong Barcelona
Budapest

Thomas Carlyle Jones, D. V. M., D. Sc.
Professor of Comparative Pathology
Emeritus, Harvard Medical School
ILSI Research Foundation
1126 Sixteenth Street, N. W., Washington, DC 20036, USA

Ulrich Mohr, M. D.
Professor of Experimental Pathology
Medizinische Hochschule Hannover
Institut für Experimentelle Pathologie
Konstanty-Gutschow-Strasse 8
W-3000 Hannover 61, Federal Republic of Germany

Ronald Duncan Hunt, D. V. M.
Professor of Comparative Pathology
Harvard Medical School
New England Regional Primate Research Center
One Pine Hill Drive, Southborough, MA 01772, USA

ISBN 3-540-54044-X Springer-Verlag Berlin Heidelberg New York
ISBN 0-387-54044-X Springer-Verlag New York Berlin Heidelberg

Library of Congress Cataloging-in-Publication Data
Eye and ear/T. C. Jones, U. Mohr, R. D. Hunt (eds.) p. cm. – (Monographs on pathology of laboratory animals) Includes index.
ISBN 3-540-54044-X (Berlin). – ISBN 0-387-54044-X (New York)
1. Eye – Histopathology. 2. Ear – Histopathology. 3. Laboratory animals – Diseases. 4. Anatomy, Pathological. I. Jones, Thomas Carlyle. II. Mohr, U. (Ulrich) III. Hunt, Ronald Duncan. IV. Series RE66.E94 1991 617.7'1-dc20 91-15514

Reproduction of the Illustrations: Gustav Dreher, Württembergische Graphische Kunstanstalt GmbH, Stuttgart
Typesetting, Printing, and Binding: Appl, Wemding
23/3130-543210 – Printed on acid-free paper

Foreword

The International Life Sciences Institute (ILSI) was established in 1978 to stimulate and support scientific research and educational programs related to nutrition, toxicology, and food safety, and to encourage cooperation in these programs among scientists in universities, industry, and government agencies to assist in the resolution of health and safety issues.

To supplement and enhance these efforts, ILSI has made a major commitment to supporting programs to harmonize toxicologic testing, to advance a more uniform interpretation of bioassay results worldwide, to promote a common understanding of lesion classifications, and to encourage wide discussion of these topics among scientists. The *Monographs on the Pathology of Laboratory Animals* are designed to facilitate communication among those involved in the safety testing of foods, drugs, and chemicals. The complete set will cover all organ systems and is intended for use by pathologists, toxicologists, and others concerned with evaluating toxicity and carcinogenicity studies. The international nature of the project – as reflected in the composition of the editorial board and the diversity of the authors and editors – strengthens our expectations that understanding and cooperation will be improved worldwide through the series.

Alex Malaspina
President
International Life Sciences Institute

Preface

This book, on the eye and ear, is the tenth volume of a set prepared under the sponsorship of the International Life Sciences Institute (ILSI). One aim of this set on the pathology of laboratory animals is to provide information which will be useful to pathologists, especially those involved in studies on the safety of foods, drugs, chemicals, and other substances in the environment. It is expected that this and future volumes will contribute to better communication, on an international basis, among people in government, industry, and academia who are involved in protection of the public health.

The arrangement of this volume is based, in part, upon the philosophy that the first step toward understanding a pathologic lesion is its precise and unambiguous identification. Therefore, the microscopic and ultrastructural features of a lesion that are particularly useful to the pathologist for definitive diagnosis are considered foremost. Diagnostic terms preferred by the author and editors are used as the subject heading for each pathologic lesion. Synonyms are listed although most are not preferred and some may have been used erroneously in prior publications. The problems arising in differential diagnosis of similar lesions are considered in detail. The biologic significance of each pathologic lesion is considered under such headings as etiology, natural history, pathogenesis, and frequency of occurrence under natural or experimental conditions.

Comparison of information available on similar lesions in man and other species is valuable as a means to gain broader understanding of the processes involved. Knowledge of this nature is needed to form a scientific basis for safety evaluations and experimental pathology. References to pertinent literature are provided in close juxtaposition to the text in order to support conclusions in the text and lead toward additional information. Illustrations are an especially important means of nonverbal communication, especially among pathologists, and therefore constitute important features of each volume.

The subject under each heading is covered in concise terms and is expected to stand alone but, in some instances, it is important to refer to other parts of the volume. A comprehensive index is provided to enhance the use of each volume as a reference.

Some omissions are inevitable and we solicit comments from our colleagues to identify parts which need strengthening or correcting. We have endeavored to include important lesions which a pathologist might encounter in studies involving the rat, mouse, or hamster. Newly recognized lesions or better understanding of old ones may make revised editions necessary in the future.

The editors wish to express their deep gratitude to all of the individuals who have helped with this enterprise. We are indebted to each author and member of the Editorial Board whose name appears elsewhere in the volume. We are especially grateful to the Officers and Board of Trustees of the International Life Sciences Institute for their support and understanding. Several people have worked directly on important details in this venture. These include Mrs. Nina Mur-

ray, Executive Secretary; Mrs. Ann Balliett and Ms. Cora Moore, Editorial Assistants; Mrs. June Armstrong, Medical Illustrator; Mrs. Sydney Fingold, Librarian; Ms. Lori MacInnes, Secretary; Ms. Sharon K. Coleman, ILSI Coordinator for External Affairs; Ms. Roberta Gutman, ILSI Publication Manager, and Mrs. Sharon Weiss, Associate Director, ILSI Research Foundation, were helpful on many occasions.
We are particularly grateful to Dr. Dietrich Götze and his staff at Springer-Verlag for the quality of the published product.

September 1991

THE EDITORS
T. C. Jones
U. Mohr
R. D. Hunt

Contents

Contributors

Sally S. Atherton, Ph. D.
Associate Professor
Department of Microbiology and Immunology
University of Miami School of Medicine
Miami, Florida, USA

William W. Carlton, D. V. M., Ph. D.
Leslie Morton Hutchings Professor
of Veterinary Pathology and Toxicology
Department of Veterinary Pathobiology
School of Veterinary Medicine, Purdue University
West Lafayette, Indiana, USA

Taisan Chiu, D. V. M., Ph. D.
Senior Research Pathologist
E. I. du Pont de Nemours & Company
Haskell Laboratory for Toxicology and Industrial Medicine
Newark, Delaware, USA

Cynthia S. Cook, D. V. M., Ph. D.
Research Assistant Professor
Department of Growth and Development
University of California
San Francisco, California, USA

Pierre Duprat, D. V. M., Ph. D.
Director of Pathology
Laboratoires Merck Sharp & Dohme
Route de Marsat
Riom Cédex, France

Jeffrey I. Everitt, D. V. M.
Staff Scientist
Department of Experimental Pathology and Toxicology
Chemical Industry Institute of Toxicology
Research Triangle Park, North Carolina, USA

Heinrich Ernst, D. V. M.
Fraunhofer Institute of Toxicology and Aerosol Research
Hannover, Federal Republic of Germany

Steven R. Frame, D. V. M., Ph. D.
Staff Pathologist, E. I. du Point de Nemours & Company
Haskell Laboratory for Toxicology and Industrial Medicine
Newark, Delaware, USA

G. H. Hottendorf, D. V. M., Ph. D.
Adjunct Professor
Pathology Department, Medical University of South Carolina
Charleston, South Carolina, USA

Alexander Kast, D.V.M.
Privat-Dozent, Senior Scientist
Department of Veterinary Pathology, University Giessen
Boehringer Ingelheim Zentrale GmbH
Ingelheim am Rhein, Federal Republic of Germany

Georg J. Krinke, D.V.M.
Research Associate
Department of Toxicological Pathology, Ciba-Geigy AG
Basel, Switzerland

Seymour Levine, M.D.
Professor of Pathology
Basic Science Building, New York Medical College
Valhalla, New York, USA

Renate Lüllmann-Rauch, M.D.
Senior Lecturer in Anatomy
Department of Anatomy, University of Kiel
Kiel, Federal Republic of Germany

Yousef Matuk, Ph.D.
Associate Professor of Ocular Biochemistry
Department of Ophthalmology, University of Toronto
Gage Research Institute
Toronto, Ontario, Canada

Ulrich Mohr, Dr. med.
Professor, Institute of Experimental Pathology
Hannover Medical School
Hannover, Federal Republic of Germany

Sylvain Michel Molon-Noblot, BSc, MSc, Ph.D.
Senior Research Biologist
Laboratoires Merck Sharp & Dohme
Route de Marsat
Riom Cédex, France

Roger A. Owen, Ph.D., M.R.C. PATH, F.R.C.V.S.
Pathologist, Laboratoires MSD-CHIBRET
Centre de Reserches
Riom Cédex, France

Robert L. Peiffer, Jr., D.V.M., Ph.D., DIP ACVO Professor
Departments of Ophthalmology and Pathology
University of North Carolina
Chapel Hill, North Carolina, USA

Dean P. Porter, M.D.
Resident in Ophthalmology
Department of Ophthalmology
University of Texas Health Center
Galveston, Texas, USA

James A. Render, D.V.M., Ph.D.
Associate Professor
Department of Pathology, College of Veterinary Medicine
Michigan State University
East Lansing, Michigan, USA

Susanne Rittinghausen
Fraunhofer Institute of Toxicology and Aerosol Research
Hannover, Federal Republic of Germany

John Curtis Seely, D.V.M.
Veterinary Pathologist, Pathco, Inc.
Research Triangle Park, North Carolina, USA

John A. Shadduck, D.V.M., Ph.D.
Professor and Dean
College of Veterinary Medicine, Texas A & M University
College Station, Texas, USA

Thomas J. Van Winkle, D.V.M.
Assistant Professor of Pathobiology
Laboratory of Pathology
School of Veterinary Medicine, University of Pennsylvania
Philadelphia, Pennsylvania, USA

Herbert E. Whiteley, D.V.M., Ph.D.
Associate Professor of Pathology
College of Veterinary Medicine, University of Illinois
Urbana, Illinois, USA

The Eye

Anatomy of the Ocular Surfaces, Cornea, and Conjunctiva, Rat and Mouse

Sylvain M. Molon-Noblot and Pierre Duprat

Gross Appearance

The eyes are protected by eyelids and suspended in the orbit by ocular muscles, which are also responsible for eye movements. The eyeball is a multilayered structure: an external fibrous layer for protection, an intermediate vascular layer for nutrition, and an internal layer connected to the central nervous system (CNS) for photoreception. The other ocular structures – aqueous humor, lens, and vitreous body – are accessory visual structures.
The ocular surfaces are represented by the cornea and conjunctiva. The cornea is a circular transparent tissue covering one-sixth of the anterior surface of the eyeball; it protrudes slightly due to its smaller radius of curvature than that of the sclera. The conjunctiva covers the posterior surface of the eyelid (forming the palpebral conjunctiva) and part of the sclera, from the fornix to the sclerocorneal junction (forming the bulbar conjunctiva). Description here is limited to the palpebral conjunctiva, which represents the larger portion.

Microscopic Features

Cornea

The cornea is a dense connective tissue membrane covered with an external nonkeratinized stratified epithelium and an internal single layer of flat epithelium (endothelium) resting on a thick homogeneous basal lamina, Descemet's membrane (Fig. 1). In normal conditions, the cornea is not vascularized, but presents a dense innervation mainly located in the anterior stroma and the basal epithelium, forming infraepithelial plexuses.

Palpebral Conjunctiva

The palpebral conjunctiva consists of a nonkeratinized stratified epithelium sitting on a well-vascularized loose connective tissue (Fig. 2). From the lid margin to the fornix, it is successively represented by its marginal, tarsal, and orbital portions. The number of epithelial cell layers diminishes from the marginal to the tarsal areas. In contrast to the cornea, goblet cells are normally found in the conjunctiva. These cells function as unicellular apocrine glands secreting mucus over the ocular surface with a consistency denser than that of the lacrimal fluid (Prince et al. 1960). They are represented by tall columnar cells in the upper portion, and cells of various shapes near the fornix (Bisaria and Bisaria 1980). Topographic analysis reveals that the density and size of goblet cell clusters are greatest in the forniceal zone, with a gradual decrease toward the bulbar and orbital zones, but these cells are absent in the limbal and tarsal conjunctiva (Huang et al. 1988). At places, goblet cells are associated with superficial crypts, to form the so-called intraepithelial cysts (Weingeist 1973 a; Pfister 1975).

Ultrastructure

Cornea, Anterior Epithelium

The anterior epithelium typically includes a basal lamina, a single layer of columnar basal cells, two layers of intermediate cells, and six to ten layers of flat superficial squamous cells. Secreted by the basal cells, the basal lamina (basement membrane) is a continuous 100- to 300-Å-thick layer of faintly granular osmiophilic material separating the stroma from the basal epithelium. The basal cell layer is tightly attached to the basal lamina by hemidesmosomes

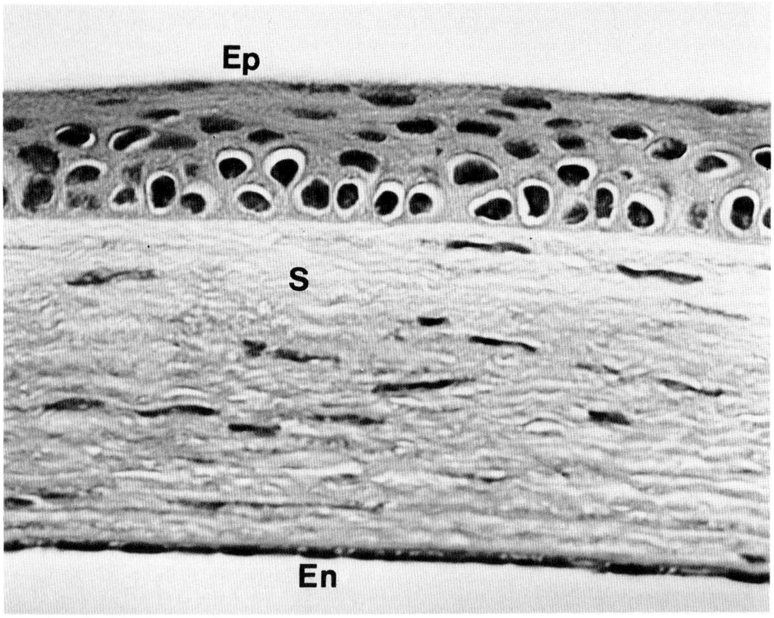

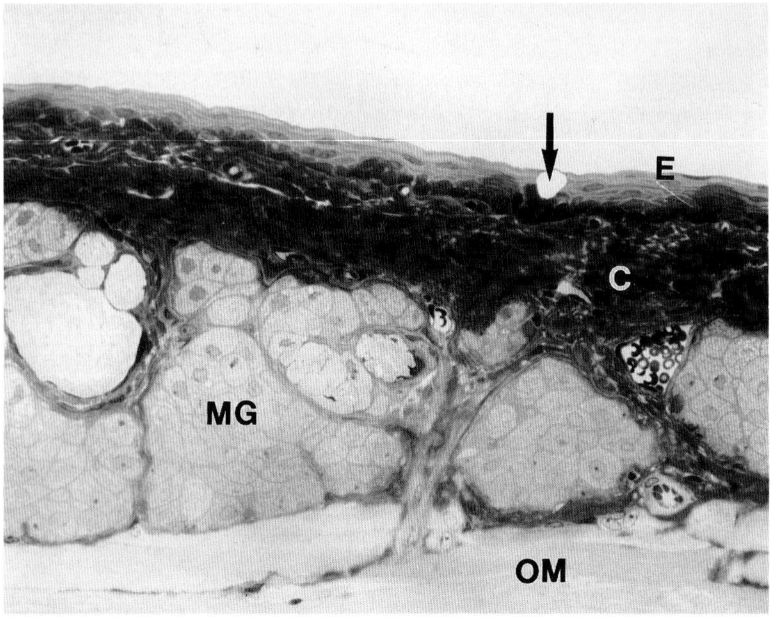

Fig. 1 *(above).* Cornea, mouse. Transverse section; note regular multilayered structure composed of a stratified epithelium *(Ep),* a dense stroma *(S)* with elongated nuclei of keratocytes, and a monostratified flat endothelium *(En)* lining adjacent to a thick basal lamina, Descemet's membrane. H & E, ×375

Fig. 2 *(below).* Lower eyelid, rat. Inner surface of the eyelid is covered with the palpebral conjunctiva consisting of a nonkeratinized stratified epithelium *(E)* resting on well-vascularized connective tissue *(C).* Several goblet cells are clustered to form an intraepithelial cyst *(arrow). MG,* meibomian gland; *OM,* orbicularis oculi muscle. Toluidine blue, ×160

represented by focal densifications of the internal layer of the plasma membrane (Teng 1961; Pedler 1962). Basal cells are tall columnar cells with a flattened base, a dome-shaped apex, and an interdigitated lateral plasma membrane (Sheldon 1956). The nucleus is roughly spherical, but it may be more or less indented (Jakus 1954). The cytoplasm contains numerous bundles of filaments, converging toward either the basal hemidesmosomes or the desmosomes located at the lateral plasma membrane of adjacent cells. Other organelles consist of a few elongated mitochondria with slightly dilated longitudinal cristae, a limited and generally

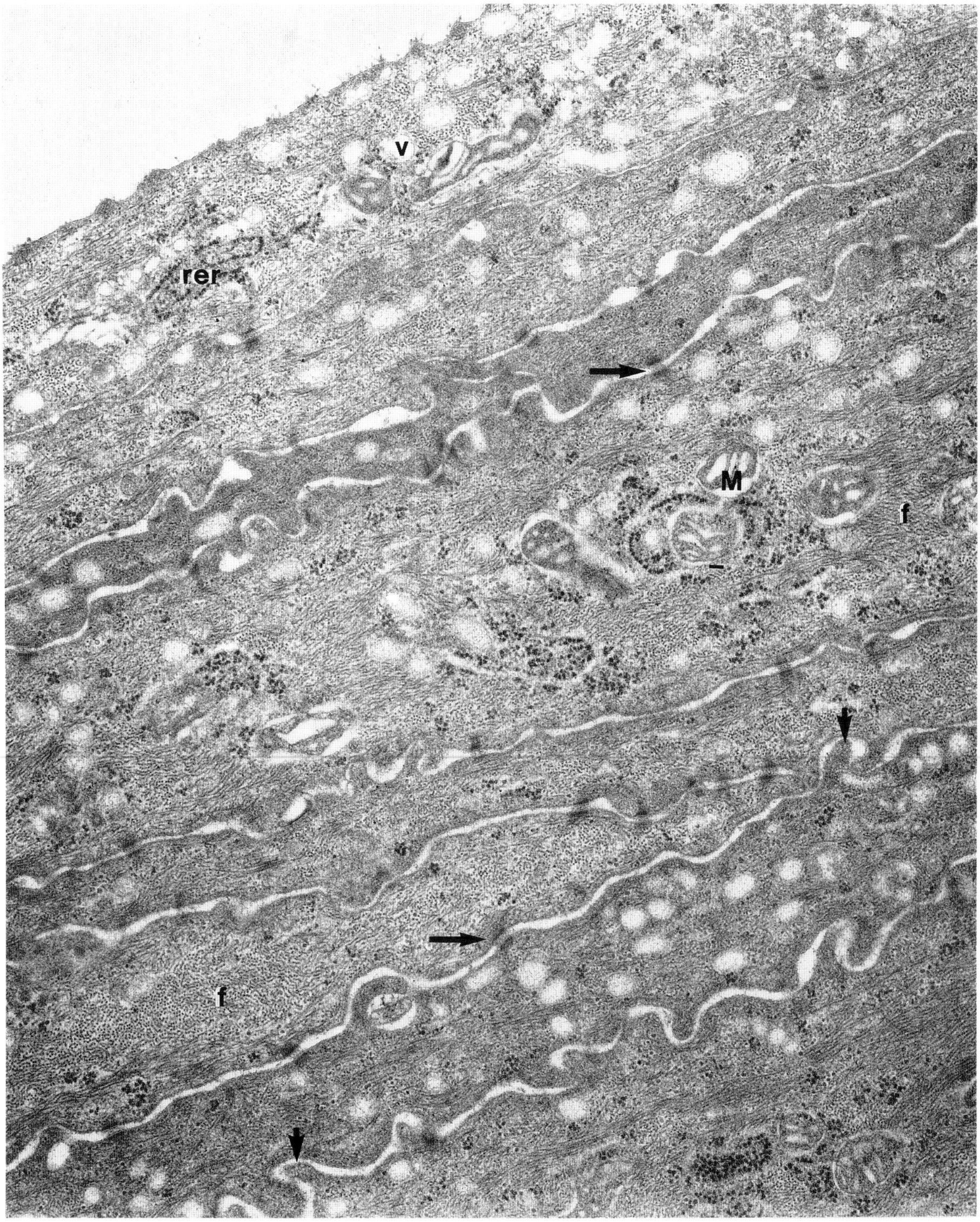

Fig. 3. Superficial corneal epithelial cells, rat. Close contact between epithelial cells results from numerous desmosomes *(arrows)* and multiple infolding of plasma membranes *(arrowheads)*. The cytoplasmic content of superficial epithelial cells consists of some mitochondria *(M)*, rare rough endoplasmic reticulum *(rer)*, and numerous filaments *(f)* and vesicles *(v)*. TEM, × 30000

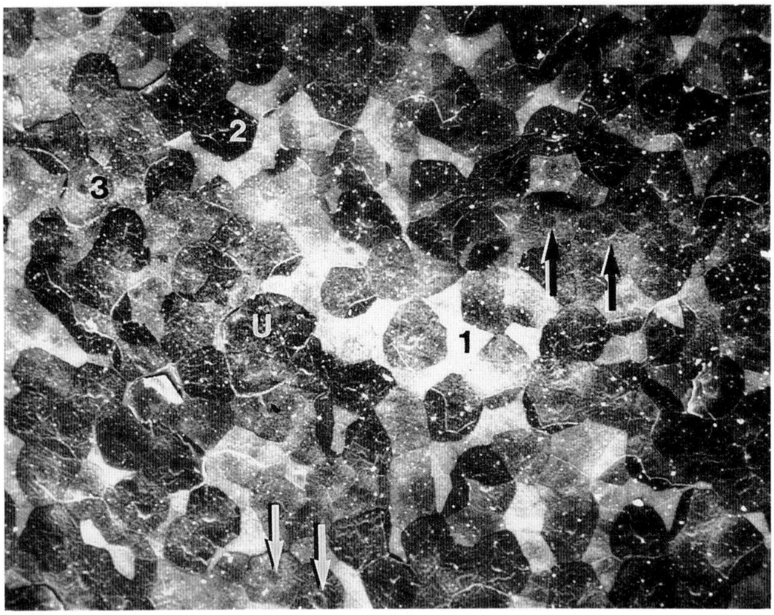

Fig. 4. Corneal epithelial surface, rat. Note the polygonal cells arranged in a mosaic pattern. Light cells *(1)*, dark cells *(2)*, and intermediate cells *(3)* can be distinguished according to their brightness under scanning illumination. Central and inconspicuous nuclei are discernable in some epithelial cells *(arrows)*. SEM, ×300

perinuclear rough endoplasmic reticulum, some round membrane-bound vacuoles, and abundant free ribosomes. The transitional zone between the basal cells and superficial squamous cells is formed by polygonal intermediate cells or wing cells. Wing cells are attached to each other by numerous desmosomes present in the deep infoldings of adjacent cell surfaces (Kaye and Pappas 1962). The ultrastructure of wing cells is similar to that of basal cells, but with fewer of organelles and a nucleus slightly elongated and oriented parallel to the corneal surface. The cytoplasm contains mainly filaments and free ribosomes. The rough endoplasmic reticulum is scarce and there are fewer mitochondria than in basal cells. The superificial squamous epithelium consists of flattened cells about 4 μm thick and 40 μm long (Fig. 3). The nucleus of superficial cells is elongated with an orientation parallel to the corneal surface. Scarce rough endoplasmic reticulum and elongated mitochondria generally occupy the perinuclear region; numerous round or oval membrane-bound vacuoles are visible between the bundles of filaments which represent the most important cytoplasmic component of superficial cells. In the interdigitations of plasma membranes, intercellular junctions are represented by desmosomes and zonula occludens, which explain the relative impermeability of the cornea (Kenyon 1979). The outer plasma membrane of superficial cells produces microvilli and microplicae covered with a thin layer rich in glycoproteins and glycolipids (Wells and Hazlett 1984).

The surface of the cornea observed by scanning electron microscopy (SEM) consists of the juxtaposition of flat polygonal cells (Fig. 4). According to their brightness under scanning illumination, epithelial cells in the rat and the mouse can be divided into light, intermediate, and dark cells. Such a description has been proposed for rabbits, cats, dogs, monkeys, and humans (Blümcke and Morgenroth 1967; Hoffmann 1972; Pfister 1973; Pfister and Burnstein 1977; Renard et al. 1983a). In the rat and the mouse, light cells are characterized by an irregular shape with a smaller surface (Table 1), and a cell membrane uniformly covered with dense microvilli measuring approximately 0.15 μm in diameter (Fig. 5). Dark cells have a slightly larger surface area than other epithelial cells, and their cell membranes bear only rare and short microvilli. Intermediate cells, which represent the majority of epithelial cells, have numerous microvilli, but the distribution is not uniform on the cell surface; cell density is generally less pronounced at the periphery and above the nuclear region. This difference in brightness is considered by most authors to be related to the length and the density of microvilli and

Table 1. Semiquantitative analysis of the cell surface of corneal epithelial cells in laboratory animals

Species	All cells (μm^2)	Light cells (μm^2)	Dark cells (μm^2)
Mouse	667 ± 246	450 ± 222	745 ± 234
Rat	718 ± 347	555 ± 272	950 ± 385
Rabbit	956 ± 297	491 ± 198	985 ± 278
Dog	1260 ± 373	580 ± 308	1300 ± 286

All figures are means ± standard deviations.

microplicae covering the surface of outer epithelial cells (Hoffmann and Schweichel 1972; Kenyon 1979; Hazlett et al. 1980; Dormans and Van Logten 1982; Pfister and Burnstein 1977). However, for others it is linked to the amount of mucosubstances visible on the cell surfaces (Renard et al. 1983b). Based on these morphologic differences between corneal epithelial cells, it has been proposed that the various cell types on the normal corneal surface are transitory stages of the same cell type, the light cells representing juvenile cells and the dark cells old degenerating cells (Hoffmann and Schweichel 1972; Pfister 1973).

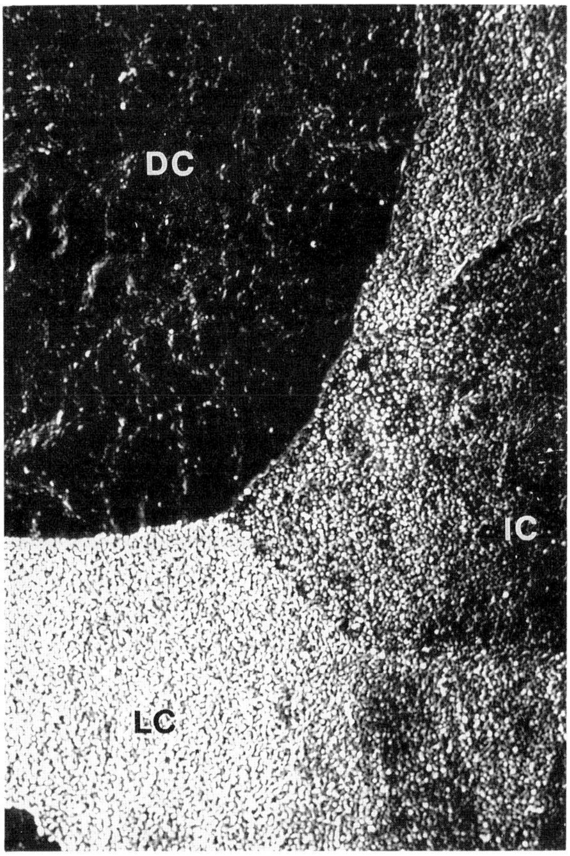

Fig. 5. Corneal epithelial surface, rat. Light cells *(LC)* are uniformly covered with dense microvilli, as opposed to dark cells *(DC)*, which have few and short microvilli. On the cell surface of intermediate cells *(IC)*, the distribution of microvilli is not uniform. SEM, × 3500

Cornea, Stroma

The stroma constitutes the major portion of the cornea, representing 80% in the rat and 70% in the mouse of the total corneal thickness. The Bowman's membrane described in man and several animal species (Pouliquen 1969; Hogan et al. 1971; Jacobsen et al. 1983) as a specialized layer of the anterior stroma has no equivalent in the rat and the mouse. In these laboratory animals, the entire stroma consists of stromal lamellae, fibroblasts (keratocytes), and matrix. Stromal lamellae are 1- to 3 µm-thick densely packed bundles of parallel collagenous fibrils (Fig. 6). Longitudinal sections of fibrils demonstrate a constant diameter of 260 Å and a banding periodicity of 640 Å. The collagenous fibrils are equally separated by an interfibrillar space filled with granular material. The bundles run in different directions, obliquely in the anterior stroma and parallel and more regularly arranged in the posterior stroma (Martin and Anderson 1981). Between lamellae, elongated fibroblasts are regularly interspersed; they have slender and long processes extending from the cell body in many directions (Kaye and Pappas 1962). These branching processes are thought to assure frequent contacts between fibroblasts (Hogan et al. 1971). Fibroblasts possess large elongated central nuclei rich in heterochromatin. The cytoplasm contains a well-developed rough endoplasmic reticulum frequently arranged in flat parallel cisternae (Fig. 6).

Other organelles are represented by a few small mitochondria, a Golgi apparatus with generally flat and lucent sacculi, and numerous filaments and free ribosomes giving the cytoplasm a homogeneous electron-dense pattern. The matrix of the stroma is rich in mucoproteins and glycoproteins. These substances fill the interfibrillar spaces and determine the exact position of stromal fibrils. This regular arrangement of lamellae and collagenous fibrils contributes to the transparency of the cornea.

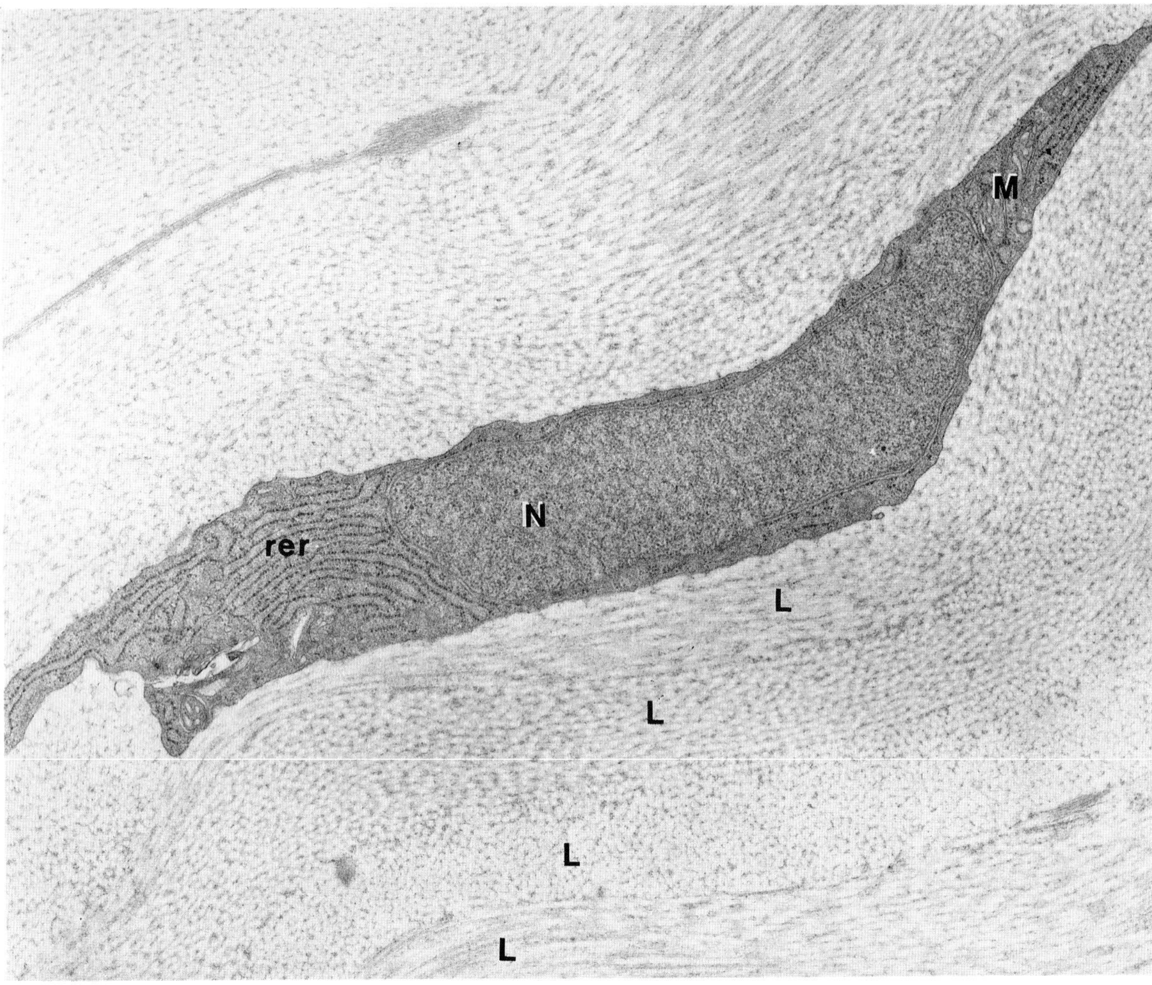

Fig. 6. Corneal stroma, rat. In the numerous superimposed collagenous lamellae *(L)*, fibrils run in the same direction, but in different lamellae orientations are varied. Elongated fibrocyte interspersed between collagenous lamellae has a prominent dense nucleus *(N)*, some round-shaped mitochondria *(M)*, and abundant rough endoplasmic reticulum *(rer)* with parallel cisternae. TEM, ×13000

Cornea, Descemet's Membrane

Descement's membrane is a 3- to 5-μm-thick homogeneous basal lamina secreted by the endothelium throughout life (Fig. 7). It contains regularly arranged fine collagenous fibrils embedded in an amorphous substance rich in mucopolysaccharides. These fibrils form layers parallel to the corneal surface and meet at nodes to form a hexagonal pattern (Jakus 1954). Ultrastructurally, the fibrillar and faintly periodic aspect is more discernable near the stroma; transitional aspects between posterior stroma and Descemet's membrane are occasionally observed, and consist of bundles of thin collagenous fibrils of Descemet's membrane interspersed between thicker stromal collagenous fibers.

Cornea, Endothelium

The endothelium consists of a single layer of flattened cuboidal cells lining the inner surface of the cornea. Endothelial cells (Fig. 7) have the typical ultrastructure of metabolically active cells: large center nuclei with peripheral heterochromatin, numerous rod-shaped mitochondria, abundant rough endoplasmic reticulum, prominent Golgi apparatus, and pinocytotic vesicles in the plasma membrane (Kaye and Pappas 1972).

The lateral cell margins are strongly infolded and intercellular junctions consist of macula adherens, zonula occludens, and macula occludens. In the rat and mouse as in other mammals, no desmosomal junction are normally

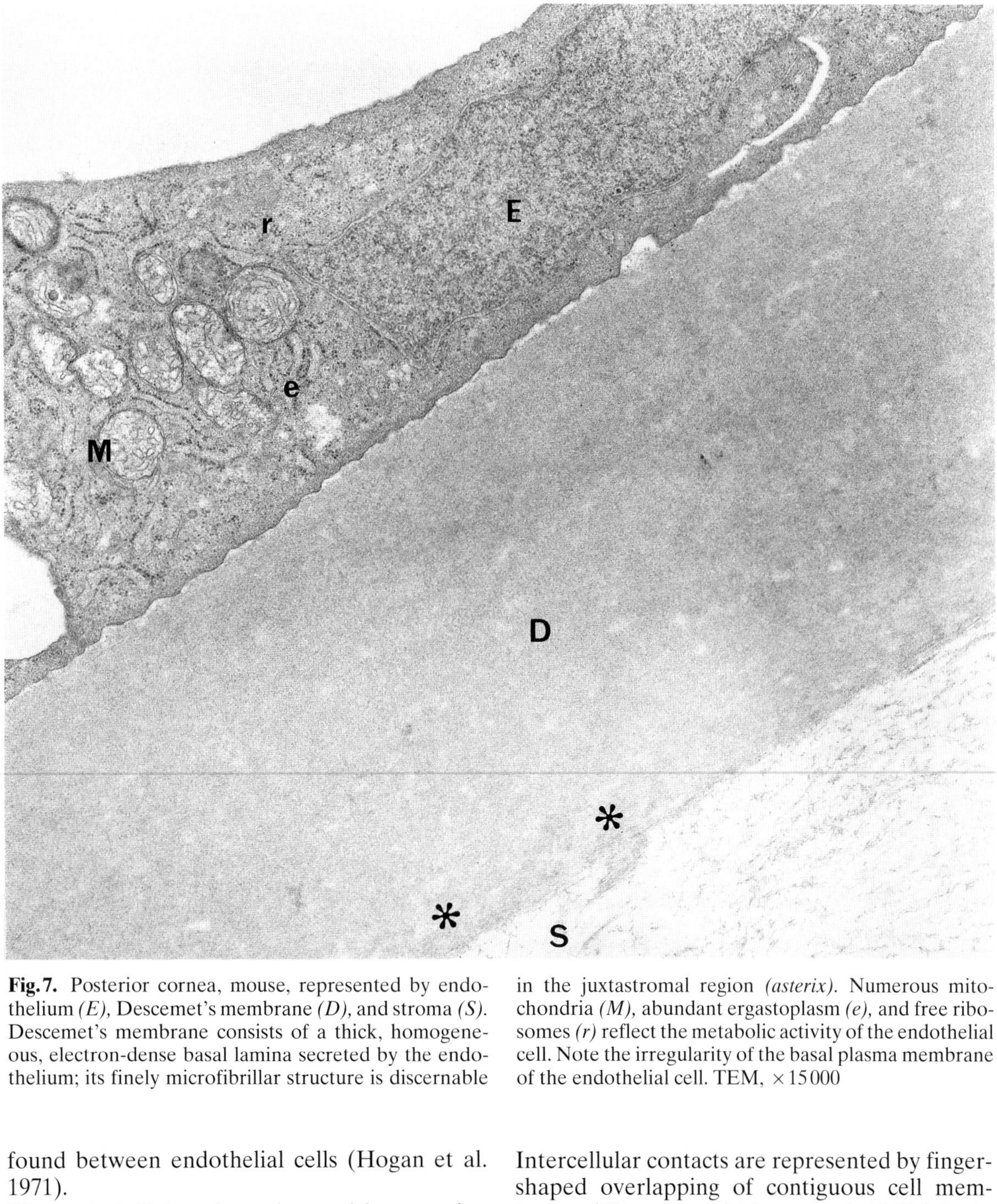

Fig. 7. Posterior cornea, mouse, represented by endothelium *(E)*, Descemet's membrane *(D)*, and stroma *(S)*. Descemet's membrane consists of a thick, homogeneous, electron-dense basal lamina secreted by the endothelium; its finely microfibrillar structure is discernable in the juxtastromal region *(asterix)*. Numerous mitochondria *(M)*, abundant ergastoplasm *(e)*, and free ribosomes *(r)* reflect the metabolic activity of the endothelial cell. Note the irregularity of the basal plasma membrane of the endothelial cell. TEM, ×15000

found between endothelial cells (Hogan et al. 1971).

The endothelial surface observed by scanning electron microscopy consists of the juxtaposition of uniformly dark polygonal cells (Fig. 8). In the rat, corneal endothelium has a high frequency of hexagonal cells with minimal variation in cell size (Meyer et al. 1988). Endothelial cells are covered by a few short microvilli randomly distributed on the cell surface; a slightly prominent round-shaped nucleus is generally visible in the central area (Hervouet et al. 1971). Intercellular contacts are represented by finger-shaped overlapping of contiguous cell membranes (Blümcke and Morgenroth 1967; Martin and Anderson 1981; Basu 1983).

Palpebral Conjunctiva, Epithelium

The palpebral conjunctival epithelium consists of cuboidal basal cells, polyhedral intermediate cells, and flattened superficial cells. Basal cells are smaller and more irregular in the conjuncti-

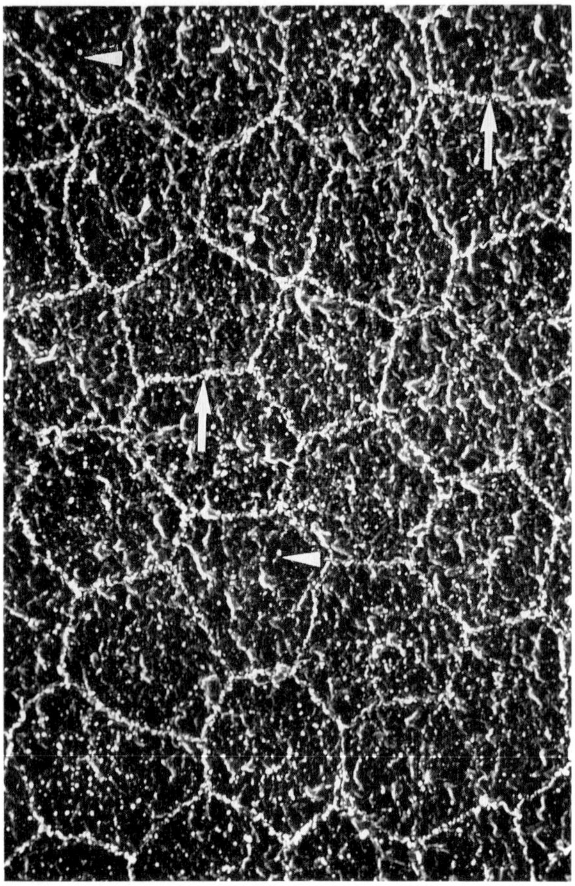

Fig. 8. Corneal endothelial surface, rat. The endothelium consists of flat uniform polygonal cells in juxtaposition. Intercellular contacts between neighboring cells are clearly visible *(arrows)*, and short microvilli are randomly distributed on the cell surface *(arrowheads)*. SEM, ×1500

va than the corresponding columnar cells of the corneal epithelium. Their basal poles contain fewer hemidesmosomes and are closely associated with the irregularities of the underlying basal lamina (Fig. 9).

The central nucleus has a prominent nucleolus and an abundant marginated heterochromatin. The cytoplasm contains numerous free ribosomes and bundle-packed filaments. In the perinuclear region a well-developed Golgi apparatus is visible together with rare mitochondria and limited rough endoplasmic reticulum. Lateral plasma membranes are markedly infolded, and intercellular junctions are represented by frequent desmosomes associated with the intracytoplasmic filaments. Between the hemidesmosomes, the basal plasma membrane often has numerous pinocytotic vesicles. The intermediate epithelial cell layers consist of slightly elongated polyhedral cells with prominent central nuclei parallel with the conjunctival surface (Fig. 10). The cytoplasm is rich in filaments as in basal cells, but mitochondria are more elongated and more numerous. Another difference is the presence of round membrane-bound vesicles with finely granular content, preferentially located in the peripheral cytoplasm and close to the Golgi apparatus. Intermediate cells are firmly attached together by desmosomal junctions; between them, adjacent cell membranes protrude short and slender digitations. The superficial epithelium consists of several layers of flattened epithelial cells, and its structure does not fundamentally differ from the corresponding portion of the cornea. Intracytoplasmic organellae are mainly represented by filaments, ribosomes, and vesicles containing homogeneous electron-dense material. These vesicles, abundant in intermediate and superficial epithelial cells, may represent mucin production from nongoblet cells of the conjunctiva (Kenyon 1979). Outer cells have microprojections, smaller than those covering the corneal surface (on flattened outer corneal cells).

The presence of goblet cells constitutes the main difference between normal conjunctival and corneal epithelium. The nucleus is compressed in the basal pole, and the apical pole is filled with small membrane-bound mucinous granules, extruding from the epithelial surface in hypermature cells. The reduced cytoplasm interspersed between the granules contains ribosomes, filaments, small mitochondriae, and scant ergastoplasm.

Scanning electron microscopic observation of the palpebral conjunctiva shows a wavy surface formed by the juxtaposition of irregular polygonal cells with marginal folds delineating the intercellular contacts (Fig. 11). At the lid margin the keratinized stratified epithelium of the skin is changed into the nonkeratinized squamous epithelium of the conjunctiva (Fig. 12) (Weingeist 1973b). In this transitional zone, orifices of the meibomian glands are observable. Based on their appearance under scanning illumination, epithelial cells of the conjunctiva can be divided into light, dark, and intermediate cells (Fig. 13). As in corneal epithelial cells, this appearance is linked to variations in microvilli and microplicae density on the cell surfaces (Pfister 1975; Kenyon 1979). These microprojections of the plasma membrane are rare or absent in dark cells, uniformly dense in light cells, and only in-

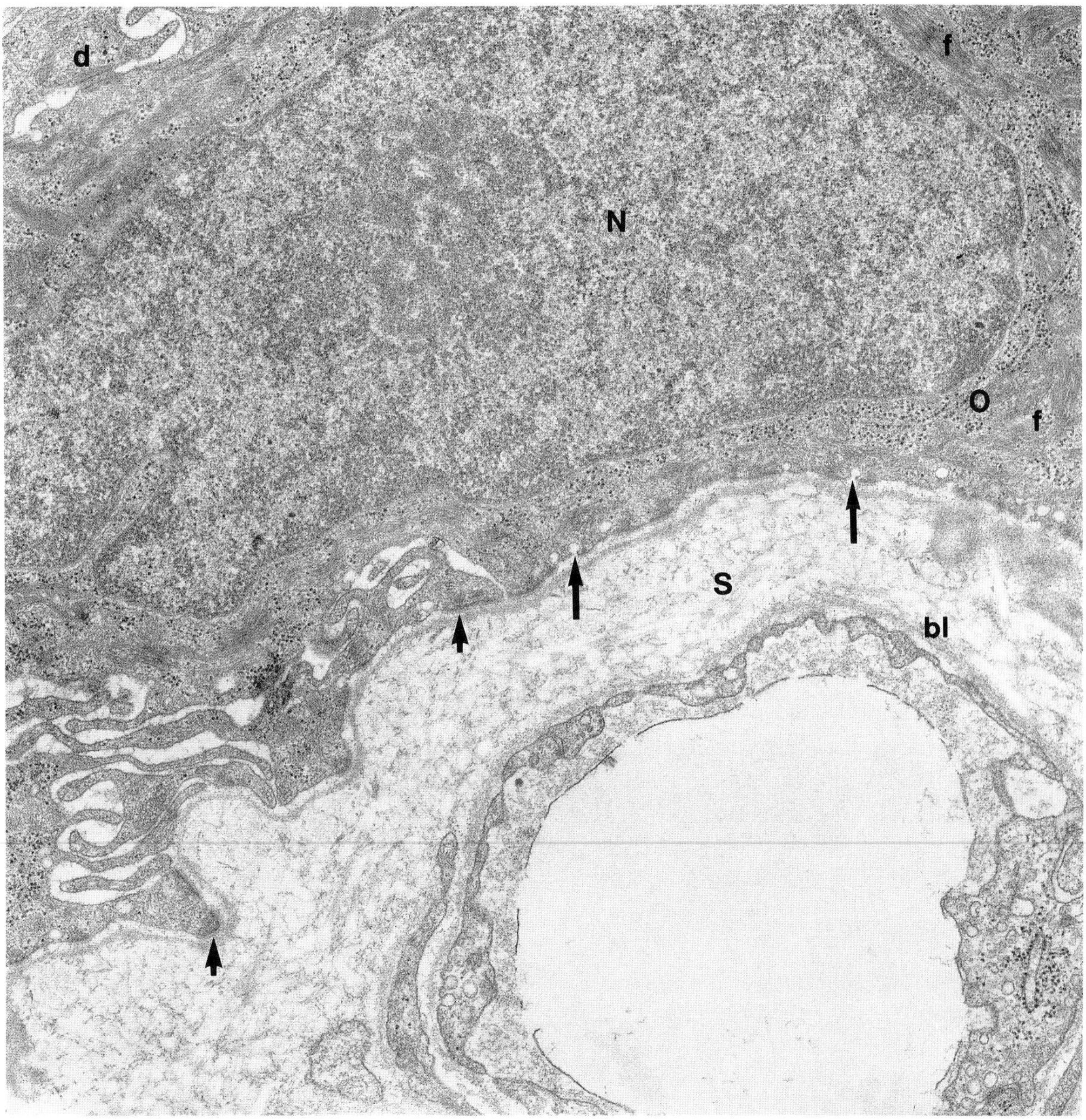

Fig. 9. Basal cell layer of the palpebral conjunctival epithelium of a rat. The cuboidal basal cell has a prominent central nucleus *(N)*, numerous intracytoplasmic bundles of tonofilaments *(f)*, and an irregular basal plasma membrane with hemidesmosomes *(arrowheads)* and pinocytotic vesicles *(arrows)*. Adjacent cells are attached to each other by desmosomal junctions *(d)*. In the stroma *(S)* a capillary with fenestrated endothelial cells is surrounded by a thin continuous basal lamina *(bl)*. TEM, ×22900

termittently present in intermediate cells with preferential locations in the perinuclear region. In the conjunctiva, the brightness of light and intermediate cells is increased by the presence of mucosubstances covering microvilli and microplicae. Randomly interspersed are goblet cell orifices. Apertures of goblet cells, some of them extruding mucus (Fig. 14), are frequently observable at the junction of three or four individual epithelial cells. Strands of mucus can also be observed on the epithelial surface.

Palpebral Conjunctiva, Lamina Propria

The lamina propria of the palpebral conjunctiva does not show the regular organization of the corneal stroma, and thus does not fundamen-

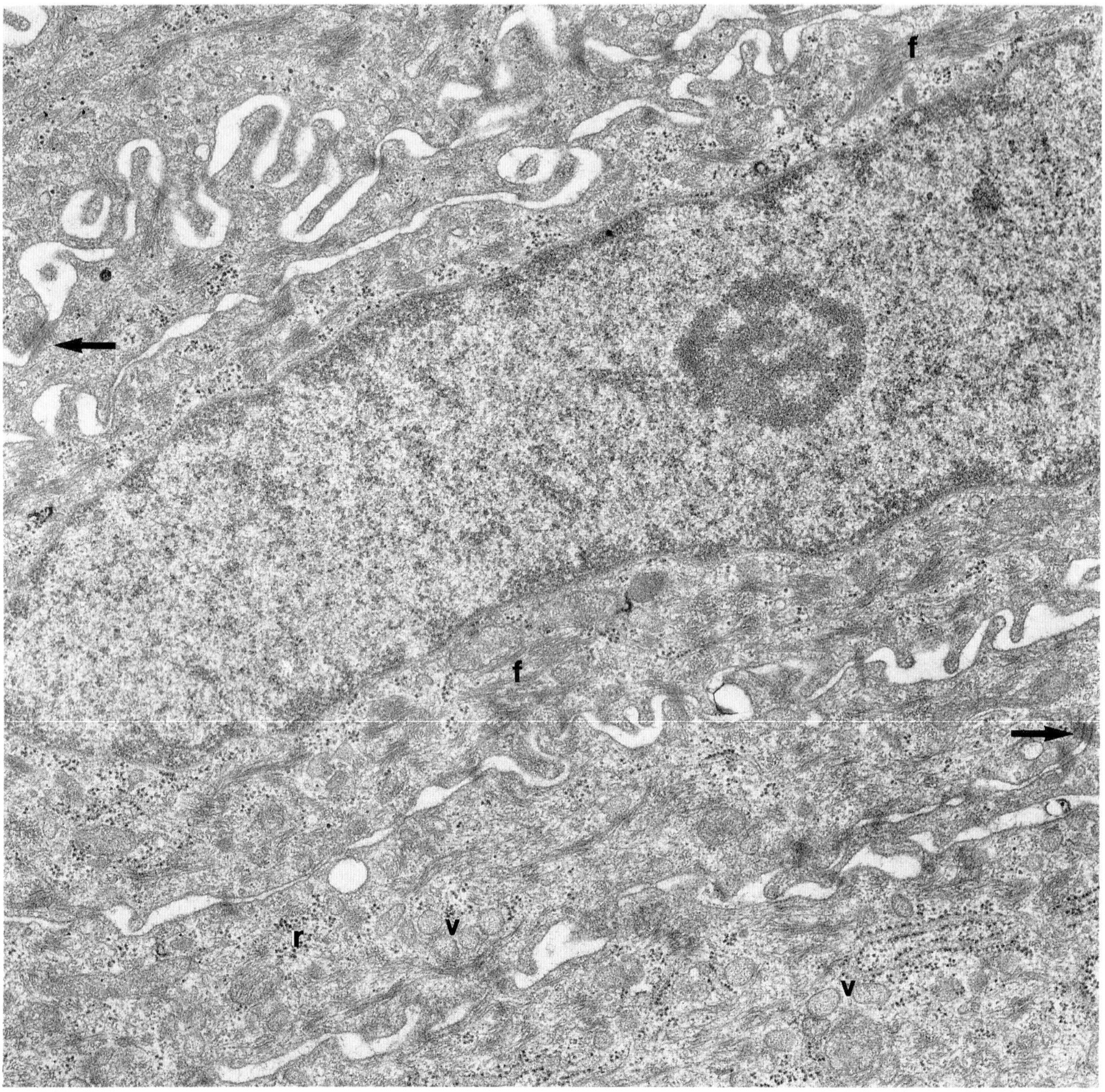

Fig. 10. Epithelial cells, palpebral conjunctiva, rat. The perinuclear cytoplasm of the elongated intermediate cells contains numerous bundles of filaments *(f)* and ribosomes *(r)* together with round membrane-bound vesicles *(v)* with finely granular content. Note interdigitations of adjacent plasma membranes and desmosomal junctions *(arrows)*. TEM, ×20000

Fig. 11 *(upper left).* Palpebral conjunctiva, rat. The epithelial surface consists of the polyhedral cells in juxtaposition and covered by variably dense microvilli; in some cells a prominent subcentral circular nucleus *(N)* is visible. Note two exfoliated cells *(EC)*. SEM, ×1000

Fig. 12 *(lower left).* Internal margin of the lower lid of a rat. *White arrows* delineate the transition from the keratinized squamous epithelium of the skin to the mucous membrane of the palpebral conjunctiva. SEM, ×750

Fig. 13 *(upper right).* Palpebral conjunctiva, mouse. Intercellular junctions *(white arrows)* separate two intermediate cells *(IC)* from a dark cell *(DC)* and a light cell *(LC)*. Density of microvilli and microplicae on the cell surface is increased in the light cell, varied in intermediate cells, and very low in the dark cell. SEM, ×5000 ▶

Fig. 14 *(lower right).* Palpebral conjunctiva, rat. Discharge of mucus *(M)* from a goblet cell located at the junction of four epithelial cells *(EC)*. SEM, ×7500

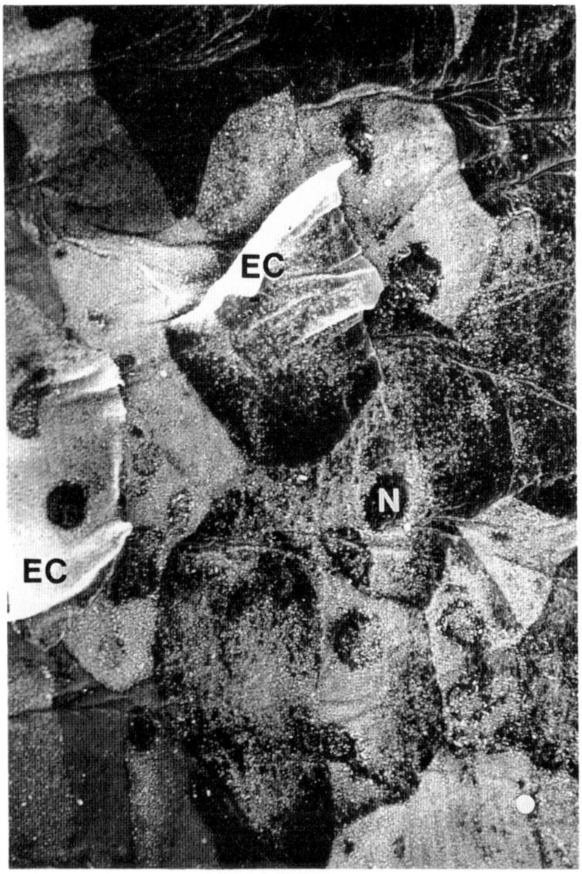
EC
N
EC

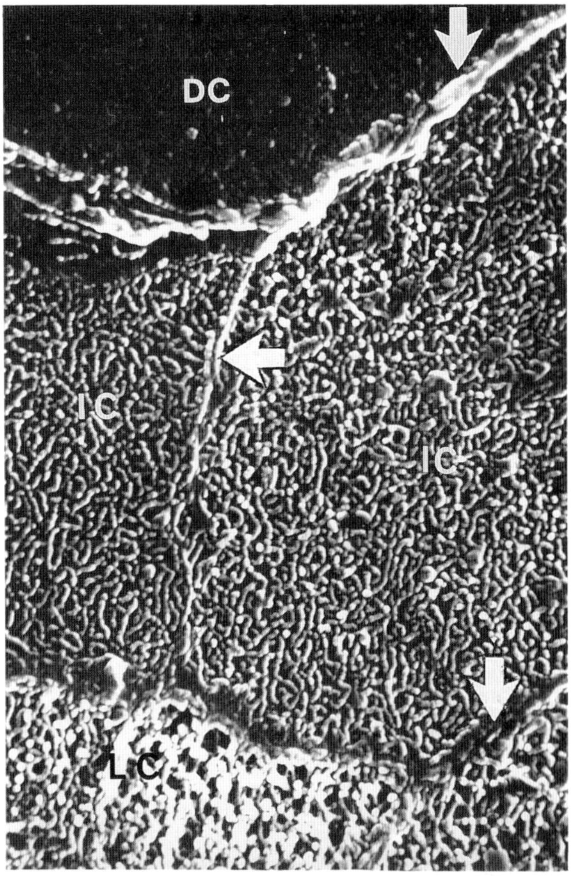
DC
IC
IC
LC

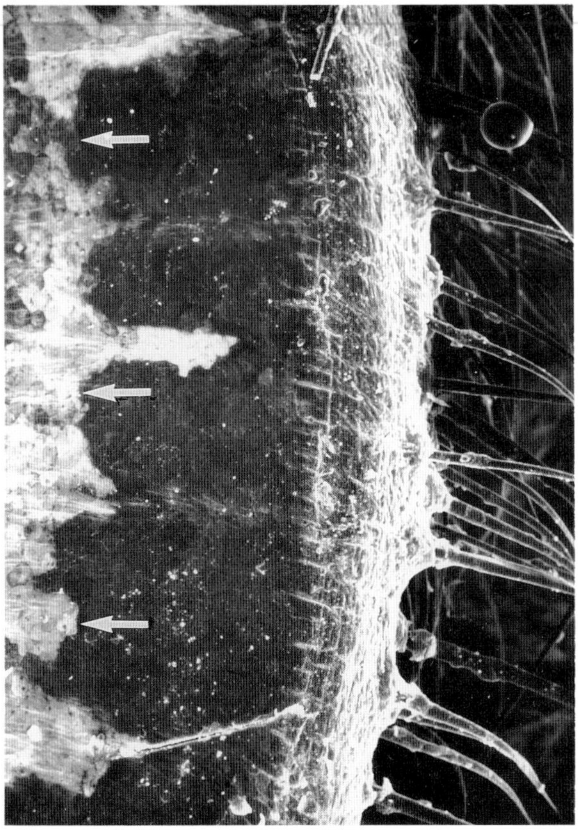

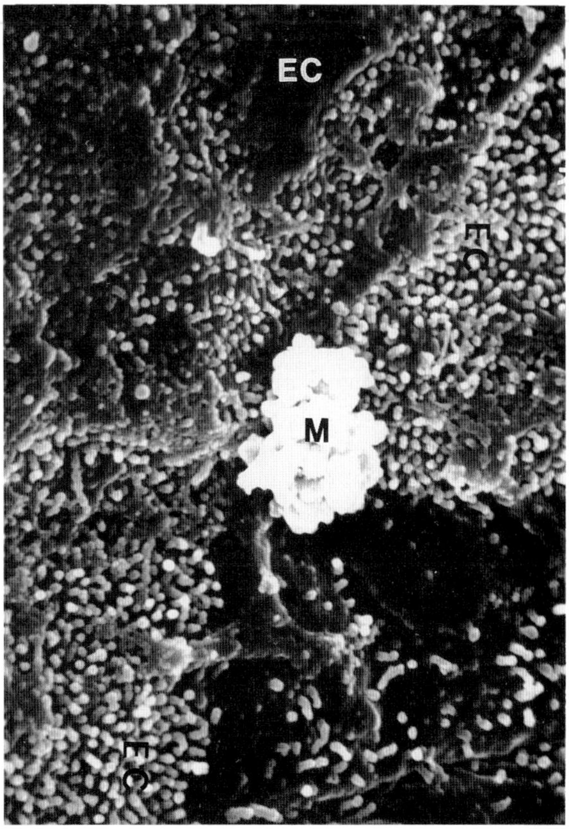
EC
EC
M
EC

tally differ from other connective tissues. It consists of an extracellular collagenous matrix with randomly oriented bundles of collagen fibrils, and a cellular component represented by fibroblasts, mast cells, lymphocytes, and occasional polymorphonuclear leukocytes and plasma cells. The stroma is richly vascularized in its deep and superficial layers by blood vessels arising from the anterior ciliary arteries (Martin and Anderson 1981). Subepithelial capillaries are limited by fenestrated endothelial cells lying on a thin continuous basal lamina (Fig. 10). Innervation of the palpebral conjunctiva arises from the lacrimal and trochlear nerves (Prince et al. 1960) and consists of myelinated and nonmyelinated fibers located in the cytoplasmic folds of Schwann cells.

Biologic Features

The movements of the eyelids (normal and reflex blinkings) are responsible for both eye protection by total eyelid closure and corneal integrity by maintaining an adequate tear film. The cornea and conjunctiva are kept permanently lubricated by ocular gland secretions and in addition abundant reflex secretion may be induced and sustained in the case of irritation. The conjunctiva is a mucous membrane involved in the production of secretions that have a significant role in the hydration and protection of the eye. In rats, the size of goblet cell clusters increases with age, but the overall density of clusters remains constant throughout life. It is thought that goblet cell development and mucin differentiation are modulated by aging processes (Huang et al. 1988). This also represents a protective mechanism, when the eyes are at risk of injury by environmental pollutants, and splash from chemicals. Covering the epithelium there is the three-layered tear film (precorneal film), consisting of an internal glycoprotein-enriched portion (next to the epithelium) produced by conjunctival goblet cells, a middle aqueous layer secreted by lacrimal glands, and an outside oily layer secreted by meibomian and other orbital glands of the eyelids. The tear film also contributes to maintaining both the integrity and optical properties of the cornea.

The structural organization of the cornea is closely related to its physiologic and physical properties. The cornea protects the inner ocular structures from external aggressions by its elasticity and resistance properties and also by its relative impermeability to noxious agents. As part of the visual system, the cornea is transparent and has an elevated refractive index (Hugues 1979). The regular arrangement of both epithelial cells and stromal collagenous bundles and lamellae explain the transparency of the cornea. Stromal hydration is regulated by ionic pumps in endothelial cells and contributes to the optical clarity of the cornea. A small excess uptake of water by an altered cornea disrupts its structural regularity, and thus transmitted light is scattered.

The cornea is not vascularized under normal conditions and its nutrition is achieved by diffusion. Therefore, drug-induced deposits (which usually do not interfere with vision but may diffract light and produce halos) are slow to clear. This has to be considered when eyes are at risk from topical or more often systemic drug exposure. Conversely, the cornea possesses a dense innervation, mainly located in its anterior portion. This innervation has been demonstrated in the rat to be greater in the periphery than at the center of the cornea (Ishida et al. 1984). Nerves from the ciliary branches of the ophthalmic nerve lose their myelin sheaths after entering the cornea. In the stroma, these nerve fibers are only surrounded by the minute cytoplasmic folds of Schwann cells, which are lost when nerve fibers enter the anterior epithelium. The infraepithelial nerves initiate the immediate reflex of blinking (and retraction of the head) upon irritation. The dense infraepithelial nerve plexuses as well as those connected with eyelashes and vibrissae contribute to the protection of the eye achieved by the closure of the eyelids.

Descemet's membrane is a strong and homogeneous basement membrane. Secreted by endothelial cells, it may be regenerated if injured. It has elastic properties and is more resistant than the rest of the cornea. In primates and carnivores, endothelial cells decrease in number but increase in size during life. In rats, aging results in a progressive decrease in cell density as well as reduced numbers of hexagonal endothelial cells (pleomorphism) and increased coefficient of variation of cell size (polymegathism) after age 34 weeks (Meyer et al. 1988). Regeneration of endothelium following injury has been demonstrated in rabbits. Nothing is known about the adaptative response of endothelium to trauma in rodents.

Table 2. Semiquantitative analysis of the form factor ($F = 4\ S/P2$) of corneal epithelial cells in laboratory animals (circular = 1.00)

Species	All cells	Light cells	Dark cells
Mouse	0.80 ± 0.15	0.69 ± 0.15	0.88 ± 0.12
Rat	0.72 ± 0.15	0.69 ± 0.16	0.75 ± 0.15
Rabbit	0.88 ± 0.14	0.64 ± 0.23	0.72 ± 0.23
Dog	0.89 ± 0.15	0.70 ± 0.18	0.78 ± 0.19

All figures are means ± standard deviations.

Comparison with Other Species

The rodent eye presents a slight and relative exophthalmia, which may explain the susceptibility of the cornea to trauma and dehydration. The cornea of rats and mice differs minimally from that of other laboratory animals. Morphometric analysis of epithelial cells (Tables 1, 2) indicates a mean cell surface of 718 μm^2 in the rat and 668 μm^2 in the mouse (Molon-Noblot and Duprat 1987), these values being close to those obtained in dogs and rabbits (Table 1). With a form factor ($F = 4\ S/P2$) of 0.72 and the rat and 0.80 in the mouse (Table 2), the corneal epithelial cell of rodents approaches the geometric hexagonal form ($F = 0.91$). Microvilli covering the surface of outer epithelial cells have a comparable diameter (about 0.15 µm) in rats, mice, rabbits, and dogs. The sole difference is the lack of Bowman's membrane, which exists in man, primates, and dogs, and has no capacity to regenerate if injured.

In rabbits, the density of goblet cells is not homogeneous in the palpebral conjunctiva, reflecting independent cycles of secretion in the marginal, tarsal, and orbital regions; globally the number of goblet cells increases with age (Pacau 1986).

References

Basu PK (1983) Application of scanning electron microscopy in ophthalmic research. Indian J Ophthalmol 31: 476–585

Bisaria KK, Bisaria SD (1980) Histological study of the glands of eyelids in the albino rat. J Anat Soc India 30: 16–20

Blümcke S, Morgenroth K (1967) The stereo ultrastructure of the external and internal surface of the cornea. J Ultrastruct Mol Struct Res 18: 502–518

Dormans JA, Van Logten MJ (1982) The effects of ophthalmic preservatives on corneal epithelium of the rabbit: a scanning electron microscopic study. Toxicol Appl Pharmacol 62: 251–261

Hazlett LD, Wells P, Spann B, Berk RS (1980) Penetration of the unwounded immature mouse cornea and conjunctiva by pseudomonas: SEM-TEM analysis. Invest Ophthalmol Vis Sci 19: 694–697

Hervouet F, George Y, Tusques J, Ertus M (1971) Aspect de differentes structures oculaires humaines au microscope a balayage. Bull Mem Soc Fr Ophthalmol 84: 603–617

Hoffmann F (1972) The surface of epithelial cells of the cornea under the scanning electron microscope. Ophthalmic Res 3: 207–214

Hoffmann F, Schweichel JU (1972) The microvilli structure of the corneal epithelium of the rabbit in relation to cell function. Ophthalmic Res 4: 175–184

Hogan MJ, Alvarado JA, Esperson Weddell J (1971) Hogan MJ, Alvarado JA, Esperson Weddell JE (eds) Histology of the human eye. Saunders, Philadelphia, pp 1–111

Huang AJ, Tseng SC, Kenyon KR (1988) Morphogenesis of rat conjunctival goblet cells. Invest Ophthalmol Vis Sci 29: 969–975

Hugues A (1979) A schematic eye for the rat. Vision Res 19: 569–588

Ishida N, Del Cerro M, Rao GN, Mathe M, Aquavella JV (1984) Corneal stromal innervation; a quantitative analysis of distribution. Ophthalmic Res 16: 139–144

Jacobsen IE, Jensen OA, Prause JU (1983) Structure and composition of Bowman's membrane. Study by frozen resin cracking. Acta Ophthalmol 62: 39–53

Jakus MA (1954) The fine structure of the rat cornea. Am J Opthalmol 38 (1/2): 40–53

Kaye GI, Pappas GD (1962) Studies on the cornea. I. The fine structure of the rabbit cornea and the uptake and transport of colloidal particles by the cornea in vivo. J Cell Biol 12: 457–479

Kenyon KR (1979) Anatomy and pathology of the ocular surface. Int Ophthalmol Clin 19: 3–35

Martin CL, Anderson BG (1981) Ocular anatomy. In: Gelatt KN (ed) Textbook of veterinary ophthalmology. Lea and Febiger, Philadelphia, pp 12–121

Meyer LA, Ubels JL, Edelhauser HF (1988) Corneal endothelial morphology in the rat. Effect of aging, diabetes, and topical aldose reductase inhibitor treatment. Invest Ophthalmol Vis Sci 29: 940–948

Molon-Noblot S, Duprat P (1987) Comparative dog and rabbit ultrastructure of the corneal surface: a quantitative scanning electron microscopic study. 15th meeting of the European Club for Ophthalmic Fine Structure, 14–15 Sept, Paris

Pacau F (1986) Les cellules muqueuses de la conjonctive du lapin. Thèse de Doctorat Vétérinaire Ecole Nationale Veterinaire de Maisons-Alfort et Faculté de Medicine de (94) Creteil, 12 June 1986

Pedler C (1962) The fine structure of the corneal epithelium. Exp Eye Res 1: 286–289

Pfister RR (1973) The normal surface of corneal epithelium: a scanning electron microscopic study. Invest Ophthalmol 12: 654–668

Pfister RR (1975) The normal surface of conjunctiva epithelium. A scanning electron microscopic study. Invest Ophthalmol 14: 267–279

Pfister RR, Burstein NL (1977) The normal and abnormal human corneal epithelial surface: a scanning elec-

tron microscope study. Invest Ophthalmol Vis Sci 16: 614–622
Pouliquen Y (1969) Atlas d'histologie et d'ultrastructure du globe oculaire. Masson, Paris, pp 1–7
Prince JH, Diesem CD, Eglitis I, Ruskell GL (1960) Anatomy and histology of the eye and orbit in domestic animals. Thomas, Springfield, pp 43–58
Renard G, Montanez-Mendoza M, Savoldelli M, Pouliquen Y (1983a) Etude en microscopie à balayage de l'épithélium cornéen. Relation de certains aspects avec le film lacrynal (abstract in English). J Fr Ophthalmol 6: 697–705
Renard G, Patey A, Savoldelli M, Montanez-Mendoza M, Pouliquen Y (1983b) Etude morphologique et quantimétrique de la surface de l'épithélium cornéen. J Fr Ophthalmol 6: 777–783
Sheldon H (1956) An electron microscope study of the epithelium in the normal mature and immature mouse cornea. J Biophys Biochem Cytol 2: 253–262
Teng CC (1961) The fine structure of the corneal epithelium and basement membrane of the rabbit. Am J Ophthalmol 51: 278–297
Weingeist TA (1973a) The conjunctiva. In: Zinn KM (ed) Ocular fine structure for the clinician. Little, Brown, Boston, pp 85–91
Weingeist TA (1973b) The conjunctiva. In: Gelatt KN (ed) Textbook of veterinary ophthalmology. Lea and Febiger, Philadelphia, pp 12–121
Wells PA, Hazlett LD (1984) Complex carbohydrates at the ocular surface of the mouse: an ultrastructural and cytochemical analysis. Exp Eye Res 39: 19–35

Calcification of the Cornea, Mouse and Rat

William W. Carlton and James A. Render

Synonyms. Band keratopathy.

Gross Appearance

Corneal calcification results in opacification, with the size of the opacity depending upon the extent of the calcification. It may appear as small, pale spots or as an opacity of geometric shape (Taradach and Greaves 1984), or it may be diffuse. Slight calcification produces a slight turbidity, more substantial focal deposits appear as gray dots beneath the corneal epithelium, and larger deposits cause the cornea to be chalky white.

In spontaneously diabetic KK mice with corneal calcification, the first change is a fine stippling of the corneal stroma just beneath the corneal epithelium. This develops into faint opacities which, later, are characteristically more dense oval-shaped opacities in the central portion of the cornea. The oval opacities consist of numerous polygonal plates (Mittl et al. 1970). The calcification appears by magnification in the living eye as aggregates of refractile bubble-like cysts that form geographic map-shaped opacities in the superficial stroma of the central cornea (Huang and Sery 1971).

In rabbits with experimental band keratopathy, the corneal lesions are seen by slit-lamp biomicroscopy as a subepithelial opacification along the interpalpebral space, either as a partial band with segments or as a complete band with fenestration (Economon et al. 1963).

Microscopic Features

The calcific deposits in the rodent cornea are generally present as basophilic extracellular granules in the corneal stroma adjacent to the corneal epithelium. The deposits may be concentrated in the interpalpebral portion of the cornea or diffusely distributed. The calcific deposits vary in morphologic features from aggregates of variable size of tiny basophilic granules (Fig. 15) within or just below the corneal epithelium to elongate cylindrical rods (Fig. 16) or plaque-shaped accumulations in epithelium or stroma (Fig. 17). In some animals, more deeply situated portions of the stroma are calcified. The calcific deposits may fracture upon sectioning and become separated from the overlying epithelium, producing artifactual separation of the corneal epithelium and its stroma. The granules may be present in a corneal stroma without other alterations, or the sites of calcification may be accompanied by such changes as edema, fibrosis, cellular infiltrates, and/or neovascularization (Fig. 18). Calcific deposits associated with granuloma formation occur in the bulbar conjunction in rats (Fig. 19).

In spontaneously diabetic KK mice, the calcium is present as extracellular deposits of fine basophilic granules or as dense strips at the junction of the epithelium and corneal stroma. More extensive calcification appears as large elongated or irregular basophilic deposits. The corneal epithelium may be thinned over the foci of calcification or it may be thickened with foci of keratinization. Older lesions tend to have neovascularization with minimal cellular infiltrate of neutrophilic and mononuclear leukocytes (Mittl et al. 1970; Huang and Sery 1971).

Ultrastructure

Experimental corneal calcification was produced by mild irradiation with a carbon dioxide laser (Fine et al. 1968). In electron micrographs, numerous spherules of fine crystals were present within the basement membrane of the corneal epithelium. The spherules appeared as concentric rings and were accompanied by conglomerates of spherules formed by fusion. Some of the calcific spherules were present within keratocytes and were lying in membrane-bound vesicles within the cytoplasm.

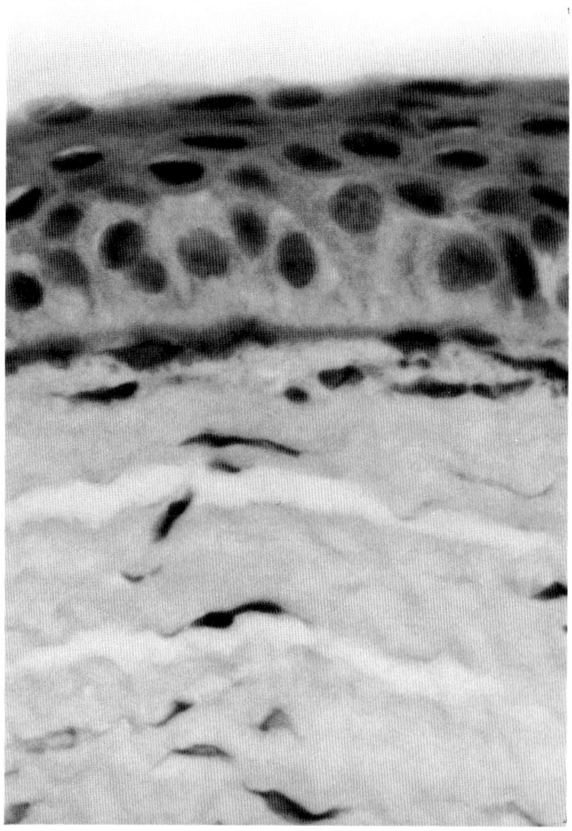

Differential Diagnosis

The distribution, size, and clinical appearance of corneal calcification are not diagnostic. Similar opacification could result from edema, lipid material, or inflammatory infiltrates in the corneal stroma. Microscopic study is sufficient to distinguish the various causes of corneal opacification. Calcium can be identified in corneal tissue by X-ray microprobe analysis. Also, in sections, deposits of calcium will be stained black by the Von Kossa silver nitrate method and red with the alizarin red S stain.

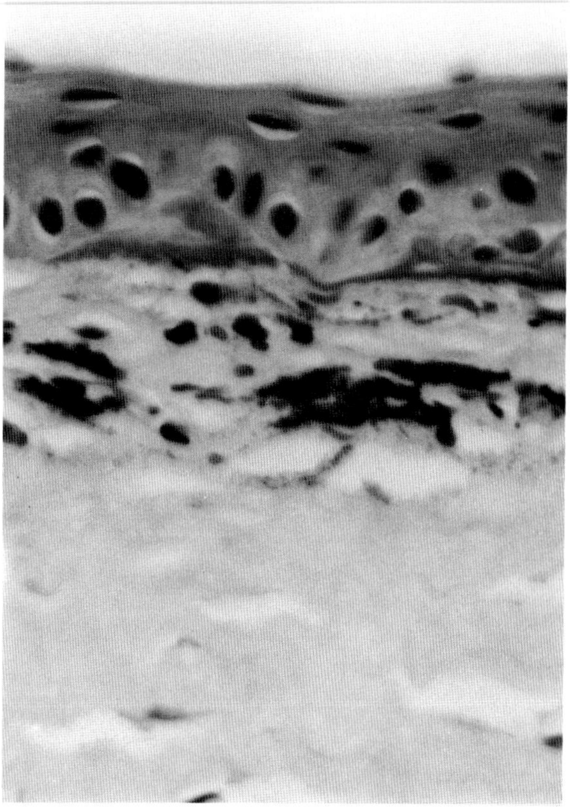

Fig. 15 *(above).* Cornea, F 344 rat. Aggregates of calcific ▸ material are seen in the corneal stroma at the junction with and just beneath the corneal epithelium. (Courtesy of Dr. C. Gries, Eli Lilly Company, United States) H & E, ×560

Fig. 16 *(below).* Cornea, F 344 rat. Fragmented calcific deposits in the corneal stroma and at the junction with the corneal epithelium. (Courtesy of Dr. C. Gries, Eli Lilly Company, United States) H & E, ×560

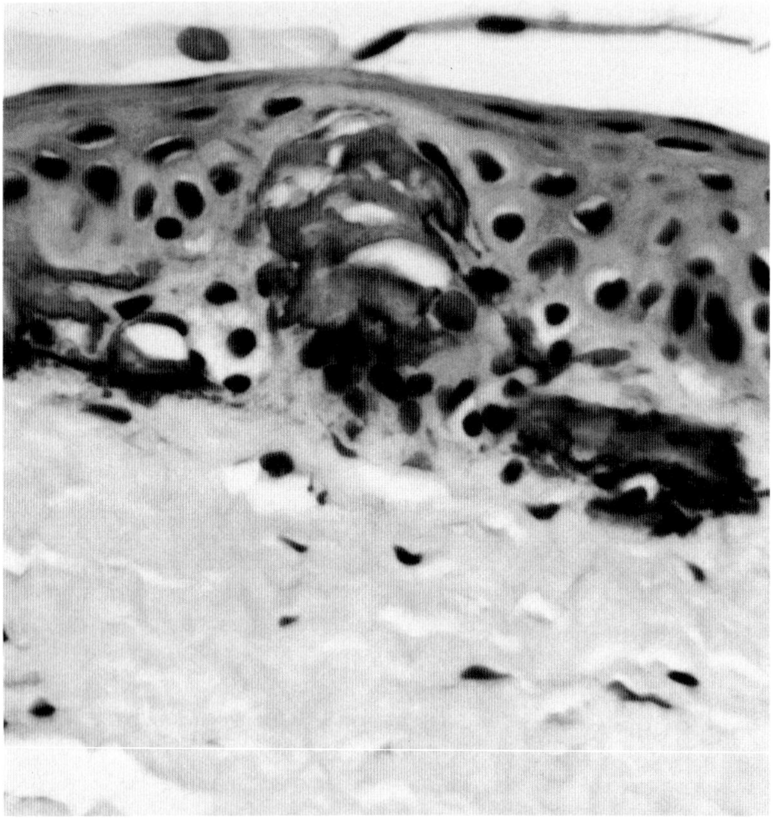

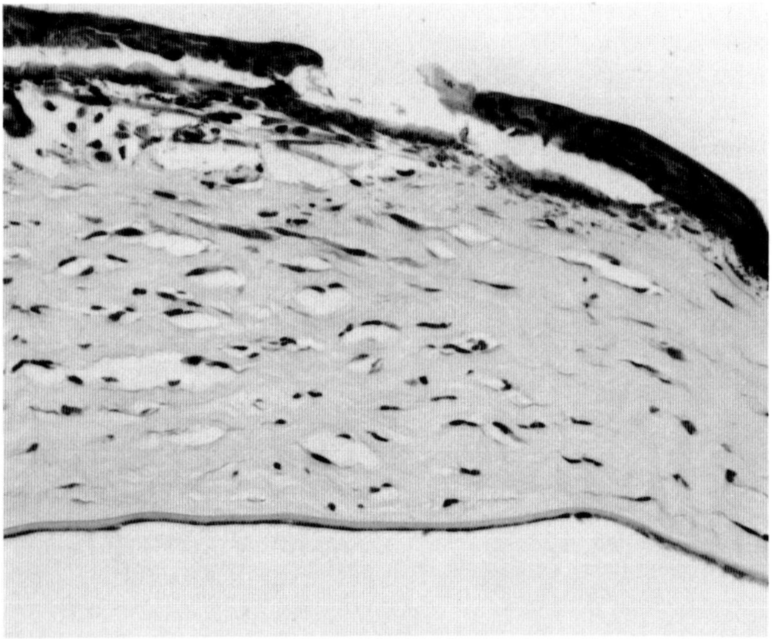

Fig. 17 *(above)*. Cornea, F 344 rat. Irregular aggregates of calcific material in the corneal stroma, in the corneal epithelium, and at the epithelial-stromal junction. Few mononuclear cells are associated with the calcific deposits. (Courtesy of Dr. C. Gries, Eli Lilly Company, United States) H & E, ×560

Fig. 18 *(below)*. Cornea, CD-1 mouse. Calcific deposits are at the junction of the corneal epithelium and stroma. The corneal epithelium is lost at one point and is separated from its stroma over a larger area. A few inflammatory cells are present about the calcific deposits and in the underlying stroma. (Courtesy of Dr. J. Long, Eli Lilly Company, United States) H & E, ×224

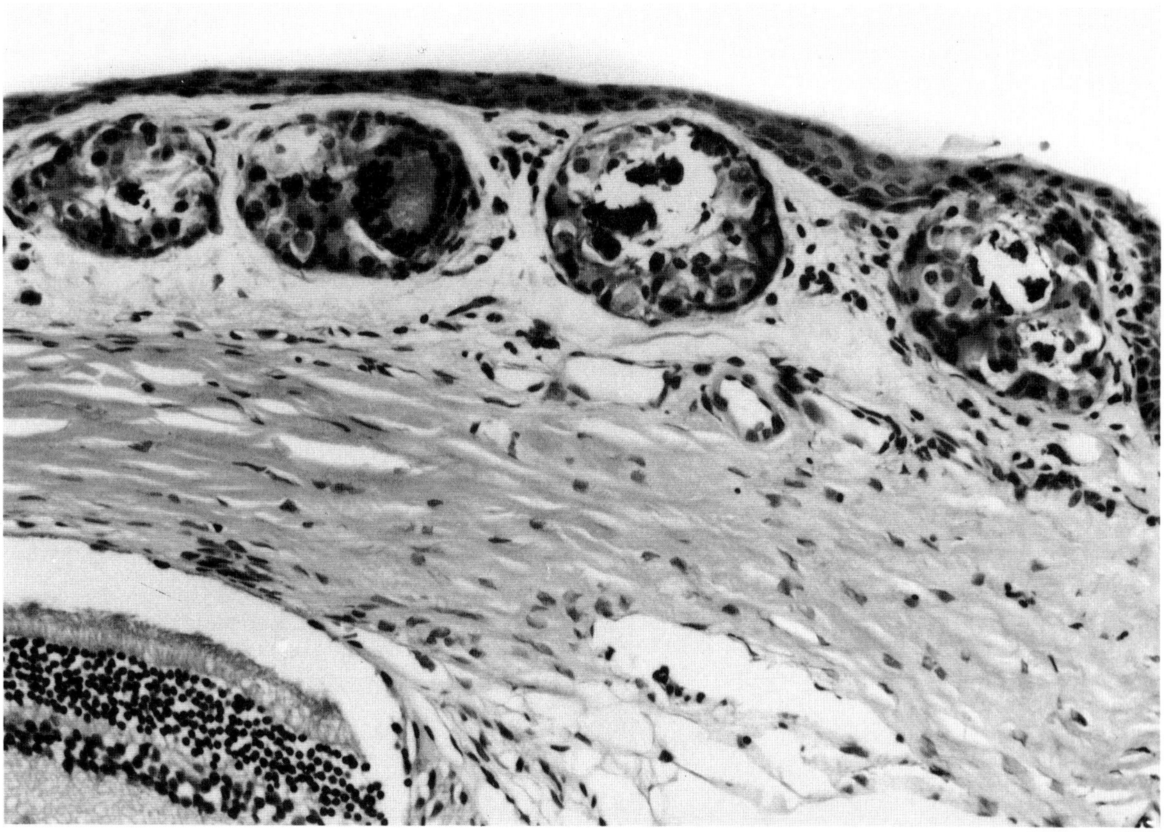

Fig. 19. Bulbar conjunctiva, F 344 rat. Multiple calcific granulomas. (Courtesy of Dr. Gries, Eli Lilly Company, United States) H & E, ×224

Biologic Features

Calcification in laboratory rodents generally follows trauma to or inflammation of the cornea. In mice with harderian gland adenoma, proptosis of the globe often leads to keratitis and subsequent band keratrophy. Mineralization of the subepithelial region of the cornea has been reported as a common lesion in breeder mice and likely was a sequela of keratitis and vascularization that followed exposure to ammonia produced by urease-positive bacteria in the bedding (Van Winkel and Balk 1986). Drying of the cornea because of evaporation is an important mechanism of induction of corneal calcification. Calcific keratopathy can be accentuated by keeping the eyelids open and it can be prevented by prolonged closure of the eyelids. Evaporation from the cornea results in supersaturation and precipitation of calcium in the superficial corneal stroma.

Calcification of the cornea has been produced in rabbits by various types of corneal injury combined with hypercalcemia produced by the administration of dehydrotachysterol. The corneal trauma includes deepithelization of the central or entire cornea, freezing of the corneal epithelium, intracameral injection of potassium permanganate, and abrasion of the endothelium. In the rat, deepithelization of the central or entire cornea was the most effective method for induction of corneal calcification (Obenberger et al. 1989), but calcification was produced by freezing of the cornea and by abrasions of the endothelium combined with hypercalcemia.

Other procedures used for the production of corneal calcification in the rat include treatment with isoproterenol, dihydrotachysterol, and 5-hydroxytryptamine (Selye et al. 1962), subcutaneous administration of morphine sulfate, and suturing the eyelids open so that they cannot be closed by the animal.

The morphine sulfate-induced corneal calcification appears related to drying of the cornea (Fabian et al. 1967) as the treated rabbits developed exophthalmos. When the marked depression and exophthalmos were reduced by nalorphine hydrochloride following the morphine sulfate, corneal calcification was prevented.

In most of the experimental procedures used to produce corneal calcification, trauma to the cornea is followed by edema and proliferation of fibroblasts. These cells are rapidly synthesizing and releasing glycosaminoglycans into the damaged regions, the area in which calcification occurs. The free anionic groups of the glycosaminoglycans bind calcium in the first phase of the calcification process (Ocumpaugh and Obenberger 1970).

Comparison with Other Species

Calcific band keratopathy occurs in human patients in association with a variety of ocular diseases including uveitis, chemical and physical injuries to the cornea, chronic glaucoma, and phthisis bulbi. In some patients, it appears as a hazy gray opacification of the cornea along the zone of the interpalpebral fissure. It may also accompany the hypercalcemia of hyperparathyroidism and vitamin D poisoning and occurs in patients with chronic renal failure (Porter and Crombie 1973). The corneal lesions in hypercalcemia are bilaterally symmetric with an associated calcification of the bulbar conjunctiva (Klintworth 1982). Histologically, band keratopathy is characterized by deposits of basophilic granular material, especially in Bowman's zone and the adjacent corneal stroma, in the interpalpebral region of the cornea.

Calcification is readily produced in the rabbit by a variety of procedures including immunogenic uveitis combined with hypercalcemia (Economon et al. 1963). Spontaneously occurring corneal calcification is rare in the rabbit. The guinea pig did not respond with corneal calcification to procedures that were successful in the rabbit and rat (Obenberger et al. 1969). Thus, the guinea pig appears much less susceptible to experimental corneal calcification than the rabbit and rat. Calcification of the cornea in domestic animals is usually an aftermath of keratitis. Calcific keratopathy as a primary disease of the cornea appears to be rare in domestic animals.

References

Economon JW, Silverstein AM, Zimmerman LE (1963) Band keratopathy in a rabbit colony. Invest Ophthalmol 2: 361–368

Fabian RJ, Band JM, Drobeck HP (1967) Induced corneal opacities in the rat. Br J Ophthalmol 51: 124–129

Fine BS, Berkow JW, Fine S (1968) Corneal calcification. Science 162: 129–130

Huang LH, Sery TW (1971) Corneal degeneration in a congenitally diabetic inbred strain of mouse. Br J Ophthalmol 55: 266–271

Klintworth GK (1982) Degenerations, depositions and miscellaneous reactions of the cornea, conjunctiva and sclera. In: Garner A, Klintworth GK (eds) Pathobiology of ocular disease. Dekker, New York, pp 1431–1475

Mittl R, Galin MA, Opperman W, Camerini-Davalas RA, Spiro D (1970) Corneal calcification in spontaneously diabetic mice. Invest Ophthalmol 9: 137–145

Obenberger J, Ocumpaugh DE, Cubberly MG (1969) Experimental corneal calcification in animals treated with dihydrotachysteral. Invest Ophthalmol 8: 467–474

Ocumpaugh DE, Obenberger J (1970) Experimental corneal calcification: a radioautographic and histochemical study. Clin Orthop 69: 1691–171

Porter R, Crombie AL (1973) Corneal and conjunctival calcification in chronic renal failure. Br J Ophthalmol 57: 339–343

Selye H, Dieudonne JM, Veilleux R (1962) A calciphylactic syndrome affecting the skeletal muscles, the salivary gland and the eyes. Exp Med Surg 20: 185–193

Taradach C, Greaves P (1984) Spontaneous eye lesions in laboratory animals: incidence in relation to age. CRC Crit Rev Toxicol 12: 121–141

Van Winkle TJ, Balk MW (1986) Spontaneous corneal opacities in laboratory mice. Lab Anim Sci 36: 248–255

Corneal Opacities, Spontaneous, Mouse

Thomas J. Van Winkle

Synonyms (and Included Conditions). Keratitis, corneal calcification, corneal dystrophy, band keratopathy, corneal keratinization.

Gross Appearance

Corneal opacities appear as unilateral or bilateral areas of white or gray opacification, haziness, or translucency. Small opacities are usually round to oval and located in the center of the cornea or slightly nasal and inferior (Fig. 20). Larger opacities may discolor the entire cornea and prevent examination of intraocular structures. The surface may be slightly roughened, granular, or dry.

Corneal opacities may be detected with the unaided eye when the cornea is illuminated with a focused light source. Small opacities and less-dense (translucent) lesions are more easily detected with direct or indirect ophthalmoscopy or slit-lamp biomicroscopy (Bellhorn 1981).

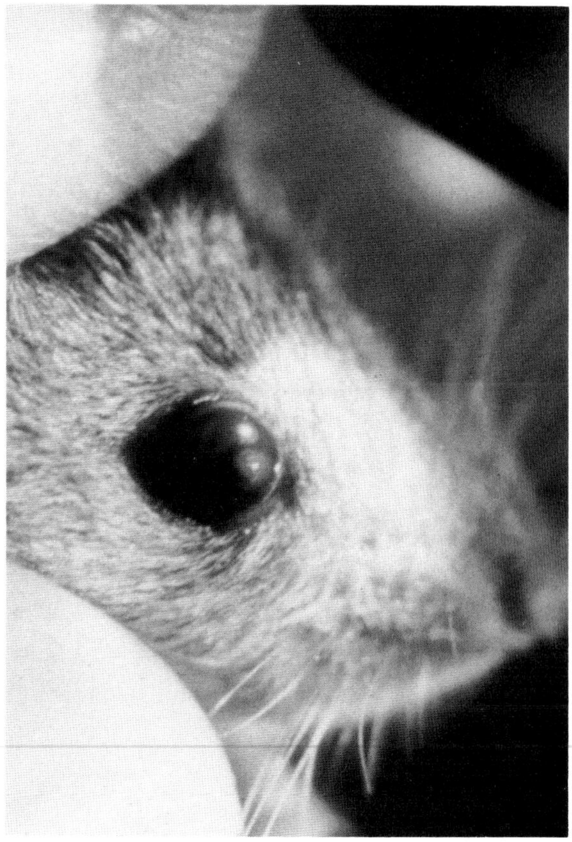

Fig. 20. Central corneal opacity, C3H mouse. There is a reflection from the light source on the superior cornea

Microscopic Features

A wide variety of morphologic alterations of the cornea can appear as corneal opacities. The microscopic appearance will depend on the cause of the opacity as well as the stage of development of the lesion during which the eye is examined. Any alteration in the corneal epithelium, stroma, or endothelium which interferes with the normal transmission of light trough these structures will cause opacification.

The most frequent reported microscopic appearance of corneal opacification in the mouse is mineralization of the anterior corneal stroma and the basement membrane zone immediately beneath the corneal epithelium (Fig. 21) with thinning of the overlying epithelium (Van Winkle and Balk 1986; Taradach and Greaves 1984; Mittl et al. 1970; see p. 16, this volume). Both calcium and ferric iron salts have been demonstrated in the mineralized areas. Other features described in opaque corneas of mice include epithelial erosion and ulceration, acute and chronic keratitis with infiltration of the cornea by inflammatory cells, anterior stromal neovascularization, stromal defects, and epithelial dysplasia, hyperplasia, and keratinization.

Differential Diagnosis

Postmortem cloudiness of the cornea and light reflections from the cornea must e differentiated from spontaneous corneal opacities. Etiologies which should be differentiated include congenital and genetic abnormalities, trauma, and infectious agents. Neoplasms involving the anterior chamber may appear as corneal opacities due to local infiltration or interference with endothelial function leading to corneal edema.

Biologic Features

The etiology and pathogenesis of many spontaneous corneal opacities in mice are undetermined. The opacities are usually observed in adult mice and few studies of the progression of

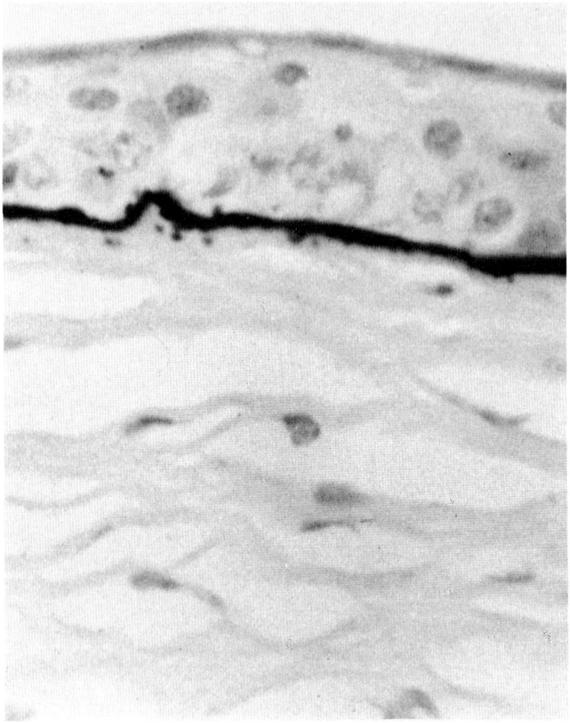

◂ **Fig. 21.** Mineralization of the corneal basement membrane in a retired breeder mouse. The overlying epithelium is flattened and dysplastic. Von Kossa, × 400

the lesion have been reported. Table 1 lists most of the reported corneal opacities and divides them into three groups. Group I are most likely true corneal dystrophies. Group II includes mice with primary abnormalities of eyelids and secondary corneal opacities due to exposure. Group III are mice with anterior stromal mineralization with or without inflammation and neovascularization.

True dystrophies of the cornea must be distinguished from other causes of corneal opacification. Dystrophies are usually bilateral, progressive, and genetically determined noninflammatory lesions involving one or more of the layers of the cornea. Three reported lesions in the mouse cornea fit these criteria (group I, Table 3). A corneal stromal defect or gap was described in a colony of C57 BL/10ChPr

Table 3. Spontaneous corneal opacities in mice

Group	Strain	% Affected	Diagnosis	Reference
I Corneal dystrophy				
	C57 BL/10ChPr	3.2	Stromal defect	Pierro and Spiggle 1967
	Rhino	100	Stromal dystrophy	Yoshida et al. 1979
	OEL	76	Keratinization	Newsome et al. 1982
II Eyelid abnormalities with secondary keratitis				
	129/RrSv (OeOe)	100	Opacity	Mackensen 1960
	C57 BL/6-ax (gpgp)	100	Opacity	Kelton and Smith 1964
III Anterior stromal mineralization with or without neovascularization and keratitis				
	KK	98	Calcification	Mittl et al. 1970
	CF1	Not given	Calcification	Saunders and Rubin 1975
	MRL/l	86	Band keratopathy	Hoffman et al. 1983
	MRL/n	89		
	DBA/2	28		
	CD-1	1.6–10.1	Dystrophy	Taradach and Greaves 1984
	MRL/Mp- + / +	5	Band keratopathy	Jabs et al. 1985
	MRL/Mp-1pr/1pr	15		
	DBA/2	29.1	Opacity	Van Winkle and Balk 1986
	C3 H	16.2	(keratitis)	
	CF1	16.2		
	BALB/c	10.0		
	C57 BL/6	4.1		
	CD-1	4.3		
	DBA-2	78	Calcification	Yamate et al. 1987

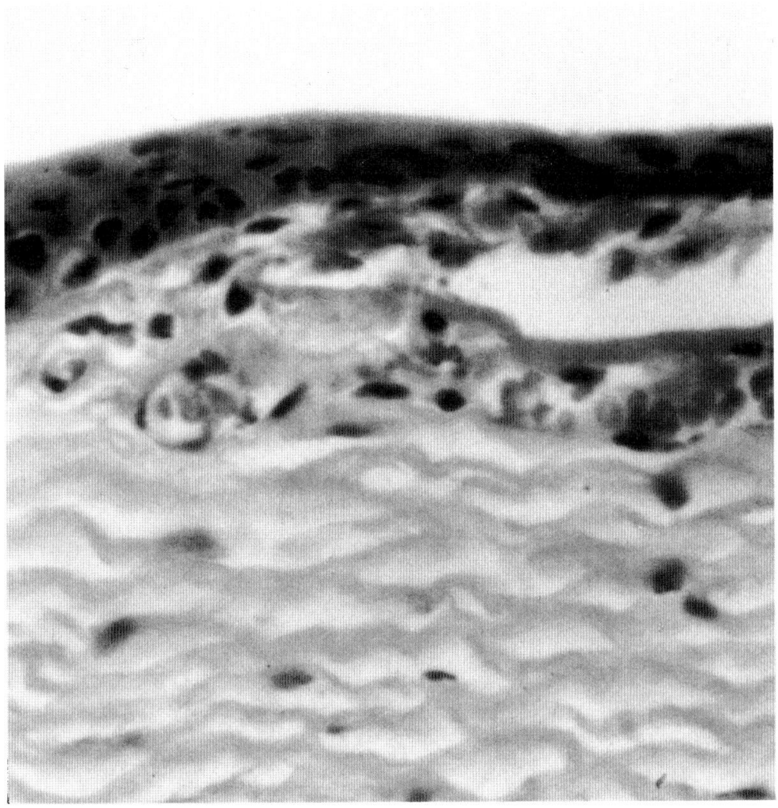

Fig. 22. Neovascularization of the anterior corneal stroma in a 6-week-old BALB/c mouse. A subepithelial cleft is bordered by a line of mineralization and surrounded by small blood vessels. The overlying epithelium is flattened. H & E, ×400

mice (Pierro and Spiggle 1967), and a stromal dystrophy followed by inflammation of the cornea was observed in the Rhino mouse (Yoshida et al. 1979). Corneal epithelial keratinization preceded by decreased corneal wetting was reported in the oel/+ mouse (Newsome et al. 1982).

Corneal opacities may be secondary to abnormalities of eyelids which lead to exposure keratitis (group II, Table 3).

These can usually be traced to a single recessive autosomal gene and 100% of homozygous mice are affected. The "gaping" gene *(gp)* was described in C57nL/6-ax mice (Kelton and Smith 1964) and the "open eyelids" gene *(oe)* was observed in 129/RrSv mice (Mackensen 1960). Similar genetically determined abnormalities of eyelids with subsequent corneal damage have been described in other mouse strains (Green 1975; Cousins et al. 1984). Keratitis has also been described in mice following exposure of the cornea during general anesthesia (Kaplun and Barishak 1976).

In group III (Table 3), the corneal opacities are characterized by mineralization of the subepithelial basement membrane and anterior corneal stroma. Keratitis with inflammatory cell infiltrates and stromal neovascularization is often present in areas of opacification. This lesion has been designated by different investigators as keratitis (Van Winkle and Balk 1986), corneal dystrophy (Taradach and Greaves 1984), corneal calcification (Mittl et al. 1970; Saunders and Rubin 1975; Yamate et al. 1987), and band keratopathy (Hoffman et al. 1983; Jabs et al. 1985). These conditions share many morphologic similarities and may have the same or a similar pathogenesis.

Spontaneous corneal opacities were observed in 205 of 1805 mice (11.4%) from barrier-reared production colonies and in 18 of 1147 axenic and gnotobiotic mice (1.6%) raised in flexible-film isolators (Van Winkle and Balk 1986). Significant differences in incidence between different strains and stocks were observed (Table 1, group III). Groups of mice with a high incidence included DBA/2 (29.1%), C3H (16.2%), CF1

(16.2%), and BALB/c (10.0%), while in CD-1 (4.3%) and C57BL/6 (4.1%) mice corneal opacities were less frequent. The microscopic appearance of the lesion was age dependent and suggested a progression from acute to chronic inflammation and eventual repair with mineralization. Epithelial necrosis, erosions, ulcers, and acute suppurative keratitis were present in 3- to 6-week-old mice. Neovascularization, epithelial flattening and dysplasia, and mineralization of the anterior corneal stroma were observed in 4- to 10-week-old mice (Fig. 22). Retired breeder mice (approximately 9 months old) had mineralization of the subepithelial stroma and an epithelial basement membrane zone with thinning of the overlying epithelium (Fig. 21).

The suspected etiology of the acute central epithelial necrosis, ulcers, and suppurative keratitis in young mice was ammonia produced in the environment from urinary urea by urease-positive fecal bacteria. Experimentally, the incidence of corneal opacities in C3H, BALB/c, and CD-1 mice was reduced (from 23.8% to 0.8%) by frequent (twice-weekly) cage cleaning. The morphologic alterations in the corneas of older mice were most likely the result of attempts to repair the more acute lesions.

The corneal calcifications in CFl (Saunders and Rubin 1975) and DBA/2 mice (Yamate et al. 1987) and the corneal dystrophy in CD-1 mice (Taradech and Greaves 1984) are morphologically similar to those described above and probably have the same pathogenesis.

Mice of the KK strain develop spontaneous diabetes mellitus and corneal opacities (Mittl et al. 1970). The corneal lesion consists of extracellular calcium deposition and infiltration of acute and chronic inflammatory cells in the anterior corneal stroma accompanied by neovascularization. The pathogenesis was not determined.

Band keratopathy has been reported in substrains of MRL mice. In MRL/l and MRL/n mice the predominate lesion was mineralization of the anterior corneal stroma and subepithelial basement membrane zone (Hoffman et al. 1983). A few mice in that study had keratitis with neovascularization and a few of the DBA/2 control mice also had band keratopathy. In another study MRL/Mp-+/+ and MRL/Mp-1pr/1pr mice were reported to have band keratopathy with neovascularization and keratitis (Jabs et al. 1985). The authors of that report suggest that the band keratopathy in their MRL substrain was due to local corneal inflammation. MRL substrains have significant uveitis as well as dacryoadenitis which may predispose them to corneal irritation.

Few details of the cage environment were given in the reports of corneal opacities in the KK mice or MRL substrains. These mice may be very sensitive to corneal irritation due to environmental factors such as ammonia levels in cages. Further studies are needed to determine if the corneal opacities listed in group III have a common pathogenesis.

Comparison with Other Species

Spontaneous corneal opacities have been reported in numerous species including the rat, hamster, rabbit, dog, cat, and man. Opacification may be due to congenital anomalies, inherited dystrophies, infectious agents, immune-mediated hypersensitivity reactions, toxins, chemical burns, nutritional deficiencies, and environmental factors (Bistner 1983). The morphology of the opacities varies depending on the etiology and stage of development. In laboratory animals one of the most common opacities is the keratitis observed in rats in association with sialodacryoadenitis virus.

References

Bellhorn RW (1981) Laboratory animal ophthalmology. In: Gelatt KN (ed) Textbook of veterinary ophthalmology. Lee and Febiger, Philadelphia, pp 664–671

Bistner SI (1983) Corneal pathology. In: Pfeiffer RL Jr (ed) Comparative ophthalmic pathology. Thomas, Springfield, pp 87–135

Cousins S, Rodrigues MM, Brown KS, Dale BA (1984) Abnormal corneal and eyelid development in the repeated epilation mouse. Lab Anim Sci 34 (2): 156–163

Green MC (1975) Mutant genes and linkages. In: Green EL (ed) Biology of the laboratory mouse. Dover, New York, pp 87–150

Hoffman RW, Yank HK, Waggie KS, Durham JB, Burge JR, Walker SE (1983) Band keratopathy in MRL/l and MRL/n mice. Arthritis Rheum 26: 645–652

Jabs DA, Alexander EL, Green WR (1985) Ocular inflammation in autoimmune MRL/Mp mice. Invest Ophthalmol Vis Sci 26 (9): 1223-1229

Kaplun A, Barishak RY (1976) Appearance of keratitis in laboratory mice: influence of azathioprine and meticorten. Lab Anim 10: 105–109

Kelton DE, Smith V (1964) Gaping, a new open-eyelid mutation in the house mouse. Genetics 50: 261–262

Mackensen JA (1960) "Open Eyelids" in newborn mice. J Hered 51: 188–190

Mittl R, Galin MA, Opperman W, Camerini-Davalos RA, Spiro D (1970) Corneal calcification in sponta-

neously diabetic mice. Invest Ophthalmol Vis Sci 9 (2): 137–145
Newsome DA, Harne LC, Brown KS, Hassell JR (1982) Corneal keratinization in the oel/+ mouse. Curr Eye Res 2: 553–560
Pierro LJ, Spiggle J (1967) Congenital eye defects in the mouse. I. Corneal opacity in C57 Black mice. J Exp Zool 166: 25–38
Saunders LZ, Rubin LF (1975) Ophthalmic pathology of animals: an atlas and reference book. Karger, Basel, pp 16–17
Taradach C, Greaves P (1984) Spontaneous eye lesions in laboratory animals: incidence in relation to age. CRC Crit Rev Toxicol 12: 121–147
Van Winkle TJ, Balk MW (1986) Spontaneous corneal opacities in laboratory mice. Lab Anim Sci 36(3): 248–255
Yamate J, Tajima M, Maruyana Y, Kudow S (1987) Observations on soft tissue calcification in DBA/2NCrj mice in comparision with CRJ: CD-1 mice. Lab Anim 21: 289–298
Yoshida M, Amemiya T, Yoshida H, Kawaji H (1979) Cornea of Rhino mouse – a model of corneal dystrophy. In: Silverstein AM, O'Connor GR (eds) Immunology and immunopathology of the eye. Masson, New York, pp 355–358

Lipidosis and Mucopolysaccharidosis of the Cornea Due to Cationic Amphiphilic Drugs, Rat

Renate Lüllmann-Rauch

Synonyms. Drug-induced corneal lipidosis and mucopolysaccharidosis; drug-induced lysosomal storage of polar lipids and of sulfated glycosaminoglycans (GAGs), as resulting from impaired degradation.

Gross Appearance

Drug-induced lipidosis and mucopolysaccharidosis in the cornea of rats have not been reported to be recognizable by the naked eye. Some lipidosis-inducing drugs (chlorphentermine, chloroquine, tilorone) cause an anterior polar cataract of the lens, which is readily visible to the unaided eye (Drenckhahn 1978; D. M. Beier and R. Lüllmann-Rauch, to be published).

Microscopic Features

Biomicroscopy

As to lipidosis, there are no reports on biomicroscopic alterations of the rat cornea. Occasionally, rats treated long-term with chloroquine show diffuse corneal clouding due to marked lipidosis and thickening of the endothelium (R. Lüllmann-Rauch, unpublished). The corneal mucopolysaccharidosis induced by long-term treatment with the experimental immunomodulatory agent tilorone (Lüllmann-Rauch 1986) is associated with fine punctate opacities (Fig. 24 a).

These can be seen under a dissecting microscope using oblique illumination. The opacities are even more readily visible in isolated cornea dissected immediately after glutaraldehyde fixation and examined under a stereomicroscope using dark-field illumination.

Light Microscopy

The diagnosis of corneal lipidosis can be made by electron microscopy only. In the case of very marked alterations, indirect indications of corneal lipidosis can be obtained by examination of semithin plastic sections of glutaraldehyde-fixed, osmicated tissues: The keratocytes, endothelium, and the basal layer of the epithelium show abnormal cytoplasmic inclusions intensely stained with toluidine blue at alkaline pH (Fig. 23 a).

Marked corneal *mucopolysaccharidosis* can be diagnosed by light microscopy. In unstained flat preparations of the glutaraldehyde-fixed cornea mounted in buffer, the keratocytes show up as large flat cells with cytoplasmic vacuolation visible by phase constrast microscopy (Fig. 24 b). When such corneal samples are incubated in 0.1% toluidine blue at pH 1 or pH 2, the keratocytes contain intensely staining cytoplasmic in-

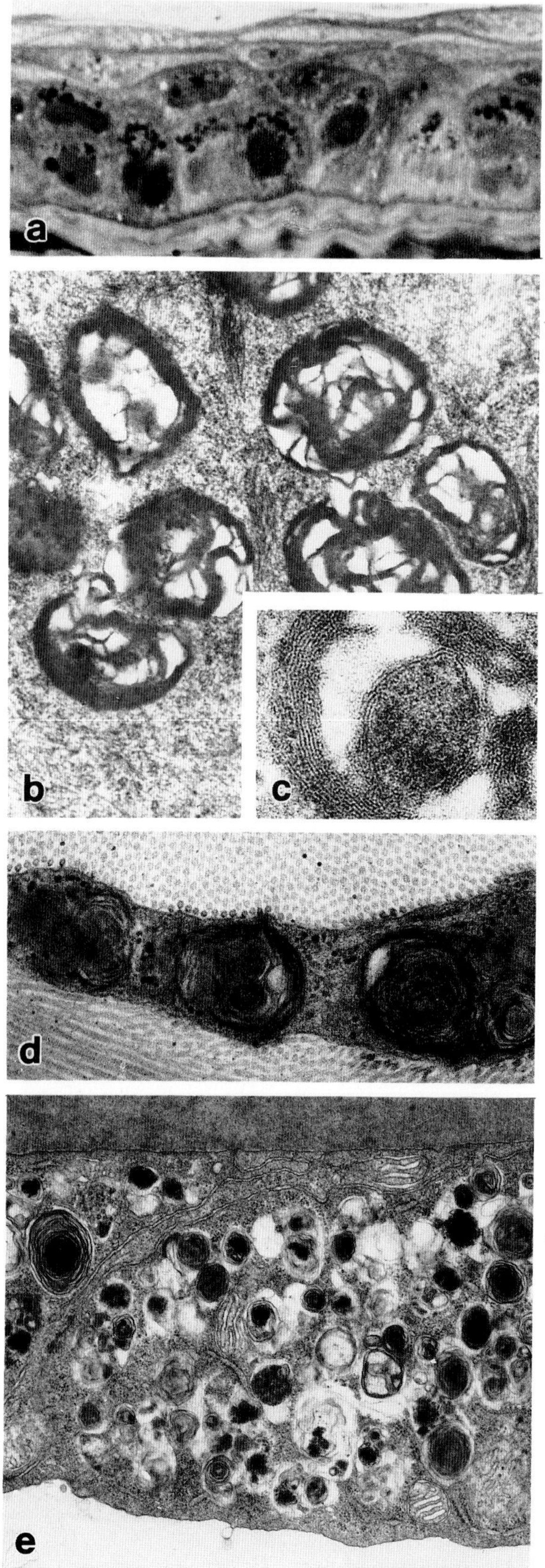

clusions (Fig. 24 c). Intense staining of the keratocytes and fine-granular staining of epithelium and endothelium is obtained when air-dried cryostat sections of unfixed ocular bulbi are incubated in toluidine blue or alcian blue at pH 1 (Fig. 24 e). In semithin plastic sections of glutaraldehyde-fixed, osmicated cornea, the keratocytes display empty cytoplasmic vacuoles (Fig. 25 a).

Ultrastructure

The ultrastructural characteristics of drug-induced lipidosis are described on p. 89 of this volume. In the case of marked corneal lipidosis, all three layers of the cornea are affected.

The epithelium (mainly the basal layer) contains lamellated inclusions (Fig. 23 b, c). In the keratocytes and in the endothelium lamellated inclusions can also be observed (Fig. 23 d, e).

Drug-induced mucopolysaccharidosis is characterized by the transformation of normal lysosomes into enlarged storage organelles which, in routine electron microscopic preparations, appear empty except for remnants of an electron-dense matrix apposed to the limiting membrane (Fig. 25). The empty spaces are a constantly occurring artifact due to the loss of the water-soluble storage material during tissue processing. When corneal mucopolysaccharidosis is fully developed, the keratocytes are greatly swollen due to numerous large vacuoles. In the endothelium and in the basal and intermediate layers of the epithelium, vacuoles with small amounts of flocculent material are found.

◂**Fig. 23. a** Drug-induced lipidosis in cornea, rat. Amiodarone (1%) topically applied for 1 week. Note dense epithelial inclusions in the supranuclear cytoplasm of the basal cells. Semithin plastic section (1 m), alkaline toluidine blue, ×960. **b** Drug-induced lipidosis in cornea, rat. Amiodarone (1%) topically applied for 1 week; epithelium with lamellated cytoplasmic inclusions. TEM, ×24000. **c** Chloroquine, 75 mg/kg per orum for 8 weeks. Note perioidic pattern of lamellar inclusion in epithelium. TEM, ×129000. **d** Chorphentermine, 50 mg/kg per orum for 11 weeks. Keratocyte with lamellated inclusions. TEM, ×34000. **e** Choroquine, 75 mg/kg per orum for 8 weeks. Endothelium is filled with lamellar inclusions. TEM, ×15000

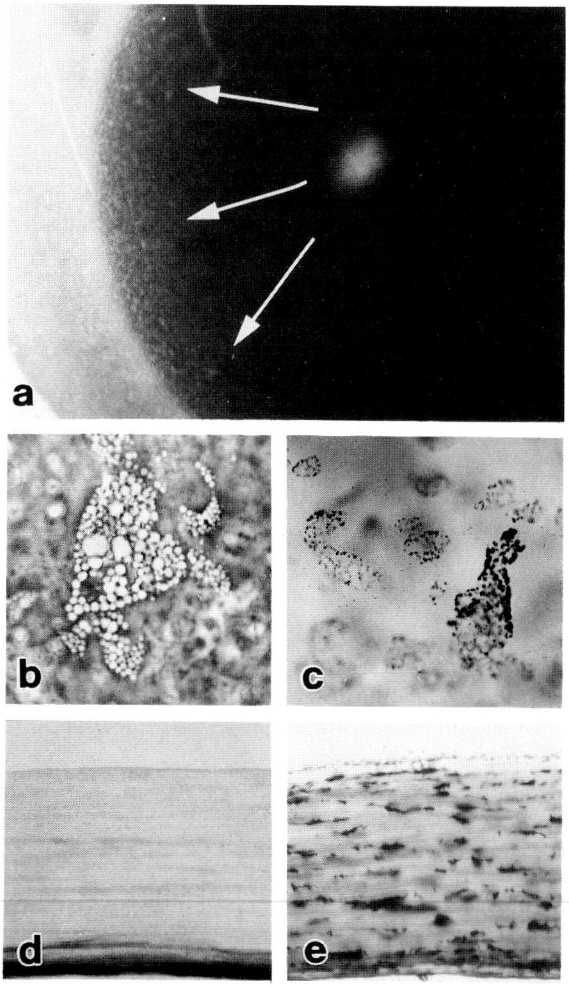

Fig. 24 a–e. Drug-induced mucopolysaccharidosis, cornea, rat. **a** Tilorone, 80 mg/kg given per orum for 15 weeks. Fine punctate opacities *(arrows)* are seen in the cornea. The lens contains an anterior polar cataract. Biomicroscopy, ×22. **b** Tilorone (2%) topically applied for 2.5 weeks. Numerous cytoplasmic vacuoles are seen in the keratocyte. Flat mount, phase contrast microscopy, ×560. **c** Tilorone (2%) applied topically for 2.5 weeks. Intensely staining inclusions are seen instead of vacuoles in the keratocyte. Flat mount toluidine blue (pH 2), ×560. **d** Untreated control rat. Cryostat section (unfixed), alcian blue (pH 1), ×140. **e** The cornea of the tilorone-treated rat (60 mg/kg per orum for 13 weeks). The keratocytes are intensely stained. Cryostat sections (unfixed), Alcian blue (pH 1), ×140

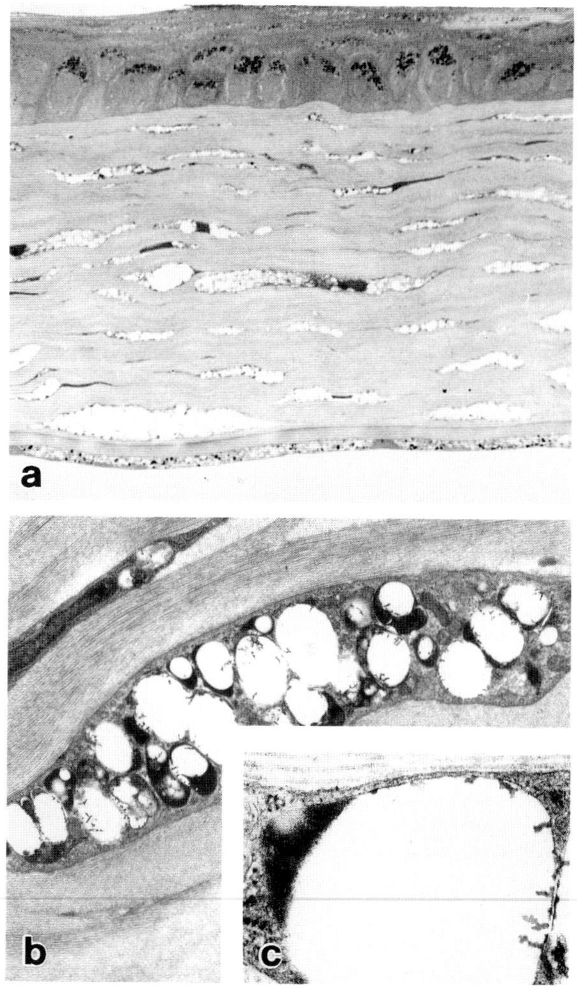

Fig. 25 a–c. Drug-induced mucopolysaccharidosis, cornea, rat. **a** Tilorone 60 mg/kg per orum for 9 weeks. Note dense inclusions in the epithelium and endothelium. The keratocytes are swollen and vacuolated. Semithin plastic section (1 m); tissue fixation with glutaraldehyde plus 1% toluidine blue; no further staining of the section, ×560. **b** Tilorone (2%) applied topically for 9 days. Note the cytoplasmic vacuoles in the keratocyte are membrane limited and appear empty apart from small amounts of an electron-dense matrix and needle-shaped structures. TEM, ×7000. **c** Vacuole in the keratocyte at higher magnification. TEM, ×32000

Differential Diagnosis

In rats, no other conditions are known to be associated with the corneal lesions described above. In untreated control rats, lysosomes of epithelium, keratocytes, and endothelium are seen as small organelles filled with a homogeneous electron-dense matrix. Care must be taken not to mistake poorly fixed, swollen mitochondria for drug-induced vacuoles.

Biologic Features

Corneal lipidosis is part of a generalized storage disease. The biologic features of drug-induced lipidosis are explained in detail on p. 90. The cationic, amphiphilic drugs so far reported to induce corneal lipidosis in rats (Bockhardt et al. 1978; Drenckhahn et al. 1983) are amiodarone (antianginal), chlorphentermine (anorectic), iprindole (antidepressant), tamoxifen (antiestrogen), and chloroquine (antimalarial). The molecular structures of selected drugs are shown in Fig. 78 on p. 90. For toxicologic studies and safety evaluation it is important to note that, upon systemic drug administration, the cornea of rats may fail to develop lipidosis, or the lipidosis may be an inconsistent occurrence; despite the fact that other ocular and extraocular tissues of the same rats consistently show marked lipidosis, and despite the fact that the particular drug may induce corneal lipidosis in other species, e.g., in man. Such species-dependent diversities have been found with amiodarone (Bockhardt et al. 1978) and chloroquine (Drenckhahn et al. 1983). As soon as the drugs were topically applied onto the rat cornea, lipidosis consistently occurred within a few days. This suggests that the distribution of the drugs throughout the ocular tissues and compartments may be different in rat and in man. Another difficulty observed with chloroquine was that the lipidosis-related alterations, if present after systemic drug administration, were not evenly distributed over the entire cornea, so that one could easily miss the alterations upon histologic examination. The examples of chloroquine and amiodarone show that negative results obtained on rat cornea after systemic drug administration may lead to false predictions concerning the cornea of man.

Corneal mucopolysaccharidosis of rats is part of a generalized storage disease which is caused, in addition to generalized lipidosis, by chronic treatment with the dicationic amphiphilic compound tilorone and several tilorone analogs (Hein and Lüllmann-Rauch 1989). These compounds were all synthesized as immunomodulatory agents. Tilorone-induced mucopolysaccharidosis is due to impaired lysosomal degradation of sulfated glycosaminoglycans (Gupta et al. 1984). The molecular mechanisms, and the molecular features of tilorone that are essential for this additional side effect, are not yet clear. As far as is known from a biochemical study on the urine and liver of tilorone-treated rats, the abnormally stored glycosaminoglycans are mainly dermatan sulfate and chondroitin sulfate (Hein et al. 1987). Histochemical studies have shown that liver, spleen, kidney, cardiac valves, cornea, and cartilage of rats are affected (Lüllmann-Rauch 1986, 1987; Lüllmann-Rauch et al. 1988). Tilorone-induced mucopolysaccharidosis has a very low tendency to recede. The corneal alterations were still present several months after discontinuation of chronic treatment (Lüllmann-Rauch 1986).

Both lipidosis and mucopolysaccharidosis of the cornea are well known to occur in the genetically determined storage diseases of man (Kenyon 1976; Berman 1982, Klintworth 1982) and of animal mutants (Shull et al. 1982; Aguirre et al. 1983; Haskins et al. 1983). With respect to corneal clouding and to the cytologic alterations, the drug-induced corneal disorders are reminiscent of the inherited storage diseases, although the molecular mechanisms are different. In any case, the corneal opacities are a result of the optical inhomogeneities caused by the accumulation of cytoplasmic inclusions or vacuoles in the corneal cells and by swelling of the keratocytes (Goldman et al. 1968; Benedek 1971).

Comparison with Other Species

In humans, chloroquine, amodiaquine, amiodarone, and perhexiline induce corneal opacities (Sandvig 1966; Grant 1974; Verin et al. 1971) that have been shown to be associated with the occurrence of numerous lamellated cytoplasmic inclusions in corneal epithelium (Toussaint and Pohl 1969; Pülhorn and Thiel 1976; D'Amico and Kenyon 1981; D'Amico et al. 1981; Chew et al 1982; Gibson et al. 1984). Furthermore, tilorone has caused corneal clouding in patients (Weiss et al. 1980). The ultrastructural examination of corneal biopsies revealed a few lamellated inclusions, which appear, however, insufficient to account for the conspicuous opacities. It is uncertain whether mucopolysaccharidosis has existed in tilorone-treated patients.

References

Aguirre A, Stramm L, Haskins M (1983) Feline mucopolysaccharidosis VI: general ocular and pigment epithelial pathology. Invest Ophthalmol Vis Sci 24: 991–1007

Beier DM, Lüllmann-Rauch R (to be published)

Benedek GB (1971) Theory of transparency of the eye. Appl Opt 10: 459–473

Berman ER (1982) Sphingolipidosis and neuronal ceroidlipofuscinosis. In: Garner A, Klintworth GK (eds) Pathobiology of ocular disease, part B. Dekker, New York, pp 897–929
Bockhardt H, Drenckhahn D, Lüllmann-Rauch R (1978) Amiodarone-induced lipidosis-like alterations in ocular tissues of rats. Graefes Arch Klin Exp Ophthalmol 207: 91–96
Chew E, Ghosh M, McCulloch C (1982) Amiodarone-induced cornea verticillata. Can J Ophthalmol 17: 96–99
D'Amico DJ, Kenyon KR (1981) Drug-induced lipidosis of the cornea and conjunctiva. Int Ophthalmol 4: 67–76
D'Amico DJ, Kenyon KR, Ruskin JN (1981) Amiodarone keratopathy: drug-induced lipid storage disease. Arch Ophthalmol 99: 257–261
Drenckhahn D (1978) Anterior polar cataract and lysosomal alterations in the lens of rats treated with the amphiphilic lipidosis-inducing drugs chloroquine and chlorphentermine. Virchows Arch [B] 27: 255–266
Drenckhahn D, Jacobi B, Lüllmann-Rauch R (1983) Corneal lipidosis in rats treated with amphiphilic cationic drugs. Arzneimittelforschung 33: 827–831
Gibson JM, Fielder AR, Garner A, Millac R (1984) Severe ocular side effects of perhexilene maleate: case reports. Br J Ophthalmol 68: 553–560
Goldman JN, Benedek GB, Dohlman CH, Kravitt B (1968) Structural alterations affecting transparency in swollen human corneas. Invest Ophthalmol Vis Sci 7: 501–519
Grant WM (1974) Toxicology of the eye: drugs, chemicals, plants, venom, 2nd edn. Thomas, Springfield
Gupta DK, Gieselmann V, Hasilik A, Figura K (1984) Tilorone acts as a lysosomotropic agent in fibroblasts. Hoppe-Seyler's Z Physiol Chem 365: 859–866
Haskins ME, Aguirre GD, Jezyk PF, Desnick RJ, Patterson DF (1983) The pathology of the feline model of mucopolysaccharidosis I. Am J Pathol 112: 27–36
Hein L, Lüllmann-Rauch R (1989) Mucopolysaccharidosis and lipidosis in rats treated with tilorone analogues. Toxicology 58: 145–154
Hein L, Lüllmann-Rauch R, Prokopek M (1987) Mucopolysaccharidosis induced by di-cationic amphiphilic drugs. Naunyn Schmiedebergs Arch Pharmacol 335 [Suppl]: R3 (abstract)
Kenyon KR (1976) Ocular manifestations and pathology of systemic mucopolysaccharidoses. Birth Defects 12: 133–153
Klintworth GK (1982) Disorders of glycosaminoglycans (mucopolysaccharidosis) and proteoglycans. In: Garner A, Klintworth GK (eds) Pathobiology of ocular disease, part B. Dekker, New York, pp 863–895
Lüllmann-Rauch R (1986) Keratopathy in rats after treatment with tilorone. Graefes Arch Clin Exp Ophthalmol 224: 377–383
Lüllmann-Rauch R (1987) Lysosomal storage of sulfated glycosaminoglycans in renal interstitial cells of rats treated with tilorone. Cell Tissue Res 250: 641–648
Lüllmann-Rauch R, Michel G, Peters A (1988) Mucopolysaccharidosis-like cellular alterations in chondrocytes of rats treated with tilorone. Exp Mol Pathol 49: 279–289
Pülhorn G, Thiel HJ (1976) Das ultrastrukturelle Bild der Chloroquin-Keratopathie. Graefes Arch Clin Exp Ophthalmol 201: 89–99
Sandvig K (1966) Chlorquine (resochin) effects on the cornea. Acta Ophthalmol 44: 355–360
Shull RM, Munger RJ, Spellacy E, Hall CW, Constantopoulos G, Neufeld EF (1982) Canine alpha-L-iduronidase deficiency. A model of mucopolysaccharidosis I. Am J Pathol 109: 244–248
Toussaint D, Pohl S (1969) Aspect histologique et ultrastructure des depots corneens dus au chlorhydrate d'amiodarone. Bull Soc Belge Ophtalmol 153: 675–686
Verin P, Gendre P, Barchewitz G, Laurent-Brochat G, Yocoubi M, Morax S (1971) Thesaurismose corneenne par amiodarone. Donnes Recentes Arch Ophtalmol (Paris) 31: 581–596
Weiss JN, Weinberg RS, Regelson W (1980) Keratopathy after oral administration of tilorone hydrochloride. Am J Ophthalmol 89: 46–53

Keratoconjunctivitis Sicca and Sequelae, Mouse and Rat

Alexander Kast

Synonyms. Purulent blepharitis, conjunctivitis, keratopathy, keratitis filiformis, dry eye syndrome, xerophthalmia, uveitis anterior, iritis, iridokeratitis, iridocyclitis, hypopyoniritis.

Gross Appearance

The first sign is dryness of the cornea observed from 5–15 min through 3 h after a single application of 75 or 106 mg/kg clonidine HCl (Fig. 26). Within 24 h, the dryness is followed by redness of the conjunctiva with a mild ramiform injection of vessels and chromodacryorrhea. On the 2nd day, small smokey rough-surfaced opacities

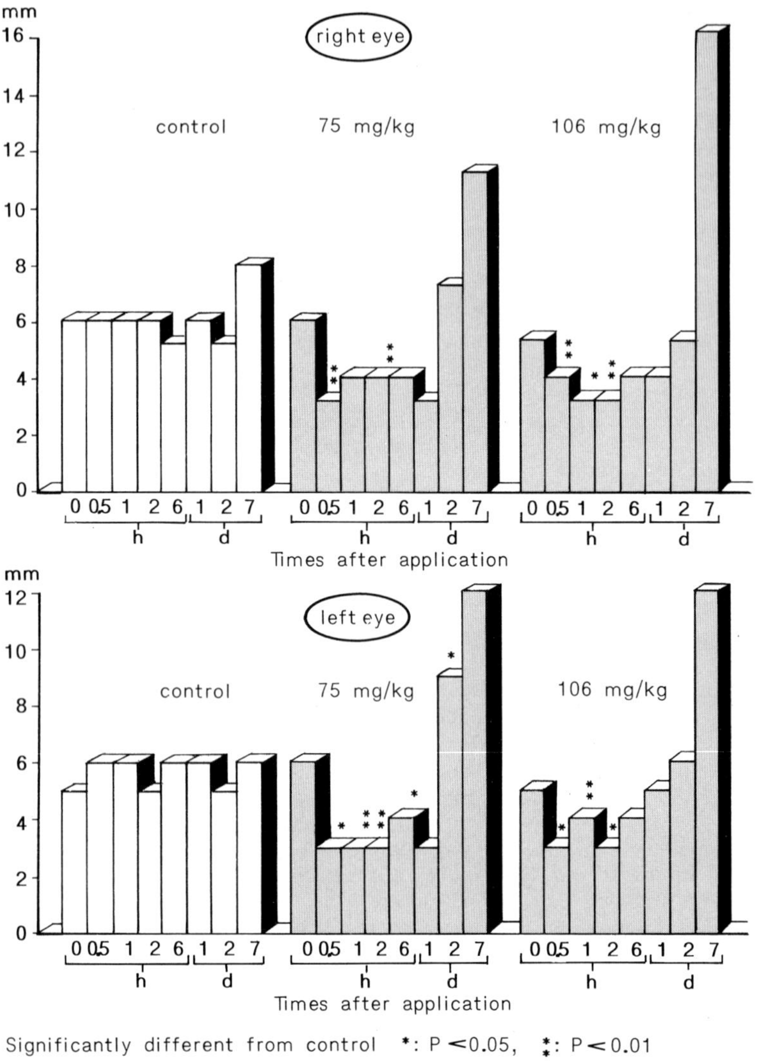

Fig. 26. Lacrimal secretion (Schirmer tear test) of male rats given a single dose of 75 or 106 mg/kg clonidine HC1 (values in millimeters per minute)

occur in the superficial layers of the central cornea. The lacrimal secretion is increased.

Sequelae. Small pustules and ulcers occur near the limbus. Pus or fibrin coagula are seen as gray-white clouds in the anterior chamber (Fig. 27). It has been assumed that sometimes coagula may precipitate during postmortem exsiccation of the eye. The effects may be unilateral or bilateral. From the 3rd to 5th day corneal ulcers and ring abscess of the cornea develop in a few animals. Most lesions heal within 7 days following a single application. In more severe cases, a chronic productive inflammation of the anterior globe and formation of a connective tissue nodule at the surface of the cornea have been observed within 2 weeks. A chronic panophthalmia is more common in rats than in mice. However, mice develop necrosis of the central cornea with a demarcation zone of leukocytes (ring abscess).

During repeated dosing for 3 months, a dry cornea has been found sporadically in rats; however, this disappeared within 5–6 h after dosing. At higher doses, the dryness of cornea has been more distinct and long-lasting, and several rats have been left with corneal opacities.

Microscopic Features

The earliest changes consist of a flattening of the superficial layers of the central cornea, first seen after 30 min–2 h (Figs. 28–30). The corneal epithelium has often desquamated to nearly half normal thickness, and single basal cells in the opaque area are ballooned. The epithelial layers appear disorganized.

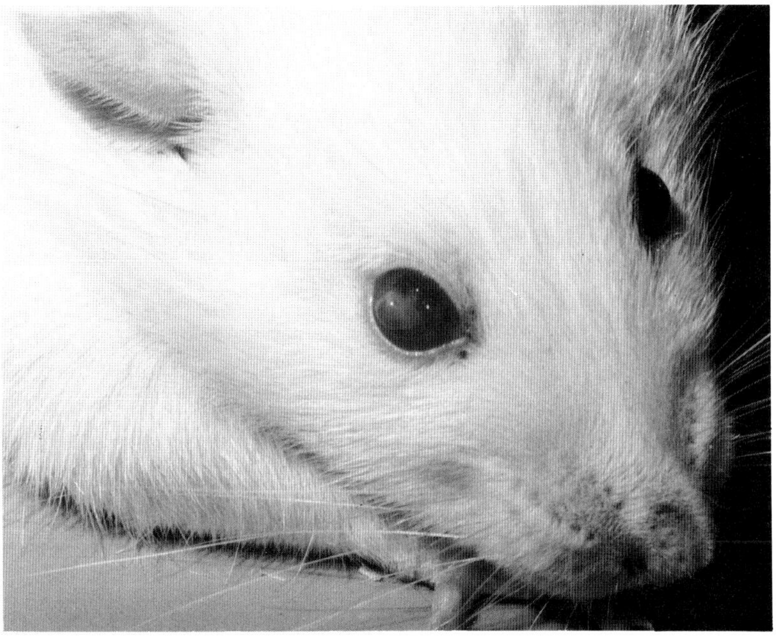

▲
Fig. 27. Male rat. Pus in the anterior chamber of the right eye 1 day after treatment

Fig. 28 *(above)*. Normal rat cornea *(left)* ▶

Fig. 29 *(below)*. Cornea, rat, 7 days after 1 mg/kg clonidine orally *(right)*. The corneal epithelium is nearly half normal thickness, with intracellular edema in single basal and wing cells. (Weisse et al. 1978) H & E, ×300

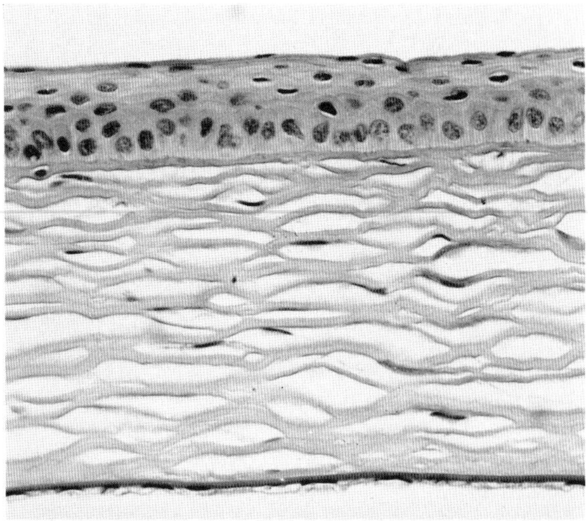

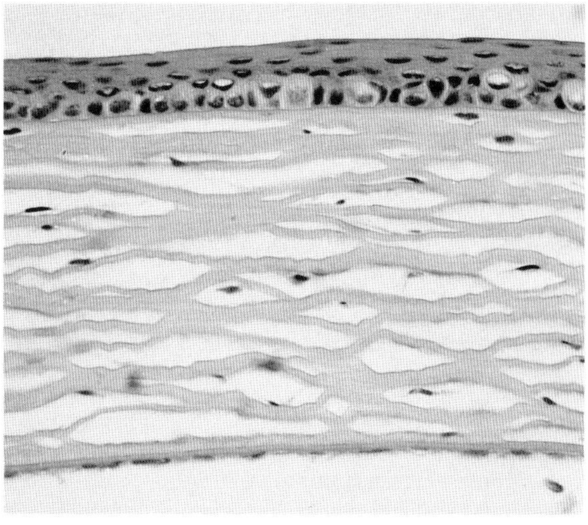

According to Gilbard et al. (1987), besides superficial epithelial cell flattening and desquamation, fine structural changes in hybrid mice are: frequent blunting and loss of surface epithelial cell microplicae, at times with frank disruption of the epithelial cell surface membrane.

Sequelae. An acute purulent conjunctivitis has been observed after 6 h, followed by ulceration and the formation of pustules predominantly near the limbus. Blepharitis is extremely rare. Within 24 h, the inflammatory process spreads from the limbus to the root of the iris, causing iridocyclitis with eosinophilia. Fibrinous leukocytic exudate from the iris floats to the iridocorneal angle outflow of the anterior chamber, where it may cause obstruction. At the same time, corneal ulceration begins, the tunica propria is infiltrated by neutrophils, and early stages of a ring abscess of the central cornea may occur. At 48 h, the lesions are fully developed, consisting of severe purulent keratoconjunctivitis, eosi-

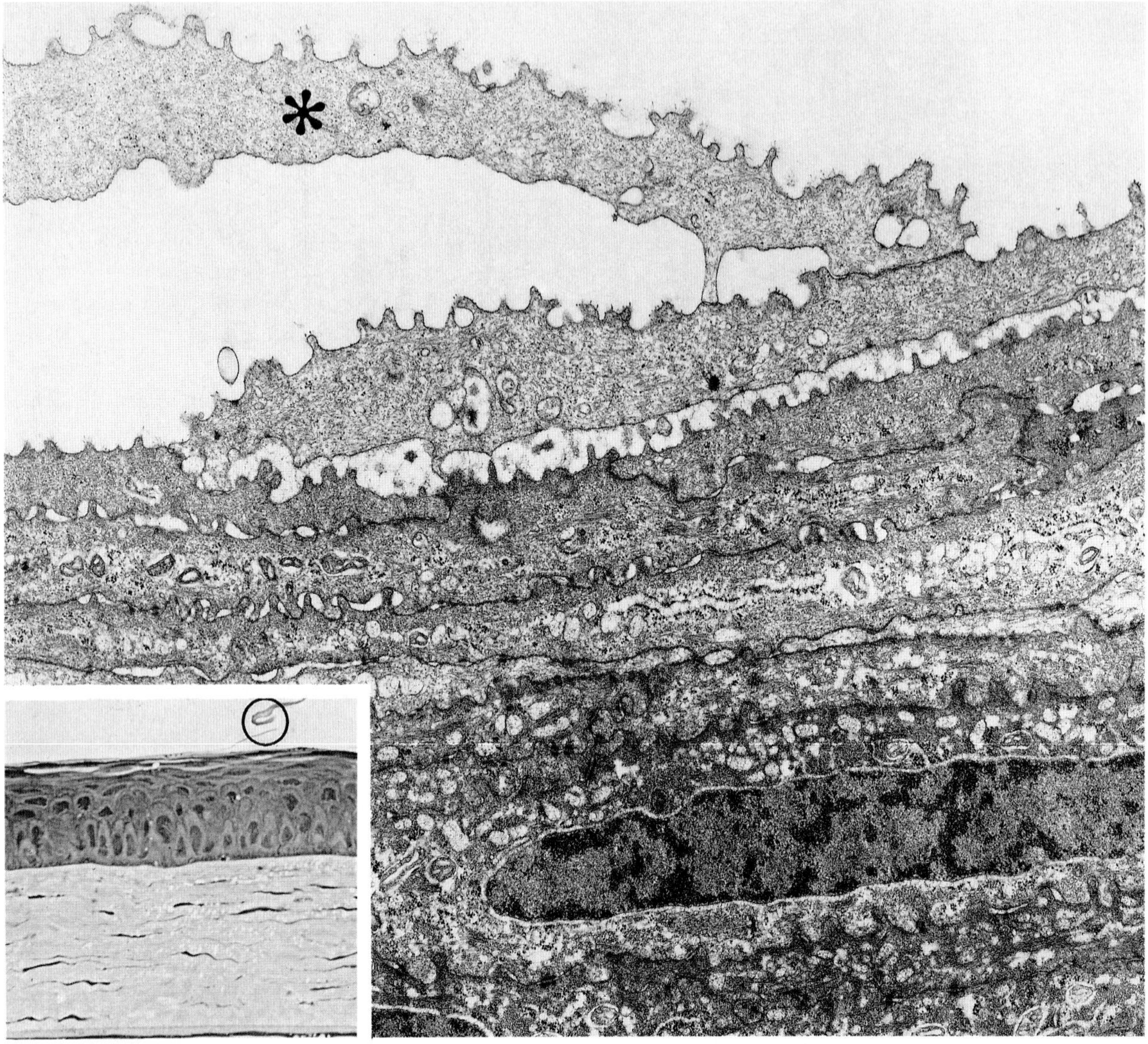

Fig. 30. Cornea, 13-week-old NZB/NZW/Fl hybrid female mouse. Superficial epithelial cells flattened and desquamated *(asterisk)*. TEM, ×13400. *Inset:* cornea of a BALB/c control mouse. Epithelium flattened and desquamated *(circle)*. (Gilbard et al. 1987) phase contrast, paraphenylenediamine, ×300

Fig. 31 *(upper left)*. Eye, male rat, 24 h after treatment. Acute conjunctivitis with pustula near the limbus. H & E, ×150

Fig. 32 *(lower left)*. Eye, male rat, 24 h after treatment. Acute keratitis with the substantia propria infiltrated by neutrophils below ulceration of the cornea, and eosinophils in Descemet's membrane. H & E, ×150

Fig. 33 *(upper right)*. Eye, male rat, 48 h after treatment. ▸ Acute iritis with leukocytes, predominantly eosinophils, and leaking of fibrinous exudate into the anterior chamber. H & E, ×300

Fig. 34 *(lower right)*. Eye, male rat, 48 h after treatment. Accumulation of leukocytes and fibrin in the angle outflow of the anterior chamber. H & E, ×150

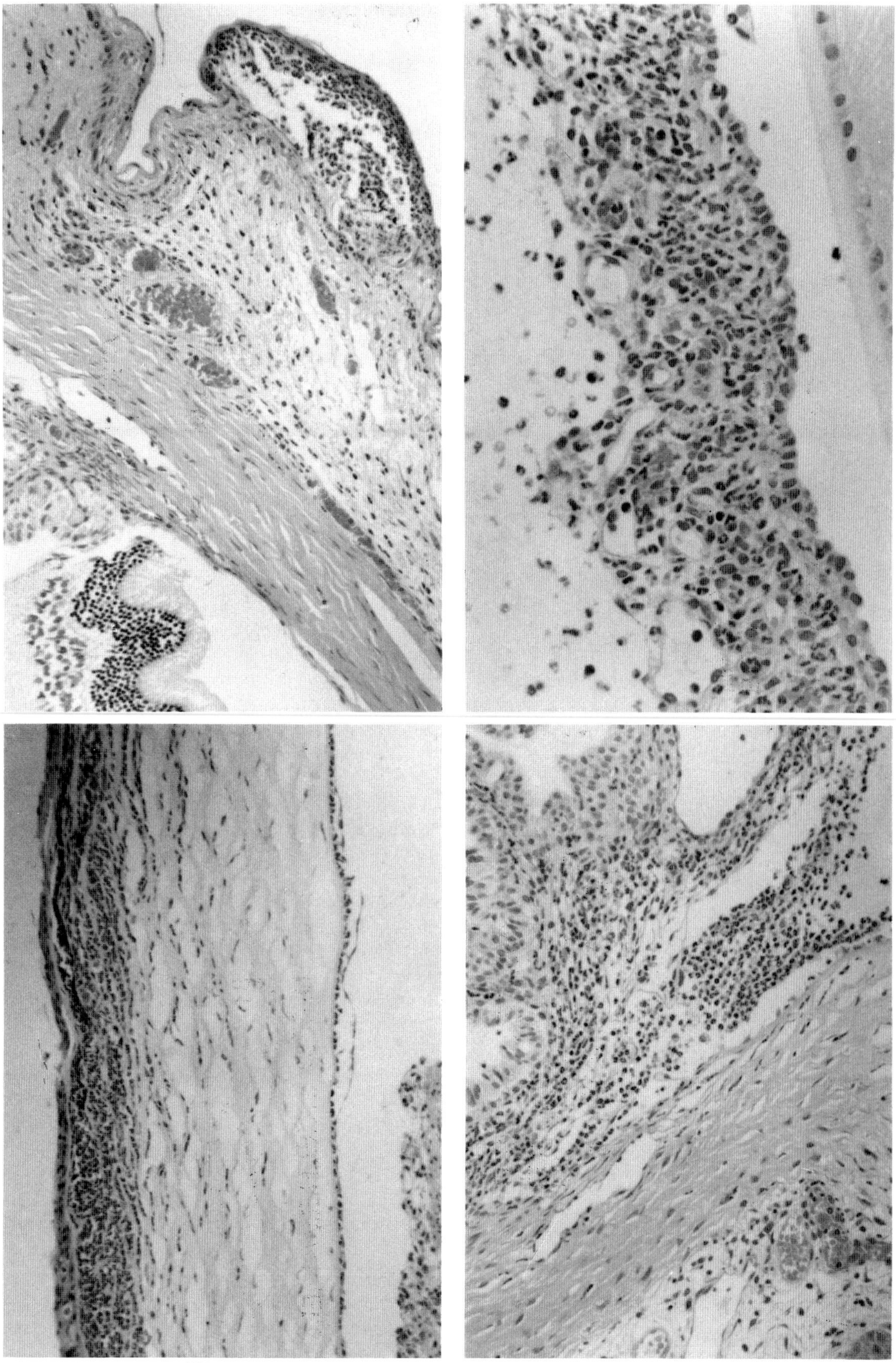

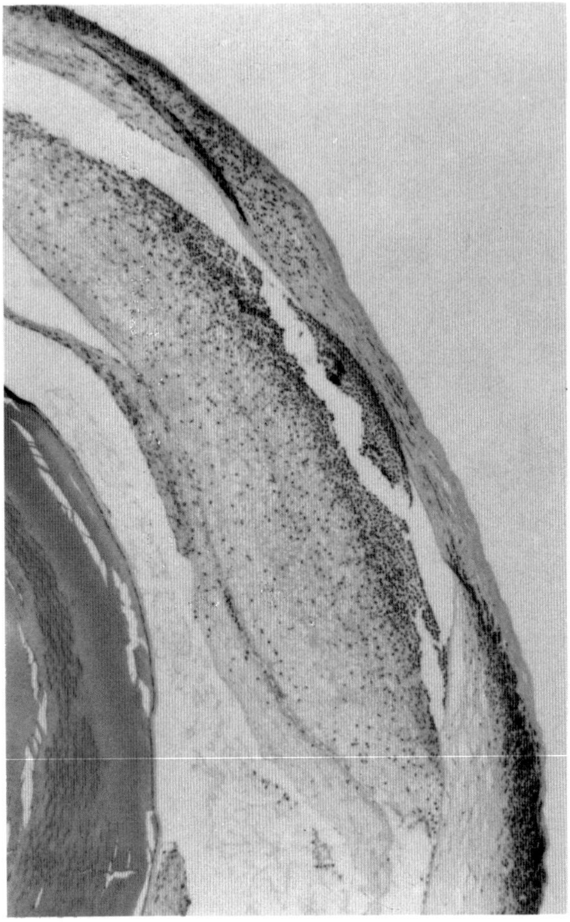

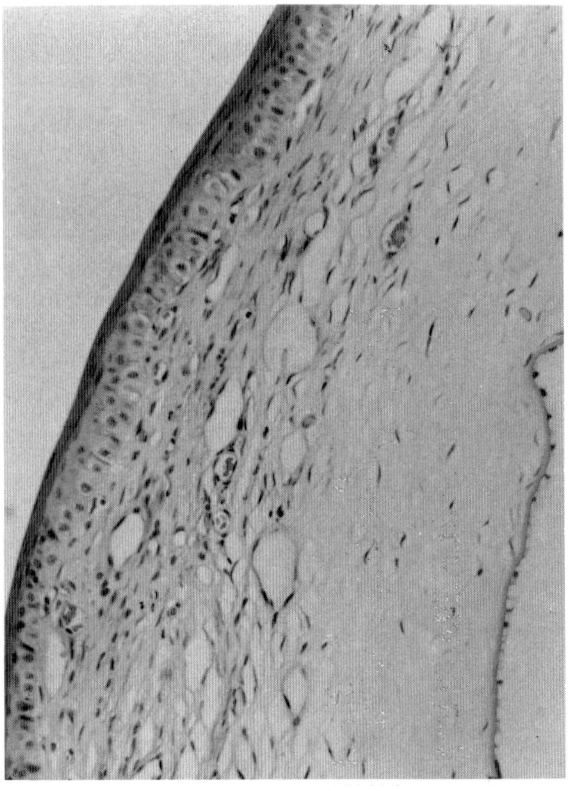

nophilic iridocyclitis, hypopyon, a blood-filled anterior chamber, a ring abscess of the central cornea, and large corneal ulcers (Figs. 31–35). The surface of the cornea may be populated with bacteria. Occasionally the iris adheres uniformly to the entire cornea (anterior synechiae). Seven days after the single application, the healing of the lesions has been essentially completed or only chronic changes remain. After 14 days, a chronic productive inflammation of the anterior globe and nodule formation at the surface of the cornea have been confirmed histologically. Sometimes one eye remains intact.

After completion of studies using repeated doses, several rats that received intermediate and high doses, including three allowed to recover, had small foci of chronic inflammation in the central cornea. These lesions included lymphocytic infiltration, a few newly formed connective tissue fibers, and the formation of small vessels (Fig. 36). Mineralization of the basement membrane and large fluid-filled bullous spaces between the corneal epithelium and anterior stroma were also observed. In two cases the inflammation resulted in adhesion between the iris and cornea (anterior synechia). In 21 rats affected only one eye contained the lesion, whereas in 8 animals both eyes were damaged.

Differential Diagnosis

Keratoconjunctivitis sicca is relatively rare in animal safety evaluation studies using systemic administration (Heywood 1985; Gopinath et al. 1987). An initial dose of narcotic analgesics, for instance morphine and 1-α-acetylmethadol, induces corneal opacities and chronic corneal changes in rats by epithelial desiccation during exophthalmos of about 3 h duration (Fabian et al. 1967; Roerig et al. 1980). The intake of the sulfonylureas carbutamide, tolbutamide, and chlorpropamide caused exophthalmos and chronic inflammation of the anterior globe in rats following 1 year of treatment (Wright 1963).

◂ **Fig. 35** *(above).* Cornea, male mouse. Ring abscess of the central cornea with hypopyon. Following a single dose of clonidine and found dead on day 2. H & E, ×15

Fig. 36 *(below).* Cornea, male rat, dosed subcutaneously with 5 mg/kg clonidine base for 3 months. Chronic keratitis parenchymatosa with corneal vascularization. H & E, ×150

Corneal opacities in rats have also occurred after organophosphate poisoning with fenthion (Baytex) according to Hikita and Ishikawa (1972). A major problem is to distinguish spontaneous from drug-related lesions (Taradach et al. 1981).

Severe inflammation of the conjunctiva in the rat is most commonly caused by sialodacryoadenitis virus (Heywood 1973; Weisbroth and Peress 1977): In this infection, ophthalmic lesions include hemorrhage into the anterior chamber, diffuse or ulcerative keratitis, anterior synechiae, hypopyon, and iridocyclitis. Keratitis and opacities of bacterial origin, for instance, caused by *Staphylococcus aureus, Pasteurella multocida,* and *Moraxella bovis,* have been reported (Foster 1958; Jones 1959; Heywood 1973; Moore 1979, Roberts and Gregory 1980; Chandler et al. 1983). As experimental infections usually failed to induce eye lesions, it has been proposed that following enzootic sialodacryoadenitis infection ophthalmic lesions are secondary to obstruction of normal lacrimal secretion (Lai et al. 1976). Panophthalmia may be caused by the orbital blood-sampling technique.

Biologic Features

According to Saunders and Rubin (1975), an inflammation of the various tissues of the anterior portion of the globe is the most common ophthalmic syndrome in young rats and is considered as a pathologic entity (Saunders 1967). Normal composition and distribution of the tear film for moistening of the mucosal surface is essential for the maintenance of the proper optical qualities of the cornea, to nourish the cornea and remove wastes; and to provide antibacterial activity. Deficiency of the tear flow may result in corneal damage (Brightman 1980; McCaa 1985). Inflammatory processes of the anterior eye are secondary and predominantly caused by infections. Ubiquitous bacteria of the normally existing conjunctival flora may be involved. The penetration of bacterial endotoxins alone into the inner eye can induce a sterile uveitis or hypopyoniritis (Kulkarni and Srinivasan 1988). The chance of an infection may also contribute to the explanation of why one eye shows severe lesions while the other does not.

The lesions induced by clonidine are interpreted as keratoconjunctivitis sicca caused by an exophthalmus of more than 60 min duration and, more important, a reduced lacrimal secretion combined with the already relatively poor tear flow and very low blinking frequency of the rat and decreased wiping or grooming. Pretreatment with the adrenergic α-blocker phentolamine has significantly reduced the appearance of corneal lesions, as has moistening of the cornea with viscous methylcellulose (Methocel) solution (Weisse et al. 1978; Kast et al. 1987).

Our investigational results have shown that clonidine at exceptionally high dosages causes a significantly diminished tear flow from 30 min through 24 h followed by an increase from day 2–7 (Fig. 26). The loss of the tear flow and its bactericidal function for up to 24 h ist the cause of secondary ocular inflammation.

The activities of clonidine stem from its stimulation of central α-adrenoceptors. Inhibitory effects of clonidine on salivary and gastric secretion involve central as well as peripheral sites of action, the latter due to an action on presynaptic α-adrenoceptors inhibiting cholinergic transmission (Hoefke 1983).

Acute toxicity testing in various animal species has revealed large differences between pharmacologically effective and toxic doses. The substance-related ocular findings in small rodents show a very good healing tendency within 1–2 weeks due to the rapid growth of the corneal epithelium from its basal cells.

In repeated dose studies, even at toxic dose levels, eye lesions are less common and seldom severe. The dose of 0.05 mg/kg has been the "no-effect level" concerning visible eye lesions. At 0.5 and 5 mg/kg clonidine, opacity of the cornea occurs from day 2 of trial, disappears during the study, or is followed by a small focal chronic keratitis.

Comparison with Other Species

The clonidine-induced changes are rodent specific, as the rabbit, the dog, and the monkey have not shown such corneal alterations (Weisse et al. 1978; Kast et al. 1987), although, following i.v. injection of clonidine, constrictions of episcleral and conjunctival vessels occur in all the animals (Baurmann et al. 1986), and in spite of the fact that the pharmacokinetic data compare rather well between the various species (Hoefke 1983). Keratoconjunctivitis sicca in rodents occurs only at high doses, far above the clinical dose of 0.005 mg/kg clonidine (transdermal therapeutic system). Clonidine and other mydriatic drugs have been used in man for more than 2 decades, often topically applied; however, such ocular lesions are unknown (Turacli 1974; Lyle and Hopkins 1977; Rangstorff and Doughty 1982).

Long-term treatment with sulfonylureas has caused similar chronic lesions of the anterior globe in rats, but not in dogs (Wright 1963). Retinal S-antigen obtained from other species can induce a T-cell-mediated uveoretinitis in rats (Rao et al. 1989).

In most cases, dogs with keratoconjunctivitis sicca have a high incidence of immune-mediated disorders including a Sjögren's-like syndrome (Kaswan et al. 1989). Sporadic cases can be attributed to drug toxicity, for instance, a variety of sulfonamides including sulfadiazine, sulfasalazine, phenazopyridine, salicylazosulfapyridine, trimethoprime, and aminosalicylic acid (Todenhoefer 1969; Aguirre et al. 1971; Slatter 1973; Bryan and Slatter 1973; Slatter and Blogg 1978; Morgan and Bachrach 1982; Sansom et al. 1985; Barnett and Joseph 1987), antispasmodic agents, and all anticholinergic compounds at high enough doses (Majeed et al. 1983, 1987; Heywood 1985). The ocular lesions are caused by an acute reduction of tear secretion and may be reversible upon withdrawal of the drug. Also in the case of sulfonamids, species susceptibility is a well-recognized phenomenon and keratoconjunctivitis sicca has not been reported as a complication in cats and man (Bryan and Slatter 1973; Sansom et al. 1985). In dogs, experimental removal of the lacrimal glands was followed by reduction of tear flow and keratoconjunctivitis sicca. Scanning electron microscopy revealed clusters of hyperplastic globlet cells on the conjunctiva in tear-deficient animals (Kern et al. 1988). In contrast to the rat, primary eye lesions of dogs are not followed by a fibrinopurulent inflammation of the anterior globe.

A keratoconjunctivitis filiformis alias sicca occurs regularly in Sjögren's syndrome (Sjögren 1933; Bruce 1941) or dry eye syndrome, the pathogenesis of which is still unknown, but there is a predilection for middle-aged women (McMonnies 1987) and a strong link with certain autoimmune disorders (Maddison 1985). Relations to severe renal disease or kidney transplants (Strempel et al. 1989), generalized xerosis in diabetic and hypertensive patients in many cases independent of drugs (Sreebny et al. 1989), altered immunoregulation-like specific autoantibodies (Maddison 1985; Pflugfelder et al. 1986; Nelson 1989), and Hashimoto's thyroiditis have been discussed. Drug-induced corneal lesions in man have been observed after isotretinoin (synthetic vitamin A, Caffery and Josephson 1988) and uncontrolled use of corticosteroids (Henkes and Canta 1973; Meier-Ruge 1973). A spontaneous animal model resembling Sjögren's syndrome exists in the NZB/NZW mouse (Baum 1975; Gilbard et al. 1987).

Keratoconjunctivitis sicca is infrequently diagnosed in other species. Infectious bovine keratoconjunctivitis is caused by several strains of *Moraxella bovis* in cattle and mice (Chandler et al. 1983). A case involving both eyes of a horse and caused by an eosinophilic granulomatous dacryoadenitis has been described by Spiess et al. (1989).

References

Aguirre GD, Rubin LF, Harvey CE (1971) Keratoconjunctivitis sicca in dogs. J Am Vet Med Ass 158: 1566–1579

Barnett K, Joseph E (1987) Keratoconjunctivitis sicca in the dog following 5-aminosalicylic acid administration. Hum Toxicol 6: 377–383

Baum J (1975) Keratoconjunctivitis sicca. Trans Am Acad Ophthalmol Otolaryngol 81: 619–623

Baurmann H, Jankolovitz M, Wirmer M, Wolter M, Anda L, Hornchen U (1986) Simultanbeobachtung okulärer Gefäßreaktionen an Vorder- und Hinterabschnitt nach Clonidin und Propranolol bei normotonen und hypertensiven Versuchstieren. Klin Monatsbl Augenheilkd 189: 467–476

Brightman AH (1980) Keratoconjunctivitis sicca. J Am Vet Med Assoc 176: 710–711

Bruce G (1941) Keratoconjunctivitis sicca. Arch Ophthalmol 26: 945–964

Bryan GM, Slatter DH (1973) Keratoconjunctivitis sicca induced by phenazopyridine in dogs. Arch Ophthalmol 90: 310–311

Caffery B, Josephson J (1988) Ocular side effects of isotretinoin therapy. J Am Optom Assoc 59: 221–224

Chandler R, Turfrey B, Smith K (1983) Laboratory model for infectious bovine keratoconjunctivitis: the pathogenicity of different strains of *Moraxella bovis*, pathology and ultrastructural observations. Res Vet Sci 35: 277–284

Fabian R, Bond J, Drobeck H (1967) Induced corneal opacities in the rat. Br J Ophthalmol 51: 124–129

Foster HL (1958) Purulent keratoconjunctivitis in laboratory rats, caused by *micrococcus pyogenes* var. *aureus*. J Am Vet Med Assoc 133: 201

Gilbard J, Hanninen L, Rothman R, Kenyon K (1987) Lacrimal gland, cornea, and tear film in the NZB/NZW Fl hybrid mouse. Curr Eye Res 6: 1237–1248

Gopinath C, Prentice D, Lewis D (1987) Experimental toxicological pathology, the eye and ear. Curr Histopathol 13: 145–155

Henkes H, Canta L (1973) Drug-induced disorders of the eye. Proc Eur Soc Drug Toxicol 14: 146–153

Heywood R (1973) Some clinical observations on the eyes of Sprague-Dawley rats. Lab Anim 7: 19–27
Heywood R (1985) Clinical and laboratory assessment of visual dysfunction. In: Hayes A (ed) Toxicology of the eye, ear and other special senses. Raven, New York, pp 61–78
Hikita H, Ishikawa T (1972) Experimental treatment of organophosphate poisoning. Inhibitory effects of GSH on corneal opacity in rats given Baytex. Jpn Rev Clin Ophthalmol 66: 832–834
Hoefke W (1983) Pharmacology of clonidine. Arzneimittelforschung [Suppl] 28: 31–64
Jones LP (1959) Purulent panophthalmitis in laboratory rats. J Am Vet Med Assoc 135: 502–503
Kast A, Tsunenari Y, Yabe T (1987) Toxicology of clonidine base in comparison with clonidine hydrochloride, acute and subacute studies in rodents. Iyakuhin Kenkyu 18: 366–391
Kaswan R, Salisbury M, Ward D (1989) Spontaneous canine keratoconjunctivitis sicca. Arch Ophthalmol 107: 1210–1216
Kern TJ, Erb HN, Schaedler JM, Dougherty EP (1988) Scanning electron microscopy of experimental keratoconjunctivitis sicca in dogs: cornea and bulbar conjunctiva. Vet Pathol 25: 468–474
Kulkarni P, Srinivasan D (1988) Cachectin: a novel polypeptide induces uveitis in the rabbit eye. Exp Eye Res 46: 631–633
Lai Y, Jakoby R, Bhatt P, Jonas A (1976) Keratoconjunctivitis associated with sialodacryoadenitis in rats. Invest Ophthalmol Vis Sci 15: 538–541
Lyle W, Hopkins G (1977) The unwanted ocular effects from topical ophthalmic drugs. J Am Optom Assoc 48: 1519–1523
Maddison P (1985) Dry eyes: autoimmunity and relationship to other systemic disease. Trans Ophthalmol Soc UK 104: 458–461
Majeed SK, Prentice DE, Heywood R (1983) A form of keratoconjunctivitis sicca in dogs treated with an antispasmodic compound. J Pathol 140: 133
Majeed SK, Gopinath C, Heywood R (1987) A report on drug-induced kerato-conjunctivitis sicca in dogs. J Comp Pathol 97: 385–391
McCaa C (1985) Anatomy, physiology and toxicology of the eye. In: Hayes A (ed) Toxicology of the eye, ear, and other special senses. Raven, New York, pp 1–15
McMonnies C (1987) Key questions in a dry eye history. J Am Optom Assoc 57: 512–517
Meier-Ruge W (1973) Eye toxicity. Proc Eur Soc Drug Toxicol 14: 133–145
Moore GJ (1979) Conjunctivitis in the nude rat. Lab Anim 13: 35
Morgan RV, Bachrach A Jr (1982) Keratoconjunctivitis sicca associated with sulfonamide therapy in dogs. J Am Vet Med Assoc 180: 432–434
Nelson J (1989) Managing the dry eye. Accurate diagnosis is the key. Postgrad Med 85: 38–41, 45–48, 55
Pflugfelder S, Wilhelmus K, Osato M, Matoba A, Font R (1986) The autoimmune nature of aqueous tear deficiency. Ophthalmology 93: 1513–1517
Rao N, Atalla L, Linker-Israeli M, Chen F, George F, Martin J, Steinman L (1989) Suppression of experimental uveitis in rats by anti-I-A antibodies. Invest Ophthalmol Vis Sci 30: 2348–2355
Rengstorff R, Doughty C (1982) Mydriatic and cycloplegic drugs: a review of ocular and systemic complications. Am J Optom Physiol Opt 59: 162–177
Roberts SA, Gregory BJ (1980) Facultative *Pasteurella* ophthalmitis in Hooded Lister rats. Lab Anim 14: 323–324
Roerig D, Hasegawa A, Harris G, Lynch K, Wang R (1980) Occurrence of corneal opacities in rats after acute administration of 1-alpha-acetylmethadol. Toxicol Appl Pharmacol 56: 155–163
Sansom J, Barnett KC, Long RD (1985) Keratoconjunctivitis sicca in the dog associated with the administration of salicylazosulphapyridine. Vet Rec 116: 391–393
Saunders LZ (1967) Ophthalmic pathology in rats and mice. In: Cotchin E, Roe F (eds) Pathology of laboratory rats and mice. Blackwell, Oxford, pp 349–371
Saunders L, Rubin L (1975) Ophthalmic pathology of animals, inflammation of the anterior segment in rats. Karger, Basel, pp 26–29
Sjögren H (1933) Zur Kenntnis der Keratoconjunctivitis sicca (Keratitis filiformis bei Hypofunktion der Tränendrüsen). Acta Ophthalmol [Suppl] 2: 1–151
Slatter D (1973) Keratoconjunctivitis sicca in the dog produced by oral phenazopyridine hydrochloride. J Small Anim Pract 14: 749–771
Slatter DH, Blogg JR (1978) Keratoconjunctivitis sicca in dogs associated with sulphonamide administration. Aust Vet J 54: 444–446
Spiess B, Wilcock B, Physick-Sheard P (1989) Eosinophilic granulomatous dacryoadenitis causing bilateral keratoconjunctivitis sicca in a horse. Equine Vet J 21: 226–228
Sreebny L, Valdini A, Yu A (1989) Xerostomia. Part II: relationship to nonoral symptoms, drugs, and diseases. Oral Surg Med Pathol 68: 419–427
Strempel I, Grueber A, Bittner K (1989) Zum Problem des trockenen Auges bei Nierentransplantierten. Klin Monatsbl Augenheilkd 195: 141–144
Taradach C, Regnier B, Perraud J (1981) Eye lesions in Sprague-Dawley rats: type and incidence in relation to age. Lab Anim 15: 285–287
Todenhoefer H (1969) Toxische Nebenwirkungen von Sulfadiazin (Debenal®, Sulfatidin®) bei der Anwendung als Geriatrikum für Hunde. Dtsch Tierärztl Wochenschr 76: 14–16
Turacli M (1974) The clonidine side effect in the human eye. Ann Ophthalmol 6: 699–710
Weisbroth S, Peress N (1977) Ophthalmic lesions and dacryoadenitis: a naturally occurring aspect of sialodacryoadenitis virus infection of the laboratory rat. Lab Anim Sci 27: 466–473
Weisse I, Hoefke W, Greenberg S, Gaida W, Stoetzer H, Kreuzer H (1978) Ophthalmological and pharmacological studies after administration of clonidine in rats. Arch Toxicol 41: 89–98
Wright HN (1963) Corneal and lenticular opacities in the eyes of rats following long-term administration of sulfonylurea derivatives. Diabetes 12: 550–554

Cyclitis Produced by Cyclophosphamide, Rat

Seymour Levine

Gross Appearance

In advanced cases of cyclitis, the eye ist hemorrhagic.

Microscopic Features

Inflammation of the ciliary body is manifested by edema which extends into the ciliary processes (Levine and Sowinski 1974a). The stroma is extended by eosinophilic fluid which may be homogeneous, granular, or vacuolated (Fig. 37) Phosphotungstic acid hematoxylin stain reveals that the fluid contains fibrin. Polymorphonuclear and mononuclear inflammatory cells are few or absent, probably because rats given cyclophosphamide are leukopenic. Small vessels sometimes contain fibrin thrombi. The overlying epithelium is attenuated, degenerated, or unchanged. Occasionally there is fluid between the two cell layers. In late stages, there is hemorrhage in the stroma. No lesion is seen in other parts of the eye.

Ultrastructure

Although cyclophosphamide cyclitis has not been studied with the electron microscope, the lesion will probably resemble that caused by this drug in the choroid plexus – namely, massive exudation of plasma with abundant fibrin and a few red cells in the connective tissue spaces between vessels and epithelium (Wenk et al. 1979). Endothelial cell junctions may be separated and some epithelial cells may be necrotic.

Differential Diagnosis

Edema and inflammation of the ciliary body can be produced in rats by endotoxin (Rosenbaum et al. 1980), but with occasional focal infiltrates of polymorphonuclear leukocytes, differing in this respect from cyclophosphamide cyclitis (Levine and Sowinski 1974a).

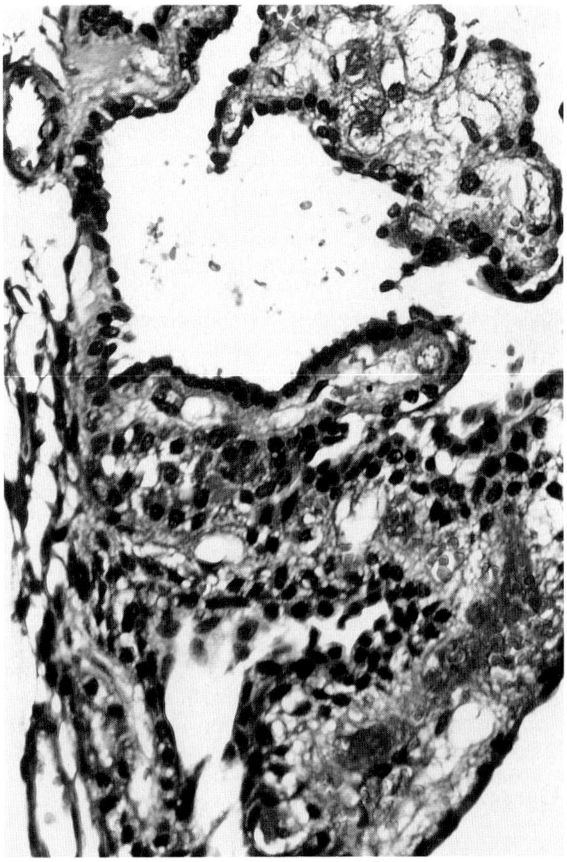

Fig. 37. Cyclitis, rat, cyclophosphamide. The stroma of the ciliary body and processes is expanded by edema fluid, which varies in appearance from dense and dark (eosinophilic) to pale and vacuolated. The epithelium is attenuated in some areas. H & E, ×300

Biologic Features

Cyclitis occurs following a large parenteral dose (250 mg/kg) of cyclophosphamide, which is lethal. The drug is activated in the liver into alkylating metabolites that damage proliferating cells in many organs and also nonproliferating cells in the urinary bladder, choroid plexus, and ciliary body. The cystitis results from the excretion of alkylating metabolites in the urine (Levine and Sowinski 1975). It is likely that the ciliary body and choroid plexus are injured during the transport of the same alkylating metabolites into aqueous humor and cerebrospinal fluid, respectively (Levine and Sowinski 1973). Indeed, the similar effects of cyclophosphamide on the ciliary body and choroid plexus provide support from experimental pathology for the close relationships already known in the anatomy and physiology of these two structures, both of neuroectodermal origin (Davson 1956). Cyclitis starts rapidly within 24 h, peaks at 48 h, and occurs less frequently than choroid plexitis. The edema is probably caused by increased permeability of the injured, vascular endothelium. The celluar infiltration that usually accompanies an injury is almost completely absent because the bone marrow is devastated by the cytotoxic drug and the rats are leukopenic. Hemorrhage is conspicuous at a later stage, due to thrombocytopenia with hemorrhages occurring in other organs (Levine and Sowinski 1974c). The occurrence of hemorrhages can be accelerated by increasing the thrombocytopenia with endotoxin (Levine and Sowinski 1974b).

Comparison with Other Species

Similar lesions have been produced in a few rabbits, cats, and dogs, but the relative frequency is unknown. Of greater interest is whether cyclitis occurs in cancer patients treated with high doses of cyclophosphamide. Many chemotherapeutic agents cause ocular complications (Griffin and Garnick 1981; Vizel and Oster 1982) but cyclophosphamide is mentioned only rarely (Kende et al. 1979). Nevertheless, the ocular effect noted after cyclophosphamide was transient blurring of vision, a complication that could be explained by cyclitis. It is possible that cyclophosphamide cyclitis is underreported because of its transient nature in man and lack of familiarity with the animal model. Also, humans are not given lethal doses, such as was the case in rats.

References

Davson H (1956) Physiology of the ocular and cerebrospinal fluids. Little and Brown, Boston

Griffin JD, Garnick MB (1981) Eye toxicity of cancer chemotherapy: a review of the literature. Cancer 48: 1539–1549

Kende G, Sirkin SR, Thomas PR, Freeman AI (1979) Blurring of vision: a previously undescribed complication of cyclophosphamide therapy. Cancer 44: 69–71

Levine S, Sowinski R (1973) Choroid plexitis produced in rats by cyclophosphamide. J Neuropathol Exp Neurol 32: 365–370

Levine S, Sowinski R (1974a) Cyclitis produced in rats by cyclophosphamide. Invest Ophthalmol Vis Sci 13: 697–699

Levine S, Sowinski R (1974b) Cyclophosphamide-induced cerebral and visceral lesions in rats. Enhancement by endotoxins. Arch Pathol 98: 177–182

Levine S, Sowinski R (1974c) A hemorrhagic diathesis with involvement of hypothalamus produced in rats by cyclophosphamide. Am J Pathol 74: 171–178

Levine S, Sowinski R (1975) Role of the kidney in development of cystitis and other toxic effects of cyclophosphamide. Invest Urol 13: 196–199

Rosenbaum JT, McDevitt HO, Guss RB, Egbert PR (1980) Endotoxin-induced uveitis in rats as a model for human disease. Nature 288: 611–813

Vizel M, Oster MW (1982) Ocular side effects of cancer chemotherapy. Cancer 49: 1999–2002

Wenk EJ, Levine S, Hoenig EM (1979) Fine structure of contrasting choroid plexus lesions caused by tertiary amines or cyclophosphamide. J Neuropathol Exp Neurol 38: 1–9

Melanoma of the Uvea, Rat

Jeffrey I. Everitt and John A. Shadduck

Synonyms. Malignant melanoma, intraocular melanoma, primary pigmented intraocular tumor.

Gross Appearance

Spontaneous uveal melanomas in rats are usually unilateral and located in the region of the ciliary body (Magnusson et al. 1978). Chemically induced tumors have originated from all parts of the uveal tract including the iris, ciliary body, and choroid. The involvement of other ocular tissues varies with the size of the neoplasm. Large tumors may fill the anterior chamber and generally result in exophthalmus and corneal opacity. Secondary glaucoma has been reported in association with uveal melanoma in the rat (Heywood 1975).

Microscopic Features

Spontaneous uveal melanomas in the rat usually consist of solid sheets of predominantly spindle shaped cells without distinct cytoplasmic boundaries. These melanomas are often well vascularized, and may exhibit a whorled or trabecular pattern (Figs. 38–40). In one series of tumors (Magnusson et al. 1978), argyrophilic fibers were consistently demonstrated, while collagen was absent. Yellowish-brown pigment, believed to be melanin, was occasionally present in spontaneous tumors of albino Sprague-Dawley rats; however, amelanotic tumors have also been described (Benson 1962; Heywood 1975; Magnusson et al. 1978).

The microscopic features of uveal melanomas induced by intraocular instillation of nickel subsulfide Ni_3S_2 in the Fischer 344 rat have been described by Albert and coworkers (1982). The neoplasms arose from the iris, ciliary body, or choroid, and were classified according to a histopathologic classification system utilized in human ophthalmic pathology (Callender 1931). Using this classification scheme, Albert described five spindle-cell tumors, two epithelioid tumors, and four mixed cell tumors. The criteria for the diagnosis of uveal melanoma were: (1) spindle-shaped or epithelioid neoplastic cells arose from the uvea; (2) spindle cells contained spindle-shaped nuclei which were cohesive with indistinct cell borders, resulting in the nuclei superficially appearing to be in a syncytium; (3) the more narrow spindle nuclei exhibited nuclear folds and the plumper spindle nuclei contained prominent nucleoli; and (4) the epithelioid cells were noncohesive cells with distinct cell borders and large oval nuclei containing prominent nucleoli. The presence of melanin pigment was not described in hematoxylin and eosin stained paraffin-embedded sections of these tumors, although several of these neoplasms stained positive by the Fontana method. Identical tumors were induced in ACI rats with intraocular instillation of crystalline nickel sulfide (NiS) (Everitt and Shadduck, unpublished data).

Kendrey and Roe (1969) described pigmented uveal melanomas induced by subcutaneous administration of urethan or *N*-hydroxyurethan to neonatal August hooded rats. These tumors were found in the iris, ciliary body, and parts of the choroid. The urethan and *N*-hydroxyurethan-induced anterior uveal melanomas consisted of round or oval tumor cells having cytoplasm filled with fine or coarse deep-brown granules. These cells generally occupied the whole iris and obliterated the normal microscopic structure. Melanosis of the ciliary body was associated with the iridal tumors, and melanin-containing cells were often found in the corneal stroma. The two posterior uveal melanomas which were induced by urethan appeared as diffuse thickenings of the choroid near the optic nerve and extended outside the globe. The cells in these choroidal tumors appeared similar to those in the tumors of the iris and contained abundant pigment within the cytoplasm. A single melanoma which was induced in the choroid by *N*-hydroxyurethan consisted of spindle-shaped and epithelial cells with little pigment and occasional mitotic figures.

Ultrastructure

No reports were found in the literature describing the ultrastructure of spontaneous uveal melanomas in rats. Albert and coworkers per-

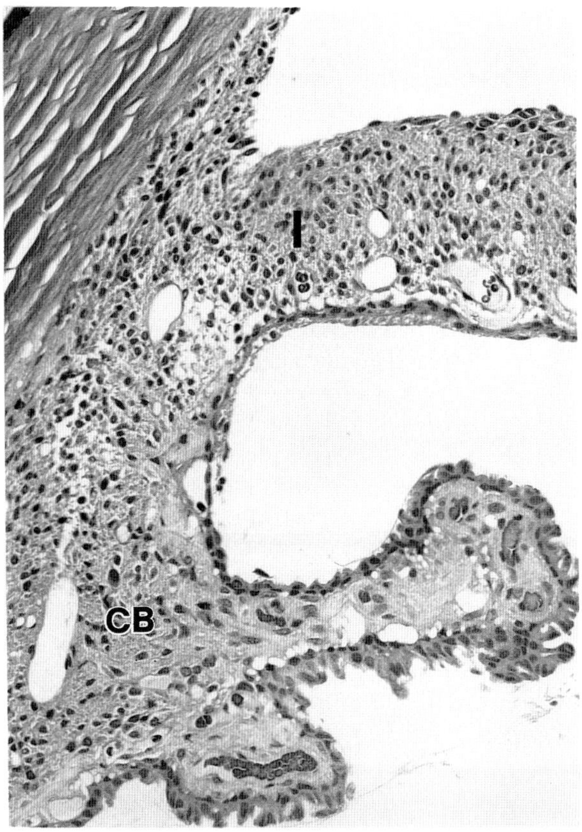

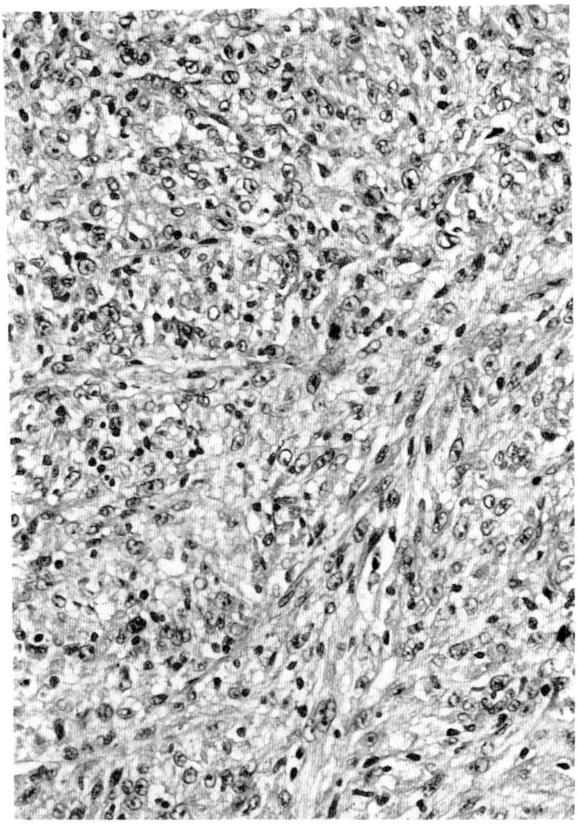

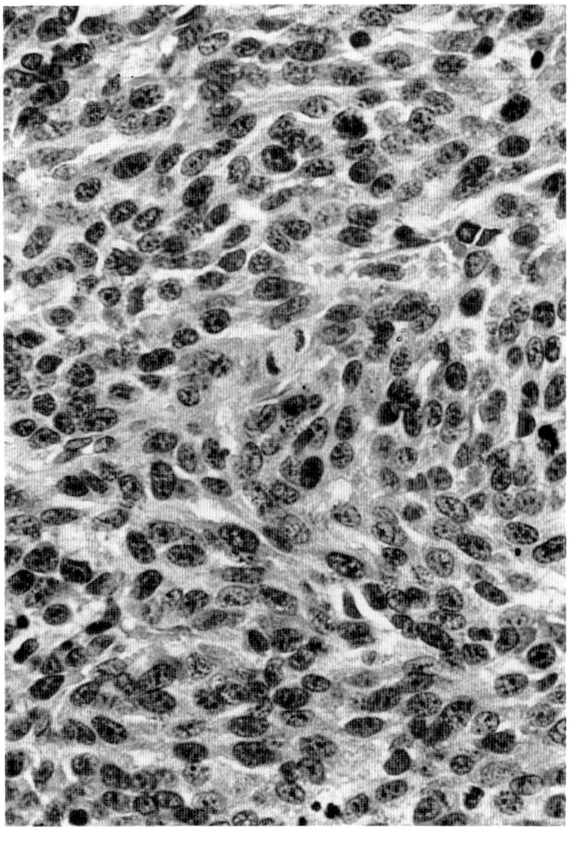

Fig. 38 *(upper left).* Spontaneous amelanotic tumor in a Fischer 344 rat. Diffuse infiltration of iris *(I)* and ciliary body *(CB)* with pleomorphic tumor cells. H & E, ×137

Fig. 39 *(upper right).* Spindle melanoma induced by nickel sulfide in an ACI rat. The neoplastic cells have a whorled pattern with indistinct cytoplasmic boundaries. H & E, ×273

Fig. 40 *(lower right).* Melanoma induced by nickel sulfide in the anterior uveal tract of an ACI rat. Note mixed spindle epithelioid appearance. Tumor cells contain prominent nucleoli. H & E, ×546

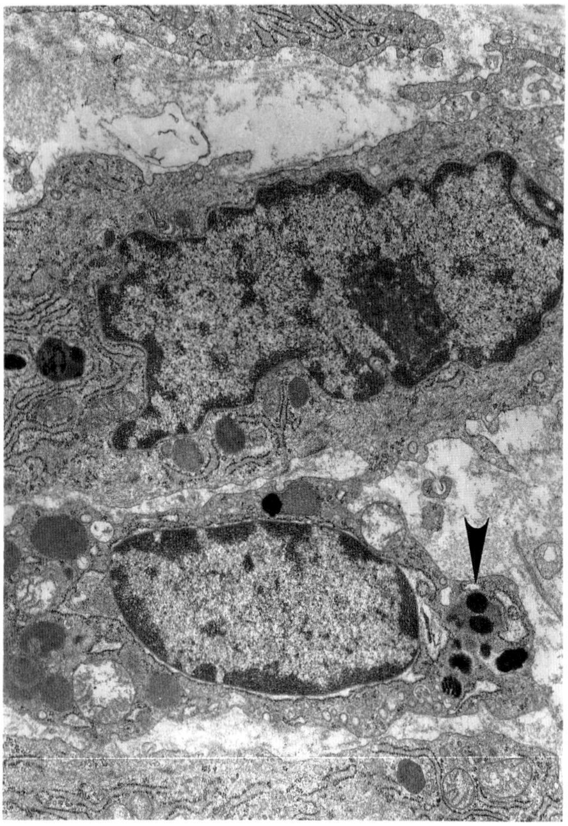

Fig. 41. Melanoma induced by nickel in an ACI rat. Marginated chromatin is present within the elongated nucleus. The upper cell contains abundant rough endoplasmic reticulum and a large nucleolus. Intracytoplasmic melanosomes are present *(arrow)*. TEM, × 11 100

formed transmission electron microscopy on four uveal melanomas induced by Ni_3S_2 in Fischer 344 rats. They confirmed the presence of combinations of the characteristic spindle and epithelioid melanoma cell types present in human intraocular uveal melanomas. Premelanosomes and melanosomes were frequently present in the cytoplasm of the melanoma cells. Similar cells were found in some intraocular uveal melanomas induced by nickel sulfide (NiS) in ACI rats.

Nickel sulfide induced melanomas in ACI rats consisted of spindle cells with elongated cell bodies containing irregular oval nuclei with marginated heterochromatin, prominent nucleoli, and abundant endoplasmic reticulum (Fig. 41). Premelanosomes and melanosomes were present in some tumor cells but were not numerous.

Differential Diagnosis

Uveal melanomas, particularly those which are amelanotic, can be extremely difficult to differentiate from other intraocular spindle cell tumors. These include neoplasms of connective tissue, vascular, neural, smooth muscle, and peripheral nerve sheath origin. Electron microscopic histochemical and immunocytochemical techniques should aid in diagnosis, but only in a few studies in rats have intraocular neoplasms been studied. Review of the National Toxicology Program Carcinogenesis Bioassay Data System for Fischer 344 rats revealed that sarcoma NOS (not otherwise specified) was the most frequently diagnosed intraocular neoplasm.

Spontaneous epithelioid anterior uveal melanomas have not been described in rats. These tumors need to be differentiated from epithelial tumors of the ciliary body in man and domestic animals, and presumably would pose similar diagnostic problems in chemically induced ocular neoplasms in laboratory animal species. Nonneoplastic melanotic lesions were described in August hooded rats treated with urethan and *N*-hydroxyurethan (Kendrey and Roe 1969) and need to be differentiated from pigmented tumors. Similar nonneoplastic pigmented nevi have been described in the uveal tract of man.

Biologic Features

Few generalizations can be made regarding the histogenesis or etiology of spontaneous or induced intraocular melanomas in rats because they are so rarely diagnosed. Intraocular neoplasms, including uveal melanomas, are infrequent findings in either control or chemically treated rats in long-term studies. A review of pathology findings in 100 000 Fischer 344 rats in the Carcinogenesis Bioassay Data Base of the National Toxicology Program (NTP) revealed only 19 intraocular neoplasms. These represented a variety of histopathologic diagnoses and reflected the difficulties involved in making a definitive diagnosis on spindle cell tumors without special studies. The true incidence of intraocular neoplasia in the rat is difficult to assess because the globe is often not examined histopathologically unless there is a gross lesion. Nevertheless, clinical ophthalmic examination would generally reveal the presence of most ophthalmic tumors and it is correct to assume that intraocular neoplasms are rare findings in most rat strains.

Table 4. Induction of melanomas in laboratory rats

Chemical	Route of administration	Strain	Incidence of melanoma	Reference
Ni_3S_2	Intraocular	F344	11/20	Albert et al. 1983
NiS	Intraocular	ACI	3/15	Everitt and Shadduck, unpublished data
Urethan	Subcutaneous	August	5/15 male 4/17 female	Kendrey and Roe 1969
N-Hydroxyurethan	Subcutaneous	August	2/21 male 0/21 female	Kendrey and Roe 1969
Platinum foil	Intraocular	N/A	N/A	Evgeneva 1972
Cellophane film	Intraocular	N/A	N/A	Evgeneva 1972
Ethionine and *N*-2-Fluorenylacetamide	Oral	Wistar	1/25	Benson 1962

Although uveal melanomas have been induced in a variety of rat strains by chemicals administered by intraocular and systemic routes (Table 4), no NTP bioassay to date has had intraocular tumors as a positive finding following treatment.

Metastasis has not been described in the few cases of spontaneous uveal melanoma reported in the rat. Pulmonary metastasis was found in a single case of uveal melanoma induced by nickel subsulfide (Albert et al. 1982). Extrascleral invasion has been noted in chemically induced uveal melanomas.

Comparison with Other Species

Melanocytic tumors, although uncommon, are the most frequent intraocular neoplasms of animals (Saunders and Barron 1958). They have been reported most frequently in dogs (Trucksa 1983) but have also been described in other domestic and laboratory species (Saunders and Rubin 1975). Clinicopathologic studies of uveal melanomas in dogs and cats have revealed several important differences from human uveal melanocytic tumors. In man, uveal tract melanomas generally arise in the posterior uvea whereas canine and feline melanomas usually arise in the anterior uvea, specifically the iris. Posterior uveal melanomas in man have a much higher metastatic potential than do human anterior uveal tract neoplasms. The histologic behavior of the canine anterior uveal melanoma is similar to that of the human anterior uveal melanoma, inasmuch as it exhibits low metastatic potential. Although there is a paucity of published cases, the feline anterior uveal melanoma may have a much greater metastatic potential (Acland et al. 1980). Insufficient numbers of uveal melanomas have been described in the rat to determine whether the biologic behavior is similar to corresponding tumors in man or domestic animal species.

References

Acland GM, McLean IW, Aquirre GD, Trucksa R (1980) Diffuse iris melanomas in cats. J Am Vet Med Assoc 176: 52–56

Albert DM, Gonder JR, Papale J, Craft JL, Dohlman HG, Reid MC, Sunderman FW Jr (1982) Induction of ocular neoplasms in Fischer rats by intraocular injection of nickel subsulfide. Invest Ophthalmol Vis Sci 22: 768–782

Benson WR (1962) Intraocular tumor after ethionine and *N*-2-fluorenylacetamide. Arch Pathol 73: 404–406

Callender GR (1931) Malignant melanotic tumors of the eye: a study of histologic types in 111 cases. Trans Am Acad Ophthalmol Otolaryngol 36: 131–142

Evgeneva TP (1972) Pigment tumors in rats caused by the implantation of platinum and cellophane films into the eye chamber. Biull Eksp Biol Med 73: 75–77

Heywood R (1975) Glaucoma in the rat. Br Vet J 131: 213–221

Kendrey G, Roe FJC (1969) Melanotic lesions of the eye in August hooded rats induced by urethan or *N*-hydroxyurethan given during the neonatal period: a histopathological study. JNCI 43: 749–761

Magnusson G, Majeed S, Offer JM (1978) Intraocular melanoma in the rat. Lab Anim 12: 249–252

Saunders LZ, Barron CN (1958) Primary pigmented intraocular tumors in animals. Cancer Res 18: 234–245

Saunders LZ, Rubin LF (1975) Ophthalmic pathology of animals. Karger, Basel

Trucksa RC (1983) Canine ocular melanocytic neoplasms. In: Peiffer RL Jr (ed) Comparative ophthalmic pathology. Thomas, Springfield

Melanoma of the Eye, Mouse

Heinrich Ernst, Susanne Rittinghausen, and Ulrich Mohr

Synonyms. Malignant melanoma, melanocytic tumor, intraocular melanoma, uveal melanoma.

Gross Appearance

A small intraocular melanoma is usually not visible with the naked eye but may be detected by ophthalmoscopy or slit-lamp biomicroscopy. Advanced tumor growth in an eye may result in macroscopic exophthalmus, opacity, or "dark spots."

Microscopic Features

The melanoma described here developed spontaneously in the choroid of the left eye of a 28-month-old female B6C3F1/Cr1BR control mouse from a chronic oral toxicity study. Histologically, the tumor appeared as a segmental convex thickening of the posterior choroid and the adjacent sclera. The continuity of the tunics, however, was not disrupted (Fig. 42). As assessed from a melanin-bleached section, the solid and well-vascularized tumor consisted of polygonal epitheloid cells with indistinct cell boundaries and moderately pleomorphic nuclei. Occasional mitotic figures were visible throughout the tumor tissue (Fig. 43). Cytoplasmic melanin pigment granules were numerous but not as frequent as seen in the melanocytes of the unaffected parts of the choroid. The pigment stained positive by Fontana-Masson (Fig. 44) and was negative for iron. The sclera bordering the tumor was infiltrated and thickened by tumor cells. There was no penetration through the sclera, however, and no extension into the anterior eye structures (Fig. 45). The artifactually detached retina had on otherwise normal appearance (Fig. 46). No distant metastases were observed.

Ultrastructure

No information is available.

Differential Diagnosis

Uveal melanoma has to be distinguished from other intraocular tumors such as pigmented or unpigmented adenoma and adenocarcinoma of the iridociliary epithelium, retinoblastoma, and medulloepithelioma. These neoplasms have been described in man (Zimmerman and Sobin 1980) and in various domestic animal species (Kircher et al. 1974; Wilcock 1985), but to our knowledge not in mice.

Biologic Features

As with cutaneous melanocytic tumors (Kanno 1989), spontaneous intraocular melanomas are exceedingly rare in mice. A single case has been reported in a JAX mouse (Cloudman 1941) and in a B6C3F1 mouse (Ward et al. 1979). They were not described in detail. Uveal melanomas may arise in the choroid, the ciliary body, or the iris. According to the cytologic composition and degree of pigmentation, uveal melanomas of other species have been classified into spindle-cell, epitheloid, or mixed-cell types (Kircher et al. 1974). In man, the mixed-cell type has a less favorable prognosis than the spindle-cell type, and the epitheloid melanoma has the worst prognosis of the three types (Zimmerman and Sobin 1980). Mixed-cell tumors are the most frequent in domestic animals (Kircher et al. 1974); data on the relative behavior of the three tumor types in animals are not available.

Comparison with Other Species

Spontaneous intraocular melanomas are rare in other animal species. Single cases have been observed in aged Sprague-Dawley (Heywood 1975; Magnusson et al. 1978), Wistar (Magnusson et al. 1978), and Chbb: THOM rats (Ueberberg and Lützen 1979). Uveal melanomas may also occur infrequently in dogs, cats, cattle, sheep, rabbits, chicken, ducks, and fish (Saunders and Barron 1958; Blodi and Ramsey 1967; Morgan 1969; Cardy 1977; Kircher 1978). In rats, ocular melanomas have been induced by administration of ethionine and *N*-2-fluorenyl-

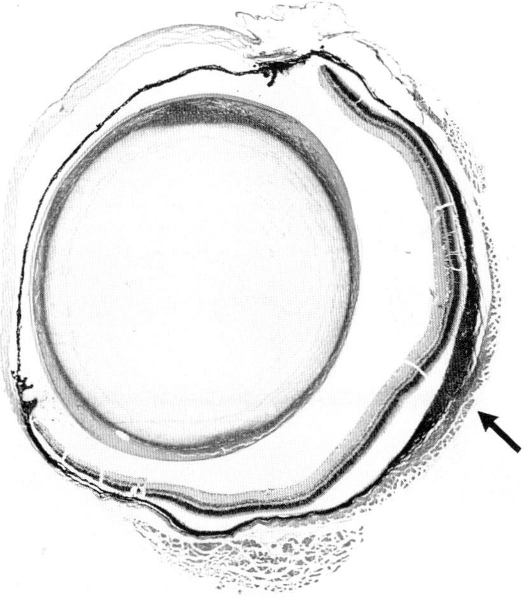

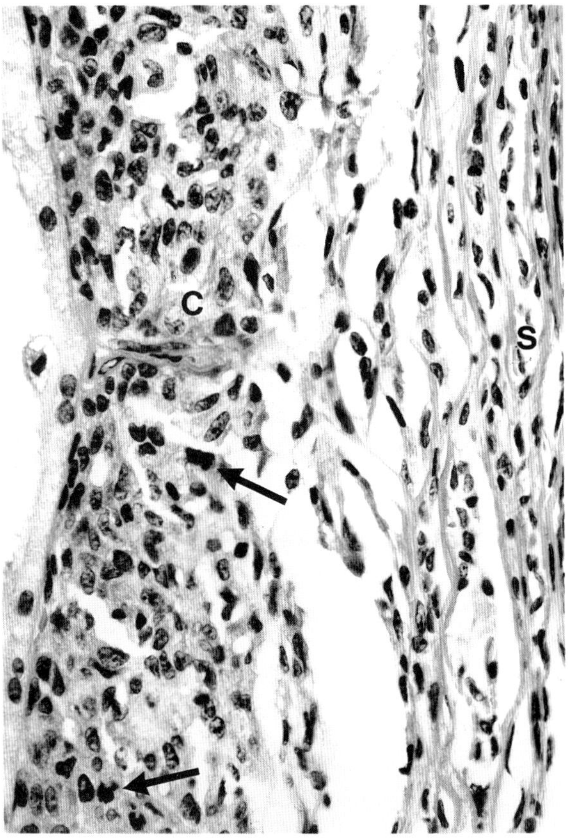

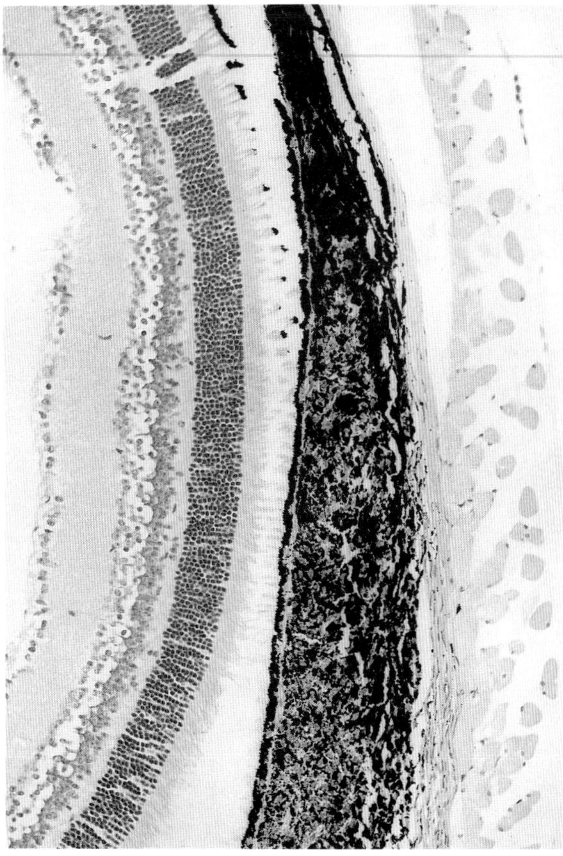

Fig. 42 *(upper left).* Eye, B6C3F1/Cr1BR untreated female mouse, 28 months of age. Melanoma of the choroid *(arrow).* H & E, ×19

Fig. 43 *(upper right).* Melanoma, choroid, mouse. Moderately pleomorphic epithelioid tumor cells within the choroid *(C)* and sclera *(S).* Occasional mitotic figures are present *(arrow).* Melanin-bleached preparation. H & E, ×476

Fig. 44 *(lower right).* Melanoma, choroid, mouse. Transition between the heavily pigmented normal choroid *(top)* and the less-pigmented, wider tumorous part of the choroid *(bottom).* Fontana-Masson stain, ×150

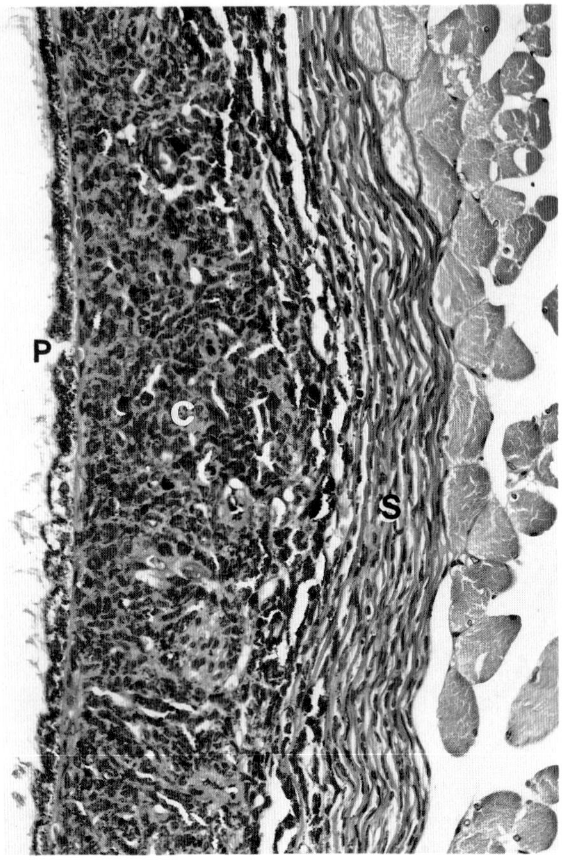

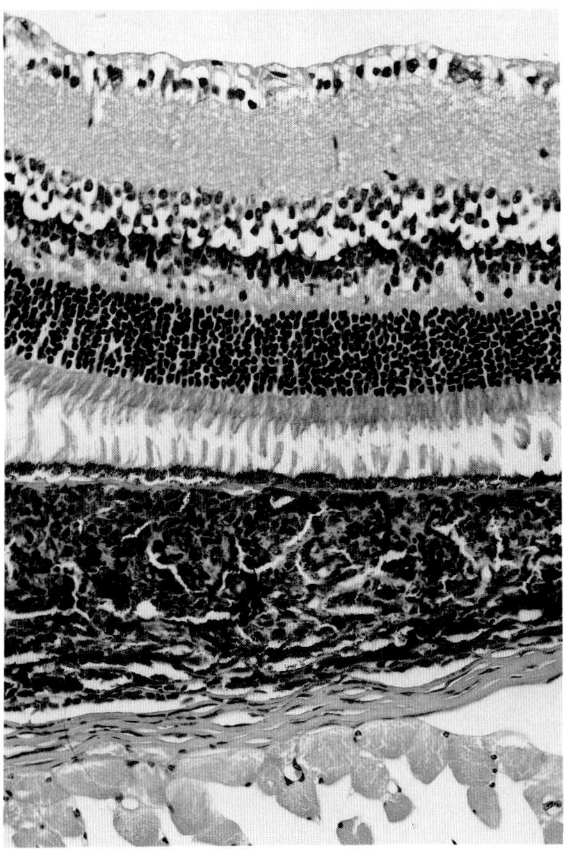

acetamide (Benson 1962), urethan and *N*-hydroxyurethan (Kendrey and Roe 1969), nickel subsulfide (Albert et al. 1982), and *N*-methyl-*N*-nitrosourea (Albert et al. 1986).

References

Albert DM, Gonder JR, Papale J, Craft JL, Dohlman HG, Reid MC, Sunderman FW Jr (1982) Induction of ocular neoplasms in Fischer rats by intraocular injection of nickel subsulfide. Invest Ophthalmol Vis Sci 22: 768–782

Albert DM, Puliafito CA, Haluska FG, Kimball GP, Robinson NL (1986) Induction of ocular neoplasms in Wistar rats by *N*-methyl-*N*-nitrosourea. Exp Eye Res 42: 83–86

Benson WR (1962) Intraocular tumor after ethionine and *N*-2-fluorenylacetamide. Arch Pathol 73: 404–406

Blodi FC, Ramsey FK (1967) Ocular tumors in domestic animals. Am J Ophthalmol 64: [Suppl] 627–633

Cardy RH (1977) Primary intraocular malignant melanoma in a Siamese cat. Vet Pathol 14: 648–649

Cloudman AM (1941) Spontaneous neoplasms in mice. In: Snell GS Roscoe B et al. (eds) Biology of the laboratory mouse, Jackson Memorial Laboratory. Dover, New York, pp 168–233

Heywood R (1975) Glaucoma in the rat. Br Vet J 131: 213–221

Kanno J (1989) Melanocytic tumors, skin, mouse. In: Jones TC, Mohr U, Hunt RD (eds) Monographs on pathology of laboratory animals, integument and mammary glands. Springer, Berlin Heidelberg, New York, pp 63–70

Kendrey G, Roe FJC (1969) Melanotic lesions of the eye in August hooded rats induced by urethan or *N*-hydroxyurethan given during the neonatal period: a histopathological study: JNCI 43: 749–762

Kircher CH (1978) Comparative pathology of ocular tumors. In: Benirschke K, Garner FM, Jones TC (eds) Pathology of laboratory animals, vol 1. Springer, Berlin, Heidelberg, New York, pp 647–662

Kircher CH, Garner FM, Robinson FR (1974) Tumors of the eye and adnexa. Bull WHO 50: 135–142

Magnusson G, Majeed S, Offer JM (1978) Intraocular melanoma in the rat. Lab Anim 12: 249–252

Morgan G (1969) Ocular tumours in animals. J Small Anim Pract 10: 563–570

◂ **Fig. 45** *(above).* Melanoma, choroid, mouse. Melanized tumor cells extend from the choroid *(C)* into the adjacent sclera *(S)* but do not penetrate it. The retinal pigment epithelial layer *(P)* appears normal. H & E, ×264

Fig. 46 *(below).* Melanoma, choroid, mouse. The retina has a normal organization and is separated from the melanoma by a distinct (Bruch's) membrane *(arrows)*. There are no pigment-containing cells in the retina except the retinal pigment epithelial cells. H & E, ×240

Saunders LZ, Barron CN (1958) Primary pigmented intraocular tumors in animals. Cancer Res 18: 234–244
Ueberberg H, Lützen L (1979) The spontaneous rate of tumors in the laboratory rat: strain Chbb: THOM (SPF). Arzneimittelforschung 29: 1876–1879
Ward JM, Goodman DG, Sqire RA, Chu KC, Linhart MS (1979) Neoplastic and nonneoplastic lesions in aging (C57BL/6N X C3H/HeN)FI (B6C3FI) mice. JNCI 63: 849–854)
Wilcock BP (1985) The eye and ear. In: Jubb KVF, Kennedy PC, Palmer N (eds) Pathology of domestic animals, vol 1. Academic, New York, pp 339–406
Zimmerman LE, Sobin LH (1980) Histological typing of tumours of the eye and its adnexa. International histological classification of tumours, no. 24. WHO, Geneva, pp 62–63

Leiomyoma of the Iris, Sprague-Dawley Rat

Roger A. Owen and Pierre Duprat

Synonyms. Benign smooth muscle tumor of the iris.

Gross Appearance

Because of their small size, intraocular location, and rarity, these tumors have not been seen grossly at necropsy. Subgrossly, they are small mesenchymal tumors confined to and distorting the iris (Fig. 47). It can be envisaged that an ophthalmologic examination would reveal a nodular growth that distorts the iris and the pupil and normal pupillary dilatation with mydriatics would be prevented. A large tumor could impede aqueous outflow, resulting in enlargement of the eye and secondary glaucoma.

Microscopic Features

The following description is based on three cases encountered in rats from our laboratory. The tumors were mainly composed of closely packed interlacing bundles of spindle-shaped cells (Fig. 48) with ill-defined eosinophilic granular cytoplasm, elongated oval nuclei, a fine chromatin pattern, and small nucleoli (Fig. 49). Mallory's phosphotungstic acid hematoxylin stain showed myoglial fibrils emerging from tumor cells and uniting to form coarse fibers at the end of bundles of cells (Fig. 50). In some areas coarse cytoplasmic vacuolation could be seen. The tumors were well vascularized with palisading of tumor cells around blood vessels. In the largest tumor, an irregular central area contained several thrombosed and congested small blood vessels. Some vessel walls were thin, necrotic, and surrounded by partly lysed fibrinous material infiltrated by a small number of neutrophils (Fig. 48). Occasional mitotic figures were found in one of the tumors.

Ultrastructure

These tumors have not been examined by electron microscopy because of lack of adequately fixed material.

Differential Diagnosis

The histomorphologic appearance and the demonstration of myoglial fibers are consistent with the diagnosis of leiomyoma of the iris as described in man (Cornand et al. 1975). This is the only important myogenic tumor of the uvea (Shields 1983). The most common iridial tumors in man are melanomas (Shields et al. 1983). Other very rare tumors described by Shields (1983) include neurilemoma, neurofibroma, choroidal osteoma, rhabdomyosarcoma, and granular cell myoblastoma. Arguably also, a benign or malignant endothelial tumor needs to be differentiated and this could be done on the relationship of the neoplastic cells to the blood-filled spaces. In vascular neoplasms, the tumor cells line vascular spaces directly without the interposition of endothelial cells.

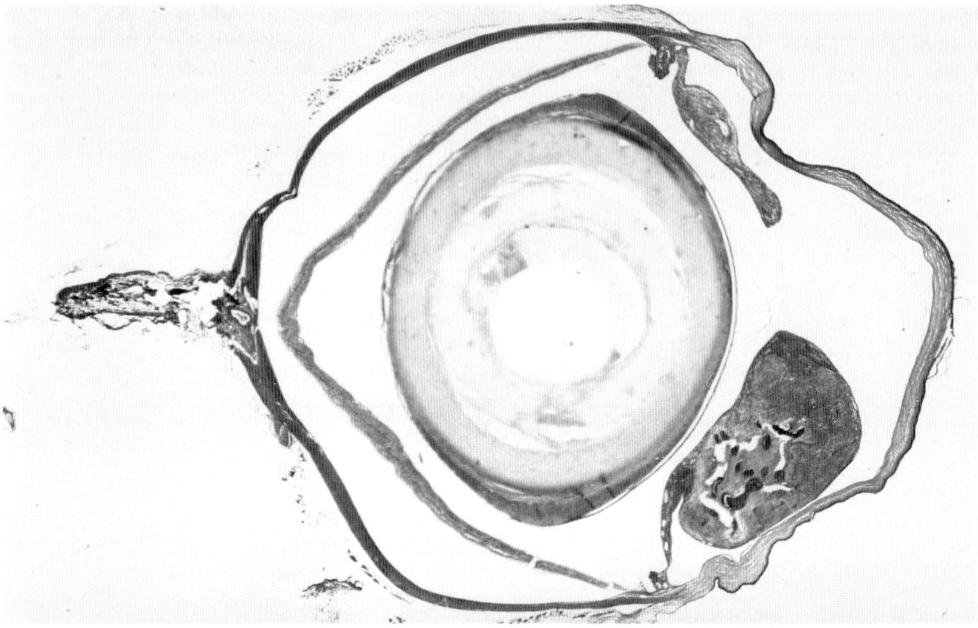

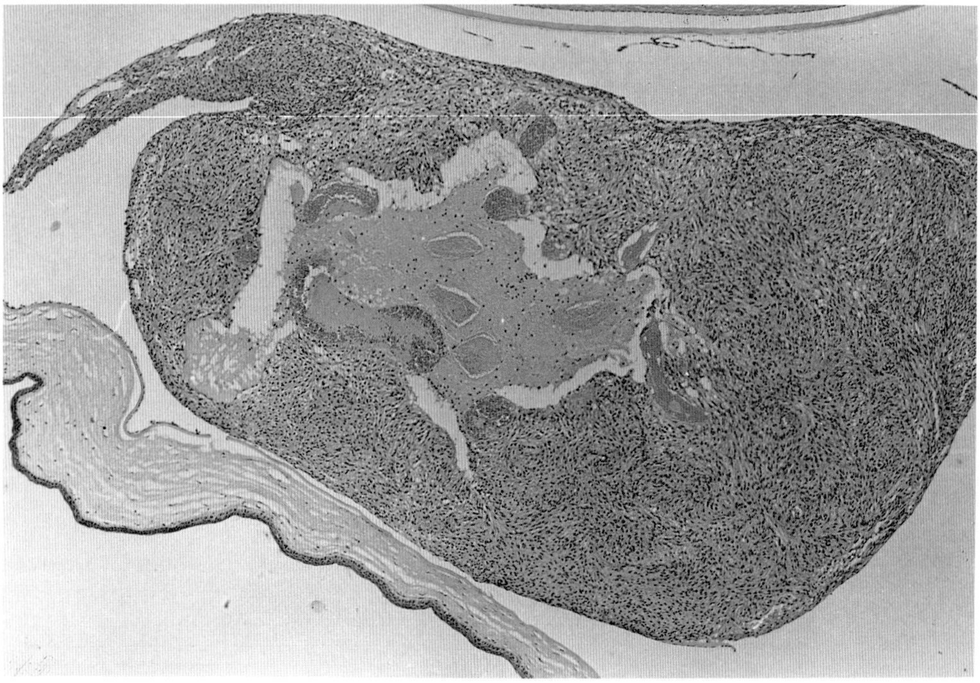

Fig. 47 *(above)*. Leiomyoma of iris in a 108-week-old Sprague-Dawley rat. Phosphotungstic acid hematoxylin (PTAH), ×8

Fig. 48 *(below)*. Leiomyoma, iris, rat. Note whorls and bundles of smooth muscle cells surrounding the blood-filled central lake. H & E, ×144

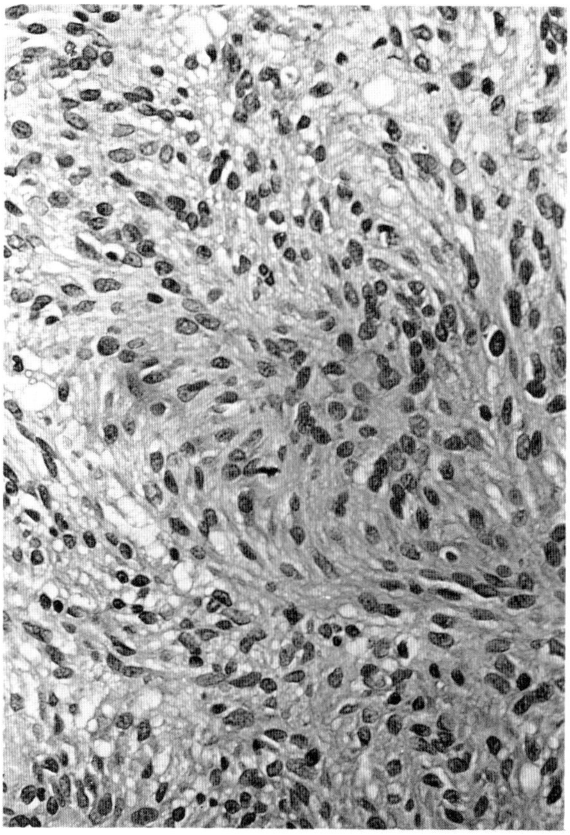

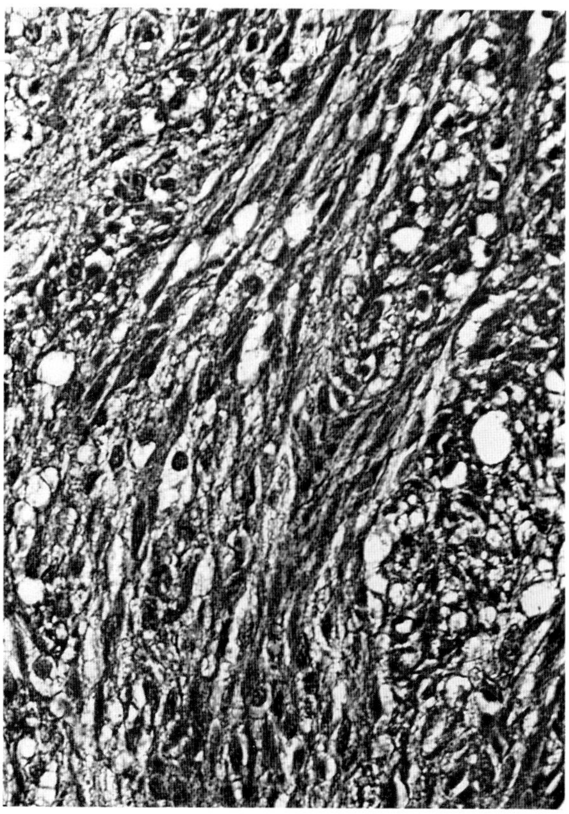

Biologic Features

These are rare tumors in any species. In the veterinary literature a leiomyoma has been reported in the iris of a dog (Barron and Saunders 1959) and another has been reported in the iris of a rat (Owen and Duprat 1987). Two other examples have been seen in our laboratory in Sprague-Dawley rats killed at the end of 2-year carcinogenicity studies. No information is available on the presence of this tumor in other strains of rat, or on the induction of this tumor in any species. A recent review of the ocular pathology of a population of rats used in long-term studies did not mention this tumor (Taradach and Greaves 1984).

References

Barron CN, Saunders LZ (1959) Intraocular tumors in animals. II. Primary non-pigmented intraocular tumours. Cancer Res 19: 1171–1174

Cornand G, Brisou B, Cozette P, Landes J, Ginoux J (1975) Un cas de leiomyome irien. Arch Ophthalmol 35: 245–252

Owen RA, Duprat P (1987) Leiomyoma of the iris in a Sprague-Dawley rat. J Comp Pathol 97: 227–229

Shields JA (1983) Myogenic, neurogenic and osseous tumors of the uvea. In: Shields JA (ed) Diagnosis and management of intraocular tumors. Mosby, St Louis, pp 360–385

Shields JA, Sanborn GE, Augsburger JJ (1983) The differential diagnosis of malignant melanoma of the iris. A clinical study of 200 patients. Ophthalmology 90: 716–720

Taradach C, Greaves P (1984) Spontanous eye lesions in laboratory animals: incidence in relation to age. CRC Crit Rev Toxicol 12: 121–147

Fig. 49 *(above).* Leiomyoma, iris, rat. Characteristic pattern of smooth muscle cell proliferation in leiomyoma. H & E, ×284 ▶

Fig. 50 *(below).* Leiomyoma, iris, rat. Myoglial fibers emanating from bundles of smooth muscle cells in leiomyoma. Phosphotungstic acid hematoxylin (PTAH), ×448

Toxic Effects of 6-Aminonicotinamide, Uvea, Rabbit

James A. Render and William W. Carlton

Gross Appearance

Bilateral iridal congestion is observed in male and female albino rabbits given intraperitoneally a cumulative amount of 6-aminonicotinamide rangig between 13 and 49 mg/rabbit (Render and Carlton 1985).

Microscopic Features

Uveal congestion with occasional ciliary edema and fibrin exudation into the ciliary stroma and the anterior chamber is observed in treated albino and pigmented rabbits (Render and Carlton 1985). Iridal hemorrhage is present in some treated albino rabbits. The principal lesion is diffuse, bilateral cytoplasmic vacuolation of the iridal and ciliary epithelium in male and female albino and pigmented rabbits (Fig. 51). Vacuolation of ciliary epithelium may be present in the absence of iridal congestion. This change varies in severity from many small vacuoles to complete replacement and nonstaining of the cytoplasm. Severely vacuolated cells may be at least twice the size of nonaffected cells. Vacuolation is observed first in the outer layer of the processes and this cell layer is most severely involved. The inner cell layer of the iridal and ciliary processes and the iris are also affected. The severity of vacuolation is generally increased following a larger number of doses. Most pigmented rabbits given at least a cumulative dose of 20 mg/rabbit have vacuolated cells in the ciliary body and iris, but a greater cumulative dose of 6-aminonicotinamide is required for induction of the lesion in albino rabbits.

The severity of cytoplasmic vacuolation of the anterior uveal epithelium varies among rabbits given a similar amount of 6-aminonicotinamide, but lesions are generally more severe in rabbits given a greater dose of 6-aminonicotinamide.

Ultrastructure

Cytoplasmic vacuolation and cellular swelling of ciliary epithelial cells causes thickening of the ciliary processes, especially the anterior processes (Render et al. 1985b). These lesions are evident in scanning electron micrographs. Cytoplasmic vacuolation and swelling of epithelial cells in posterior ciliary processes is mild. In scanning electron micrographs, surface alterations are more severe in the anterior ciliary processes. Anterior ciliary processes, especially of the ciliary crest, are thickened and flat, and individual processes are poorly defined (Fig. 52). By scanning electron microscopy of the posterior surface of the pupillary region of

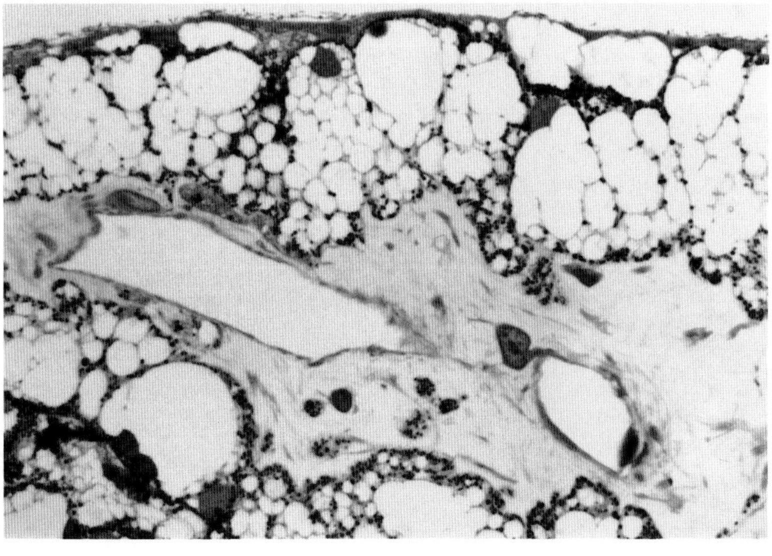

Fig. 51. Severe cytoplasmic vacuolation of ciliary epithelium of the iridal processes. H & E, ×560

the iris of control rabbits, radial ridges and furrows are variable in thickness and irregular. Radial furrows are shallow.

In transmission electron micrographs, the inner and outer epithelial cells of the anterior ciliary processes contain membrane-bound, coalescing, electronlucent vacuoles of variable size (Fig. 53, see p. 52). Some vacuoles contain membranous debris arranged in loose whorls. Other organelles are morphologically normal. Similar vacuoles are present within the iridal epithelial cells.

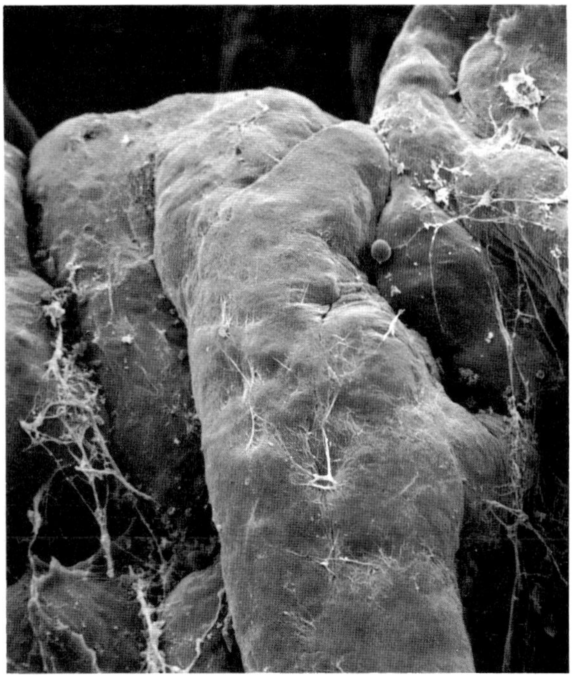

Fig. 52. Thickened and flattened anterior ciliary processes. SEM, ×280

Differential Diagnosis

Vacuolation of the epithelium of the anterior uvea is not a change unique to the toxicosis of 6-aminonicotinamide. Vacuolar change, detectable ultrastructurally in the anterior uveal epithelium, has been described following administration of naphthalene (Matsuura 1968). Vacuolar change recognized by light microscopy has been reported under several conditions such as after freezing of the ciliary processes and after administration of colchicine (De Ocampo 1966). Cytoplasmic vacuolation of ciliary epithelium has been observed in ruminants and horses and similar changes in the inner nuclear layer of sheep have been reported after the ingestion of locoweed (Van Kampen and James 1971). Lacy vacuolation of epithelium in the iridal outer layer has been described in people with diabetes mellitus (Yanoff et al. 1970). The vacuoles produced by these various methods have varied in intravacuolar content and some have disappeared spontaneously. The contents of the vacuoles produced by 6-aminonicotinamide or naphthalene (Matsuura 1968) or by freezing (De Ocampo 1966) are not stained by periodic acid Schiff reagent. However, the contents of the vacuoles present in diabetic patients (Yanoff et al. 1970) or rabbits given colchicine are stained by the periodic acid Schiff method. The vacuoles produced in the anterior uveal epithelium of rabbits by 6-aminonicotinamide are not positive for lipids by the oil red 0 method.

Intracytoplasmic vacuoles, often with dilated intercellular spaces, have been produced in the outer ciliary epithelium of rabbits by administration of *Shigella* sp. endotoxin (Pappas and Smelser 1958), by the intraocular injection of mineral oil (Pappas and Smelser 1958), after freezing of the ciliary processes (De Ocampo 1966), and after colchicine administration (De Ocampo 1966). Both layers of the ciliary epithelium of rabbits are vacuolated after dosing with naphthalene (Matsuura 1968). In naphthalene and 6-aminonicotinamide toxicosis in rabbits, vacuoles represent distentions of the cytocavitary network.

Cytoplasmic vacuolation of inner ciliary epithelial cells has been reported in animals with storage diseases. Inner ciliary epithelial cells, as well as iridal epithelial cells, uveal endothelial cells, uveal perithelial cells, and uveal fibroblasts, contain distended lysosomes in goats with β-mannosidosis. Cats with mucopolysaccharidosis I have membrane-bound intracytoplasmic vacuoles in both inner and outer ciliary epithelial cells, iridal epithelial cells, and uveal fibroblasts (Haskins et al. 1983). Intracytoplasmic vacuoles are present in uveal fibroblasts and the inner ciliary epithelial cells of cats with mucopolysaccharidosis VI (Aguirre et al. 1983).

Biologic Features

The biochemical mechanism for the development of the lesion in rabbits is unknown, but it appears to be related to a nicotinamide deficiency. Simultaneous administration of nicotinamide prevented iridal congestion in rabbits

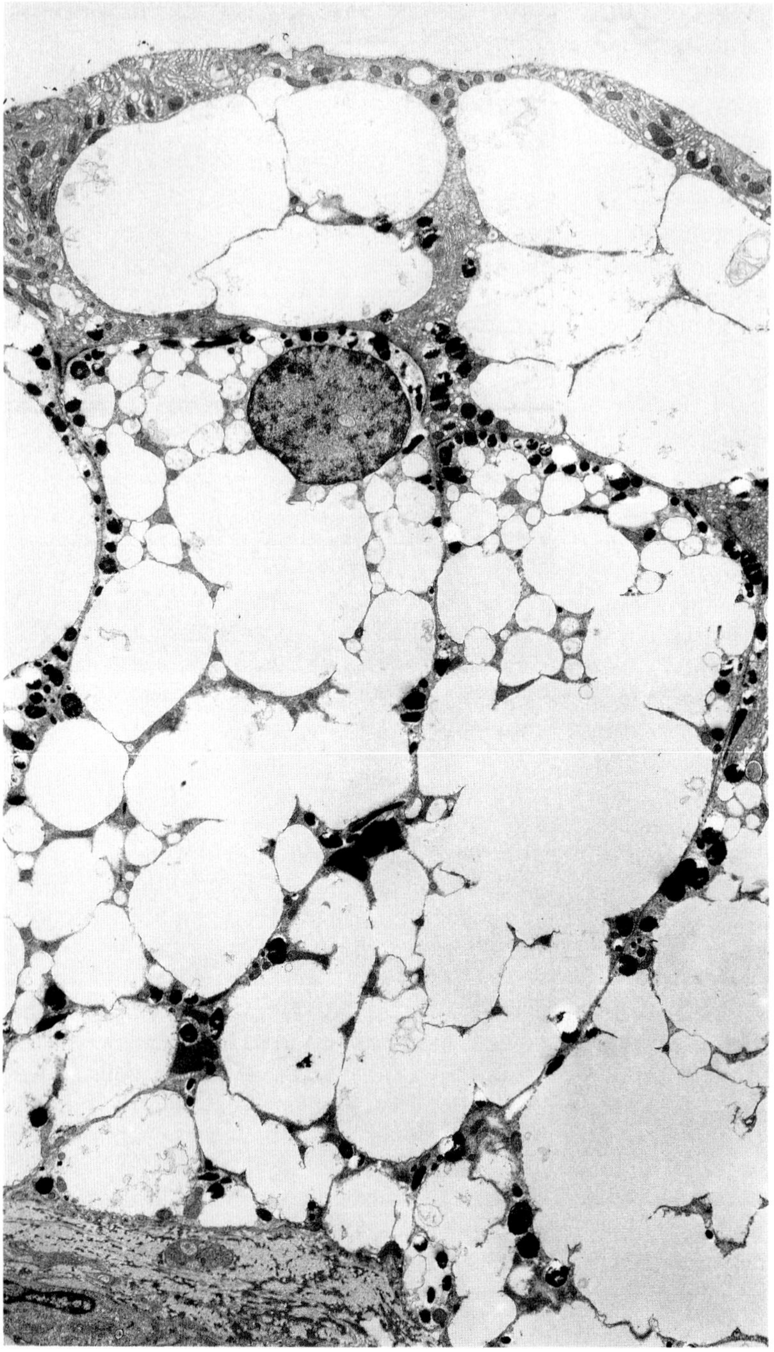

Fig. 53. Inner and outer ciliary epithelial cells containing numerous, coalescing, electronlucent intracytoplasmic vacuoles. TEM, ×2000

given 6-aminonicotinamide (Render and Carlton 1985). 6-Aminonicotinamide is an antimetabolite that replaces nicotinamide in metabolic pathways (Herken 1971) and is biosynthetically converted into more complex compounds, such as 6-aminonicotinamide adenine dinucleotide phosphate. Such nucleotide complexes of 6-aminonicotinamide interfere with specific reactions, like those that involve nicotinamide adenine dinucleotide phosphate-dependent enzymes, and biologic processes such as transport through membranes may be inhibited.

Such a mechanism may account for the accumulation of fluid in the ocular epithelial cells that produced the observed vacuolar change. Lesions are produced by 6-aminonicotinamide in several tissues, including the central nervous and digestive systems and the testis (Render et al. 1985 a). Daily doses of 6-aminonicotinamide given by intraperitoneal injection produce ataxia of the hind limbs progressing to an ascending paresis, anorexia, diarrhea, and death in male and female albino and pigmented rabbits. Light microscopic lesions include atrophy and necrosis of the white lobe of Harder's gland and atrophy of seminiferous tubules with cellular necrosis, vacuolation, and the presence of multinucleated giant cells. Cytoplasmic vacuolation is observed in epithelial cells from many tissues, usually in the basal portion of the cells. Spongiosis and gliosis are seen in certain parts of the central nervous system. Ultrastructural alterations in the gallbladder epithelium consist of distention of intracellular space, mild distention of perinuclear space, and coalescing, intracytoplasmic, membrane-bound vacuoles, a few of which contain membranous debris. Additional ocular alterations consist of microscopic vacuolation of the retinal pigment epithelium which ultrastructurally are seen to be distended intracellular spaces. Electronlucent, membrane-bound vacuoles are present in the photoreceptor cells of the outer plexiform layer. A few vacuoles are observed in the inner and outer nuclear layer.

Comparison with Other Species

6-Aminonicotinamide has been used experimentally as a teratogen (Kochhar and Larsson 1977), a neurotoxin (Sasaki 1982), and a cancer chemotherapeutic drug (Shapiro et al. 1957) in animals. 6-Aminonicotinamide, a potent antagonist of nicotinamide (Johnson and McColl 1955), has been used clinically in human medicine for the treatment of disseminated neoplasia (Herter et al. 1961; Perlia et al. 1961; Taylor et al. 1958) and psoriasis (Zackheim 1975, 1978) but not without toxic side effects. Among neurologic, oral, and gastrointestinal signs and symptoms, ocular side effects, including excessive tearing, angular blepharitis, conjunctivitis, and uveitis have been reported in human cancer patients treated systemically with 6-aminonicotinamide (Herter et al. 1961; Perlia et al. 1961; Taylor et al. 1958). Human patients treated topically with 6-aminonicotinamide complained of an ocular burning sensation, a temporary "haziness of vision", and periocular cutaneous lesions (Zackheim 1975, 1978).

Ocular lesions associated with the administration of 6-aminonicotinamide have been reported in rats. Astrocytosis, axonal degeneration, and demyelination were found in the optic nerves of rats given 6-aminonicotinamide (Meyer-Konig 1973). Astrocytic swelling results from a distention of the perinuclear cisternae and endoplasmic reticulum. This occurs in the orbital portion of the optic nerve and results in eventual scar formation and accumulation of fibrous astrocytes. Distention of the endoplasmic reticulum also occurs in oligodendrocytes which is accompandied by myelin splitting. These changes occur in the cerebral portion of the optic nerve and the orbital tracts, but they are followed by myelin breakdown and eventual axonal degeneration of the whole optic nerve.

Alterations in lenticular and retinal development in fetal rats and rabbits have been reported (Chamberlain and Nelson 1963; Sandor et al. 1978, 1981; Schardein et al. 1967). Ocular alterations consist principally of vacuolation of lens fibers, lack of differentiation of the retina (Chamberlain and Nelson 1963), and vacuolation of the retinal pigment epithelium due to distention of perinuclear cisternae (Sander et al. 1978). Vacuolation of uveal epithelial cells in rats and species other than rabbits has not been studied.

References

Aguirre G, Stramm L, Haskins M (1983) Feline mucopolysaccharidosis VI: general ocular and pigment epithelial pathology. Invest Ophthalmol Vis Sci 24: 991–1007

Chamberlain JG, Nelson MM (1963) Congenital abnormalities in the rat resulting from single injections of 6-aminonicotinamide during pregnancy. J Exp Zool 153: 285–299

De Ocampo G (1966) Inhibition of reaction to freezing injury of the ciliary body by colchicine. J Philipp Med Assoc 42: 573–598

Haskins ME, Aguirre GD, Jezyk PF, Desnick RJ, Patterson DF (1983) The pathology of the feline model of mucopolysaccharidosis I. Am J Pathol 112: 27–36

Herken H (1971) Antimetabolic action of 6-aminonicotinamide of the pentose phosphate pathway in the brain. In: Aldridge WN (ed) Mechanisms of toxicity. St Martin, New York, pp 189–203

Herter FP, Weissman SG, Thompson HG Jr, Hyman G, Martin DS (1961) Clinical experience with 6-aminonicotinamide. Cancer Res 21: 31–37

Johnson WJ, McColl JD (1955) 6-aminonicotinamide – a potent nicotinamide antagonist. Science 122: 834

Kochhar DM, Larsson KS (1977) Alterations in the metabolism of GAG and collagen. In: Wilson JG, Fraser F (eds) Handbook of teratology, vol. 2, Plenum, New York, pp 256–257

Matsuura H (1968) Electron microscopic studies of lens and ciliary body of rabbits with experimental naphthalene cataract. Acta Soc Ophthalmol Jpn 72: 1708–1732

Meyer-Konig E (1973) Ultrastruktur der Glia und Axonschädigung durch 6-Aminonicotinamid (6-AN) am Sehnerv der Ratte. Acta Neuropathol (Berl) 26: 115–126

Pappas GD, Smelser CK (1958) Studies on the ciliary epithelium and the zonule. I. Electron microscopic observations on changes induced by alteration of normal aqueous humor formation in the rabbit. Am J Ophthalmol 46: 299–318

Perlia CP, Kofman S, Sky-Peck H, Taylor SG III (1961) Clinical use of 6-aminonicotinamide in patients with disseminated neoplastic disease. Cancer 14: 644–648

Render JA, Carlton WW (1985) Ocular lesions of 6-aminonicotinamide toxicosis in rabbits. Vet Pathol 22: 72–77

Render JA, Carlton WW, Hinsman EJ, Turek JJ (1985a) Pathology of 6-aminonicotinamide toxicosis in the rabbit. Food Chem Toxicol 23: 795–803

Render JA, Turek JJ, Hinsman EJ, Carlton WW (1985b) Ultrastructural ocular lesions of 6-aminonicotinamide toxicosis in rabbits. Vet Pathol 22: 475–482

Sandor S, Amels D, Checiu M (1978) 6-aminonicotinamide induced eye defects in rats. Morphol Embryol (Bucur) 24: 311–323

Sandor S, Checiu M, Fazakas-Todea I (1981) Regeneration of retinal pigment epithelium damage in rat foetuses by 6-aminonicotinamide. Morphol Embryol (Bucur) 27: 11–13

Sasaki S (1982) Brain edema and gliopathy induced by 6-aminonicotinamide intoxication in the central nervous system of rats. Am J Vet Res 43: 1691–1695

Schardein JL, Woosley ET, Peltzer MA, Kaumb DH (1967) Congenital malformations induced by 6-aminonicotinamide in rabbit kits. Exp Mol Pathol 6: 335–346

Shapiro DM, Dietrich LS, Shils ME (1957) Quantitative biochemical differences between tumors and host as a basis for cancer chemotherapy v. niacin and 6-aminonicotinamide. Cancer Res 17: 600–604

Taylor SG III, Kofman S, Sky-Peck HH, Perlia C (1958) 6-aminonicotinamide in disseminated human cancer. J Lab Clin Med 52: 950

Van Kampen KR, James LF (1971) Ophthalmic lesions in locoweed poisoning of cattle, sheep, and horses. Am J Vet Res 32: 1293–1295

Yanoff M, Fine BS, Berkow JW (1970) Diabetic lacy vacuolation of iris pigment epithelium. Am J Ophthalmol 69: 201–210

Zackheim HS (1975) Treatment of psoriasis with 6-aminonicotinamide. Arch Dermatol 111: 880–882

Zackheim HS (1978) Topical 6-aminonicotinamide plus oral niacinamide therapy for psoriasis. Arch Dermatol 114: 1632–1638

Inherited Cataracts, Mouse

Robert L. Peiffer, Jr.

Synonyms. Genetic cataract.

Gross Appearance

Gross detection of cataracts in mouse eyes is made difficult by the lesions having to be distinguished from fixation artifact; this is particularly true in regard to localized cataractous change. With intumescent cataracts the lens will be larger than normal; with hypermaturity the cortex will liquefy; and with partially resorbed cataracts the lens will be smaller, with wrinkling of the lens capsule. Areas of calcification or fibrous metaplasia will appear as dense white opacities. With posterior lenticonus an axial protrusion will be noted extending into the vitreous cavity, and if the lens capsule is ruptured free cortical material will appear as flocculent opacities in the anterior or posterior chambers.

Histologic Appearance

While the lesions of cataracts are nonspecific, inherited cataracts will frequently be characterized by temporal and spatial features that are suggestive of inherited cataract in a particular strain. Inherited mouse cataracts that have been reasonably well defined are summarized in Table 5. Increasing numbers of mutant strains are currently being identified, with inherited cataracts occurring as an isolated finding or associated with multiple acular anomalies. Features of those that have been studied morphologically will be summarized below.

A dominant mode of inheritance has been reported for the cataracts in the *Fraser mouse* strain (Fraser and Schabtach 1962; Hamai and Kuwabara 1975). Cataracts begin at 14 days embryonically and continue to mature throughout life. Initially, the cell fiber nuclei in the deep cortex become pyknotic; degeneration of cytoplasm follows. Two weeks postnatally, the anterior epithelium undergoes unusual mitotic activity with the formation of multiple cell layers that infiltrate into the abnormal fibers of the anterior cortex. The anterior capsule thickens and its abnormal basement membrane ist produced by the aberant epithelial cells. Cells at the equatorial region retain their ability to differentiate until complete hydration of the lens occurs after 1 year of age. Degeneration of elongated older cells takes place by the breakdown of the nuclear membrane. Swelling of the apical ends of lens fibers at the anterior suture zone has been demonstrated (Zwaan and Williams 1968a, b, 1969; Sakuragawa et al. 1975).

The *Nakano mouse* cataract develops as an autosomal recessive trait which appears clini-

Table 5. Inherited cataracts in the mouse

Strain	Age of onset	Appearance/location	Genetics
Fraser (shriveled)	3–4 weeks	Anterior cortical	Autosomal intermediate
Deer	2 months to 1 year	Posterior/subcapsular	Autosomal recessive
Nakano	2–3 weeks	Nuclear	Autosomal recessive
Philly	5–6 weeks	Anterior/subcapsular/nuclear	Autosomal recessive
Emory	6–8 months	Posterior, cortical	Autosomal dominant
Swiss	3 weeks +	Anterior, equatorial	Autosomal dominant
Robertsonian	3 weeks +	Nuclear/posterior with capsular rupture	Undetermined
NOP	3 weeks +	Anterior, nuclear	Autosomal dominant
House mouse	Congenital	Subcapsular	Autosomal dominant

cally as a small nuclear "pinhead" opacity 3 weeks after birth (Iwata and Kinoshita 1971). The opacity is accompanied by marked morphologic alterations in the lens and decreased protein synthesis (Fukui et al. 1976). Six days postnatally the denucleation process of developing lens fibers is impaired. This is followed by swelling at the distal portion of the lens fibers in the deep posterior suture area of the perinuclear zones (Hamai et al. 1974).

The *Philly mouse* develops hereditary cataracts visible to the casual observer 5–6 weeks after birth (Kador et al. 1980 a, b). In cytologic studies the lens cells maintain normal function until 7 days postnatally, followed by loss of differentiating ability and swelling of the posterior lens fibers (Uga et al. 1980). Two weeks after birth, enlargement of the lens bow nuclei is noted. By the 4th week, posterior lens fibers are swollen, and degenerating cells and large intercellular spaces are present in the superficial bow cortex. Between 5 and 6 weeks, epithelial cells at the equator become elongated, with reduced mitosis. The cells in the posterior cortex become degenerate, causing a widening of the posterior sutures. Clinically at this stage the lenticular nucleus becomes markedly opaque.

A progressive, hereditary autosomal recessive cataract has been investigated in the *Deer mouse* (Burns and Feeney 1975). Based on genetic studies the cataracts are of two types: type I (early onset) and type II (late onset). The opacification process in type I is associated with abnormal closure of the fetal fissure and hyaloid vascular abnormalities. There is abnormal posterior migration of disrupted lens bow cells before lens opacity is apparent. Posterior subcapsular cataracts subsequently develop and spread centrally and inferionasally to the equatorial area and then to the entire equator; the nuclear opacities are clinically evident either as a "shell" pattern or as isolated dots. Histologically, abnormal migration and proliferation of lens epithelium and the enlargement und vacuolar degeneration of basal process of cortical lens fibers occur (Burns et al. 1980; Feeney-Burns et al. 1980). Type II cataracts follow the same developmental pattern but are rarely associated with extensive hyaloid vascular abnormalities and progress more slowly.

The *Emory mouse* cataract is a late-appearing (6–8 months) cataract inherited as an autosomal dominant trait (Kuck et al. 1981). Morphologic features include thickening of the lens capsule, loss of lens bow nuclei, and basophilic particles observed within cortical fibers in the early stages, these equatorial changes being accompanied by posterior subcapsular bladder cells and fiber vacuolization. With progression, the posterior capsule thickens and acquires a serrated edge. In advanced cataracts, cortical fibers are vacuolated superficially and calcified in deeper zones.

The autosomal dominantly inherited cataract in *Swiss mice* described by Tissot and Cohen (1972) is characterized by rapid loss of nuclei by primary lens fibers first noted embryologically on the 14th day. Secondary lens fibers have an irregular array; the fibers subsequently degenerate with vacuolization. The anterior epithelium in the advanced cataract is multilayered and vascularized (Davidorf and Eglitis 1966).

Histologic features of the *NOP mutant,* a congenital autosomal dominantly inherited nuclear cataract (Graw et al. 1984), and the *Robertsonian mouse* cataract (K. Munger 1986, personal communication) have not been described; in the latter we have observed a spectrum of changes including spontaneous rupture of the posterior capsule with extrusion of cortex. A cataract has been described in the *house mouse* (Paget et al. 1961) as a subcapsular lesion appearing at birth and inherited as an autosomal dominant condition (Table 5).

Ultrastructure

Transmission electron microscopy of *Fraser cataract* in its early developmental stages demonstrates degenerating ectodermal cells in the invaginating optic cup. Primary lens fibers contain increased dilated rough endoplasmic reticulum, vacuoles, and mitochondria and decreased crystalline substance and polysomes. By the 13th and 14th fetal day, the apical portions of these cells begin to swell with subsequent degeneration (Hamai and Kuwabara 1975).

Hamai et al. (1974) studied the *Nakano mouse cataract* using the transmission electron microscope (TEM) and found affected lens fibers to contain coarse granular substance and an abundance of microorganelles. In the *Philly mouse cataract,* dense particles are seen in the young lens fibers; older fibers degenerate with swelling, the accumulation of dense amorphous or granular cytoplasmic substances, and the appearance of extracellular droplets (Uga et al. 1980). The earliest ultrastructural changes in *deer mice cataract* are loss of fiber cell hexagonal

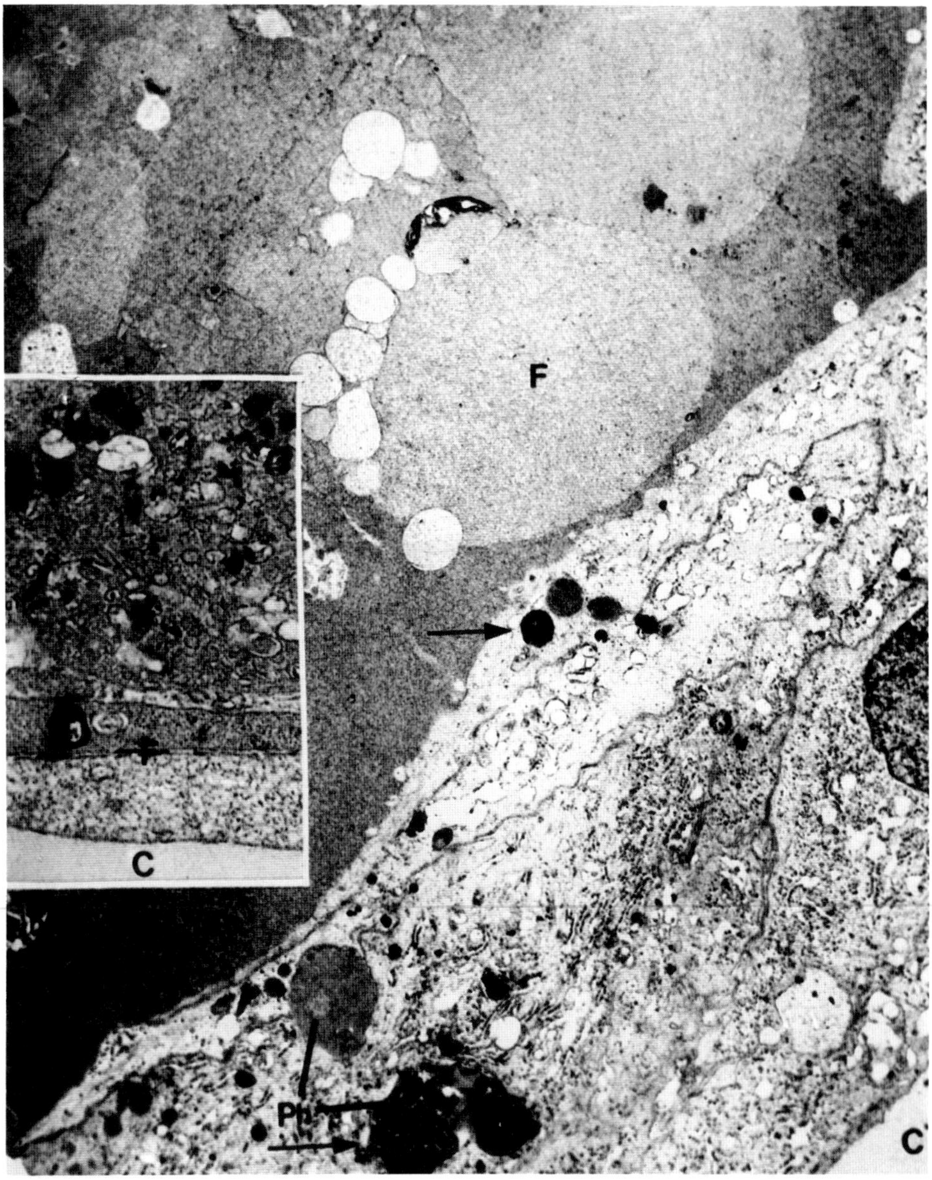

Fig. 54. Early posterior subcapsular cataract in a 7-week-old *deer mouse.* Phagosomes *(ph)* are seen in the cytoplasm of migrated epithelial cells and contain proteins released by degenerating lens fiber cells *(F)*. Posterior capsule is designated as *C*. A positive acid phosphatase reaction is apparent in some phagolysosomes *(arrows)*. TEM, ×6500. *Inset:* Multiple small lysosomes in subcapsular fiber cells of a posterior cataract in a 12-week-old *deer mouse.* (From Feeney-Burns et al. 1980) TEM, ×27000

packing, cell fusion, and formation of fiber cell syncytia in the posterior subcapsular region. Osmophilic densities are present on the plasma membrane at sites of cell confluency, and larger osmophilic whorls are located at ball and socket interlocking cell junctions in more advanced cataract. Epithelial cells migrate posteriorly, where they phagocytize lens proteins, incorporating them into acid-phosphatase positive lysosomes (Figs. 54, 55) (Feeney-Burns et al. 1980). Morphologic changes in cortical fiber cell membranes of the developing *Emory mouse cataract* were studied with scanning, transmission, and freeze-fracture electron microscopy (Lo and Kuck 1987). The major changes noted are the formation of extensive ridge patterns of fiber cell membranes in the outer cortical region (Figs. 56, 57).

In the *Robertsonian mouse* the cataracts are manifest by posterior fiber degeneration and

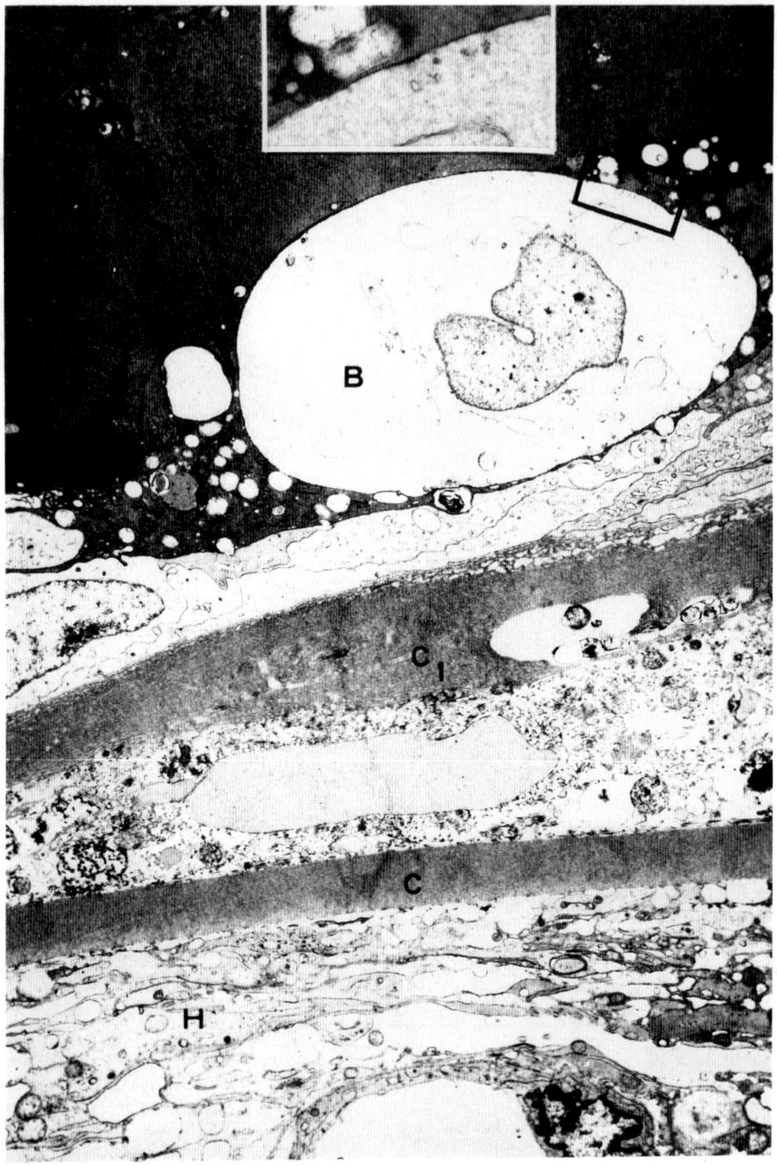

Fig. 55. Posterior subcapsular cataract in a deer mouse. Fiber cells are ruptured, a bladder cell *(B)* lies amid cell debris, connective tissue is present between duplicated capsule *(C, C1)*, and a persistent hyaloid vascular system is present. TEM, ×4200. *Inset* shows granularity of bladder cell cytoplasm. (From Feeney-Burns et al. 1980) TEM, ×16000

thinning of the posterior capsule with extrusion of fibers (Fig. 58).

Differential Diagnosis

Cataracts in mice tend to be the common end-stage process of a variety of insults to the lens and as such are difficult to differentiate in regard to etiology. While features may be characteristic of a certain type of cataract (inherited versus noninherited, inherited in one strain versus another), diagnosis of etiology based upon morphology alone is usually somewhat speculative, especially with advanced cataract.

Biologic Features

Natural History

Although the natural history of inherited cataracts in mice is not well documented in each strain, in general they tend to be progressive to total opacification over variable records of time.

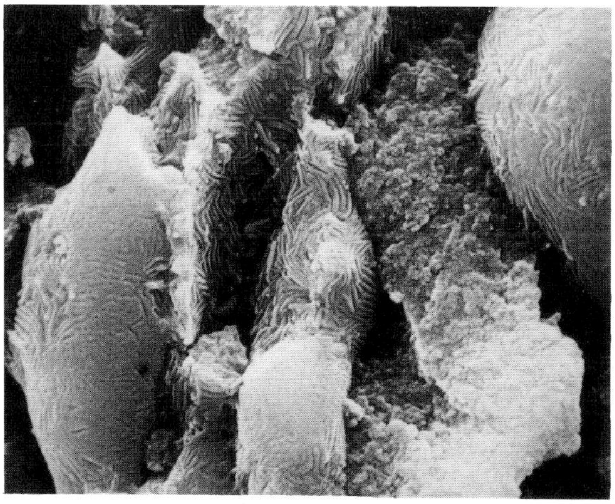

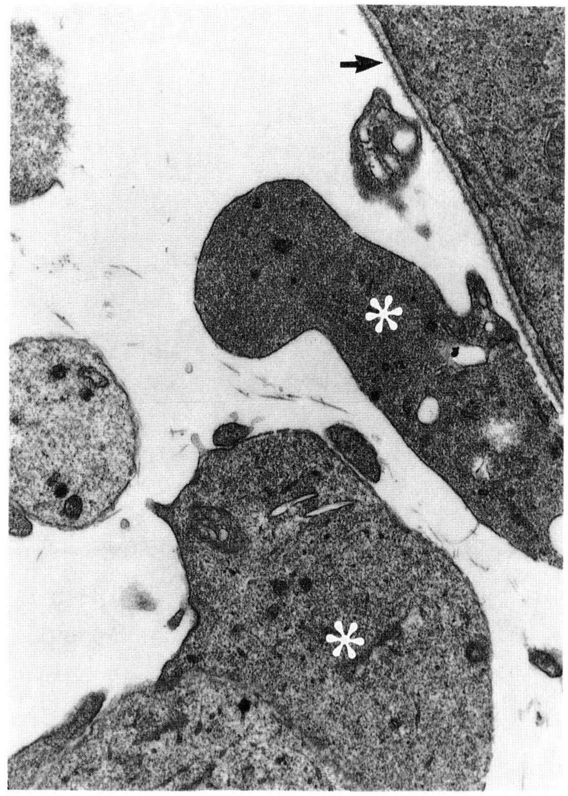

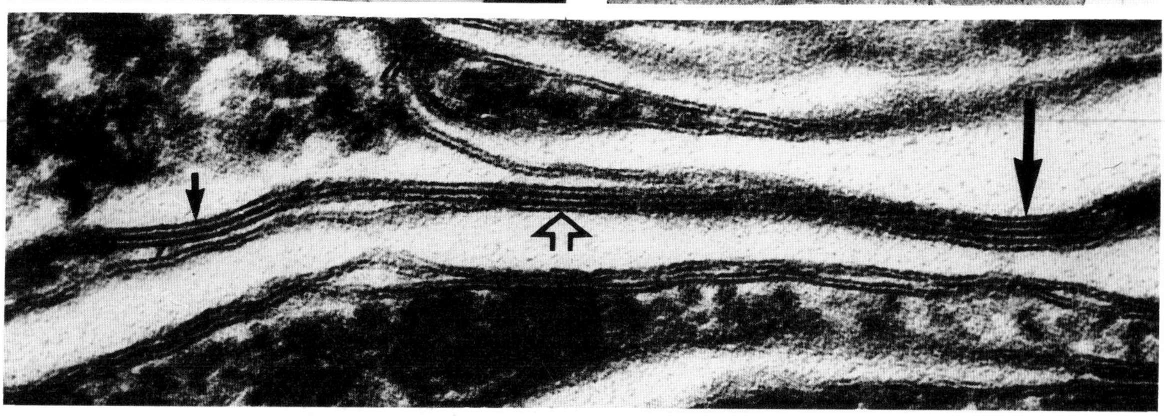

Fig. 56 *(upper left).* Outer cortical fibers about 60 nm deep from the capsule surface from an *Emory mouse* lens 15 months of age. Large globular structures representing swollen and distorted fibers are observed at the posterior suture; surfaces are occupied by shorter, less prominent ridges. (From Lo and Kuck 1987) SEM, ×5000

Fig. 57 *(below).* Outer cortical fiber cell membranes in the cell breakdown areas of *Emory mouse* cataract, 15 months of age. An adhesion process between membranes is evident; a 13-nm pentalamellar profile *(short arrow)* is adhered with a unit membrane below at the *open arrow* to form a 19.5-nm heptalamellar structure which is further adhered with another unit membrane, a portion of which is cut tangentially, to form a 0.26-mm nonolamellar profile *(large arrow).* (From Lo and Kuck 1987) TEM, ×150000

Fig. 58 *(upper right). Robertsonian mouse* cataract, posterior lens. The capsule *(arrow)* is thinned and fiber cells (*) are located within the retrolental vitreous. TEM, ×16000

Etiopathogenesis

Mechanisms of cataractogenesis are poorly understood; however, biochemical alterations have been studied and defined in several of the inherited mouse cataracts.

The *Fraser* and *Philly mouse cataracts* are suspected to be osmotic cataracts, based on morphologic evidence. Alterations in membrane permeability and lens protein synthesis have been demonstrated in the latter (Kador et al. 1980 a, b; Shinohara and Piatigorsky 1980). The *Nakano mouse cataract* is also an osmotic cataract due to the inhibition of membrane-bound Na^{+}–K^{+} ATPase (Fukui et al. 1978).

Biochemical changes associated with the *Emory mouse cataract* include the conversion of soluble to insoluble protein, depression of glutathione, and increases in calcium and free phosphate in affected lenses (Kuck and Kuck 1983). Graw et al. (1984) describe reduced protein, increased oxidized glutathione, and reduced enzyme activity in cataractous NOP mouse lenses.

Frequency

Incidence of affected offspring from parents of known clinical and/or genetic features is predictable based on described genetic patterns (Table 5).

Comparison with Other Species

Inherited cataracts have been described in rats, dogs, sheep, cattle, and turkeys. The majority are autosomal recessive traits, each with its own distinctive clinical, morphologic, and biochemical features.

References

Burns RP, Feeney L (1975) Hereditary cataracts in deer mice *(Peromyscus maniculatus)*. Am J Ophthalmol 80: 370–378

Burns RP, Anderson RS, Feeney-Burns L (1980) Cataract-webbed traits in *Peromyscus*. II. Biomicroscopy and histology of eyes. Invest Ophthalmol Vis Sci 19: 31–42

Davidorf F, Eglitis I (1966) A study of a hereditary cataract in the mouse. J Morphol 119: 89–100

Feeney-Burns L, Burns RP, Anderson RS (1980) Ultrastructure and acid phosphatase activity in hereditary cataracts of deer mice. Invest Ophthalmol Vis Sci 19: 777–788

Fraser FC, Schabtach G (1962) "Shrivelled": a hereditary degeneration of the lens in the house mouse. Genet Res 3: 383–387

Fukui HN, Obazawa H, Kinoshita HJ (1976) Lens growth in the Nakano mouse. Invest Ophthalmol Vis Sci 15: 422–425

Fukui HN, Merola LM, Kinoshita JH (1978) A possible cataractogenic factor in the Nakano mouse lens. Exp Eye Res 26: 477–485

Graw J, Kratochvilova J, Summer KH (1984) Genetical and biochemical studies of a dominant cataract mutant in mice. Exp Eye Res 39: 37–45

Hamai Y, Kuwabara T (1975) Early cytologic changes of Fraser cataract. An electron microscopic study. Invest Ophthalmol Vis Sci 14: 517–527

Hamai Y, Fukui HN, Kuwabara T (1974) Morphology of hereditary mouse cataract. Exp Eye Res 18: 537–546

Iwata S, Kinoshita JH (1971) Mechanism of development of hereditary cataract in mice. Invest Ophthalmol Vis Sci 10: 504–512

Kador P, Fukui HN, Fukushi S, Jernigan HM Jr, Kinoshita JH (1980 a) Philly mouse: a new model of hereditary cataract. Exp Eye Res 30: 59–68

Kador P, Uga S, Piatigorsky J (1980 b) The Philly mouse hereditary cataract. In: Regnault F, Hockwin O, Courtois Y (eds) Aging of the lens. Cellular and biochemical aspects. Elsevier, Amsterdam, pp 157–170

Kuck JFR, Kuck KD (1983) The Emory mouse cataract. Loss of soluble protein, glutathione protein sulfhydryl and other changes. Exp Eye Res 36: 351–362

Kuck JFR, Kuwabara T, Kuck KD (1981) The Emory mouse cataract: an animal model for human senile cataract. Curr Eye Res 1981–82 1: 643–649

Lo WK, Kuck JF (1987) Alterations in fiber cell membranes of Emory mouse cataract: a morphologic study. Curr Eye Res 6: 433–44

Paget OE, Baumgartner-Gamauf M, Gama FM (1961) Histologische Untersuchungen an einer dominant erblichen Form einer Cataract bei der Hausmaus. Zool Anx 166: 55–69

Sakuragawa M, Kuwabara T, Kinoshita JH, Fukui HN (1975) Swelling of the lens fibers. Exp Eye Res 21: 381–394

Shinohara T, Piatigorsky J (1980) Persistence of crystallin messenger RNAs with reduced translation in hereditary cataracts in mice. Science 210: 914–916

Tissot RG, Cohen C (1972) A new congenital cataract in the mouse. J Hered 63: 197–201

Uga S, Kador PF, Kuwabara T (1980) Cytological study of Philly mouse cataract. Exp Eye Res 30: 79–92

Zwaan J, Williams RM (1968 a) Morphogenesis of the eye lens in a mouse strain with hereditary cataracts. J Exp Zool 169: 407–421

Zwaan J, Williams RM (1968 b) Studies in the development of a hereditary cataract in the house mouse. Anat Rec 160: 456–457

Zwaan J, Williams RM (1969) Cataracts and abnormal proliferation of the lens epithelium in mice carry the cat_{Fr} gene. Exp Eye Res 8: 161–169

Cataract Due to Tryptophan Deficiency, Rat

James A. Render and William W. Carlton

Synonyms. None.

Gross Appearance

The lenses from tryptophan-deficient rats are smaller than lenses from control rats (McAvoy et al. 1979; Bunce et al. 1978) and have changes in the fibers of the cortex. The refractive index differs between the cortex and nucleus (von Sallmann et al. 1959). Posterior, subcapsular, saucer-shaped opacities and discrete, anterior, subcapsular haze occurs in rats fed a tryptophan-deficient diet (Koch et al. 1982). Initially, an apparent difference in the optical sensity of the lens occurs in the form of a concentric cortical band or ring (Totter and Day 1942). Eventually, lenticular opacification develops and is progressive in the perinuclear area (von Sallmann et al. 1959). This progressive opacification involves the anterior and posterior cortex and gives the cataract a shell-shaped appearance (Totter and Day 1942). The diameter of this shell appears to be approximately two-thirds of the total lenticular diameter. With time, rats given a tryptophan-deficient diet have lenses which are partially or entirely white and opaque. Sometimes, a peripheral rim of clear lens fiber exists (Totter and Day 1942). Some young rats fed a diet deficient in both tryptophan and vitamin E develop either unilateral or bilateral cataracts of variable size (Bunce and Hess 1976). These lenticular opacities are central and nuclear. The anterior and posterior cortex is clear. The area of opacity expands as the central lesion expands.

Microscopic Features

Alterations involve the lenticular fibers and changes in the number, distribution, and morphology of nuclei in the nuclear bow region (McAvoy and Van Heyningen 1976). Nucleated lenticular fibers extend deep into the lens and the nucleated cells are two to three times more numerous in the lens of deficient rats than in the lens of control rats (McAvoy et al. 1979; von Sallman et al. 1959). Lenticular cells vary in shape and have nuclei with abnormal morphologic features. The cells are thicker or larger than normal lenticular cells, especially in the anterior and posterior cortex, and form irregular rows. Hydropic swelling involves the subcapsular ends of fibers which have nuclei at the lenticular bow and occurs first at the ends of fibers, particularly at the sutures (von Sallmann et al. 1959). Later, hydropic change with vacuole formation is present in the fibers of the deeper cortex and spreads along the sutures toward the surface. This change eventually leads to lenticular fiber degeneration around the anterior pole, resulting in the formation of an amorphous, granular, wedge-shaped lesion extending anteriorly along the suture (von Sallmann et al. 1959). The cells in the equatorial region and the lenticular epithelial cells have normal microscopic features despite severe changes in the cortex.

Ultrastructure

No description of the ultrastructural features of lenticular cataract produced by tryptophan deficiency was found.

Differential Diagnosis

Cataractous changes produced by tryptophan deficiency may or may not be difficult to distinguish from lesions produced by other causes. Lenticular opacities have been described in rats given diets deficient in one of several essential amino acids, including phenylalanine (Bowles et al. 1947), valine, and histidine (Hall et al. 1948; Ferraro and Roizin 1947), but the frequency, course, and morphology of the lenticular changes have been studied most completely in rats given tryptophan-deficient diets. The cataract produced by a tryptophan deficiency is quite unlike the cataracts produced by administration of xylose or galactose, the feeding of a riboflavin-deficient diet (Totter and Day 1942), those induced by orthovoltage irradiation (Pfeiffer et al. 1981), and some inherited cataracts (Gelatt and Das 1984). The posterior subcapsular cataractous changes in rats due to tryptophan deficiency could possibly be confused with those observed in aging Wistar rats (Gorthy 1977) or those associated with hereditary retinal dystrophy in Royal College of Surgeons rats (Gelatt and Das 1984, p. 92, this volume).

Corneal vascularization also occurs in rats fed a tryptophan-deficient diet but this lesion may be due to other nutritional deficiencies. These include vitamin A (Stephenson and Clark 1920), riboflavin (Pirie 1948), lysine (Totter and Day 1942), methionine (Sydenstricker et al. 1946), protein (Sydenstricker et al. 1946), sodium (Follis et al. 1941), and zinc (Follis et al. 1942). The corneal vascularization produced by a tryptophan deficiency is similar to that produced by a lysine deficiency but different from that produced by a riboflavin deficiency (Totter and Day 1942). In the latter, the vessels simultaneously invade the cornea from all of the periphery and the cornea is often opaque. The vascularization of the cornea in the young rat fed a tryptophan-deficient diet is well advanced by the time of cataract development. The vessels are predominantly superficial in the cornea, but, in advanced cases, the vessels are present in the deeper portions of the stroma, associated with an inflammatory cell infiltrate (Buschke 1943).

Biologic Features

Rats given diets deficient in tryptophan lost weight, became emaciated, and were hunchback with a rough haircoat (Ferraro and Roizin 1947; Totter and Day 1942). Many developed alopecia, particularly of the face. Corneal changes associated with a tryptophan deficiency (Pirie 1948) consisted of vascularization. The vascularity occurred in a clear cornea (Totter and Day 1942). The vessels grew anteriorly toward the center of the cornea from the lateral canthus. Corneal vascularization was not detected in rats fed diets deficient in tryptophan and vitamin E (Bunce and Hess 1976) and did not occur in young male rats fed a diet low enough in tryptophan to induce cataract (Bunce et al. 1978).

Supplementation of deficient diets with 0.1% or 0.2% tryptophan prevents the lenticular changes in rats (Bunce and Hess 1976) and guinea pigs (von Sallmann et al. 1959). Smaller quantities of tryptophan added to the diet delay the onset of changes.

The cataractous changes are partially reversible within 18 months after discontinuing a tryptophan-deficient diet (Koch et al. 1982). New lens fibers form, grow, and cause the formation of a zonular cataract by making the opaque layer in the lens recede.

Rats deficient in tryptophan have lenses with lower dry weights and a slight increase in water compared with lenses from control rats of the same age (Koch et al. 1982). The differentiation of the lenticular fibers appears normal and the water-insoluble lenticular proteins are not altered. However, the β-crystallins and individual β-subfractions are markedly altered (Koch et al. 1982).

Comparison with Other Species

The gross and histopathologic changes in the lenses of tryptophan-deficient rats are similar to those changes in the lenses of tryptophan-deficient guinea pigs (von Sallmann et al. 1959). The experimental production of this cataract in other rodent species apparently has not been reported. A search of the literature reveals no citation of the occurrence of tryptophan deficiency cataract in human patients.

The cataract produced by a tryptophan deficiency is quite unlike lenticular opacities resulting from xylose or galactose feeding, or riboflavin deficiency (Totter and Day 1942). Protein changes in tryptophan-deficient rats differ from those in other types of experimental cataracts (Russell et al. 1979). Rats fed a tryptophan-deficient diet have lenses with an increased wet weight, increased insoluble protein, and disappearance of the β-crystallins (Bunce et al. 1978). In the Nakano strain of congenitally cataractous mice, the water-insoluble proteins are predominantly increased and the γ-crystallins are decreased. In experimental galactose cataracts, the α-crystallins are increased and the γ-crystallins are decreased (Ocken et al. 1977).

References

Bowles LL, Sydenstricker VP, Hall WK, Schmidt HL Jr (1947) Cataracts resulting from a deficiency of phenylalanine in the rat. Proc Soc Exp Biol Med 66: 585–586

Bunce GE, Hess JL (1976) Lenticular opacities in young rats as a consequence of maternal diets low in tryptophan and/or vitamin E. J Nutr 106: 222–229

Bunce GE, Hess JL, Fillnow GM (1978) Investigation of low tryptophan induced cataract in weanling rats. Exp Eye Res 26: 399–405

Buschke W (1943) Classification of experimental cataracts in the rat. Recent observations on cataract associated with tryptophan deficiency and with some other experimental conditions. Arch Ophthalmol 30: 735–750

Ferraro A, Roizin L (1947) Ocular involvement in rats on diets deficient in amino acids. I. Tryptophan. Arch Ophthalmol 38: 331–341

Follies RH Jr, Day HG, McCollum EV (1941) Histological studies of the tissues of rats fed a diet extremely low in zinc. J Nutr 22: 223–237

Follis RH Jr, Orent-keiles E, McCollum EV (1942) Histologic studies of the tissues of rats extremely low in sodium. Arch Pathol 33: 504–512

Gelatt KN, Das ND (1984) Animal models for inherited cataracts: a review. Curr Eye Res 3: 765–778

Gorthy WC (1977) Cataracts in the aging rat lens. Ophthalmic Res 9: 329–342

Hall WK, Bowles LL, Sydenstricker VP, Schmidt HL (1948) Cataracts due to deficiencies of phenylalanine and histidine in the rat: a comparison with other types of cataracts. J Nutr 36: 277–296

Koch HR, Ohrloff C, Bours J, Riemann G, Dragomirescu V, Hockwin O (1982) Separation of lens proteins in rats with tryptophan deficiency cataracts. Exp Eye Res 34: 479–486

McAvoy JW, Van Heyningen R (1976) Changes in the cells of the lens bow and epithelium of tryptophan deficient rats. Biology of the epithelial lens cells. INSERM (Inst Natl Sante Rech Med) Colloq 60: 245–250

McAvoy JW, Palfrey LJ, van Heyningen R (1979) A light microscope study of the lens of the tryptophan-deficient rat. Exp Eye Res 28: 533–538

Ocken PR, Fu SCJ, Hart R, White JH, Wagner BJ, Lewis KE (1977) Characterization of lens proteins. I. Identification of additional soluble fractions in rat lenses. Exp Eye Res 24: 355–367

Peiffer RL Jr, Wright W, Steinbok P, Mahaley MS (1981) Long-term study of the ocular effects of orthovoltage irradiation in rats. Am J Vet Res 42: 1598–1605

Pirie A (1948) Comparison of eye changes in riboflavin deficiency and in tryptophan deficiency in the rat. Br J Nutr 2: 14–20

Russell P, Smith SG, Carper DA, Kinoshita JH (1979) Age and cataract related changes in the heavy molecular weight proteins and gamma crystallin composition of the mouse lens. Exp Eye Res 29: 245–255

Stephenson M, Clark AB (1920) A contribution to the study of keratomalacia among rats. Biochem J 14: 502–521

Sydenstricker VP, Hall WK, Hock CW, Pund ER (1946) Amino acid and protein deficiencies as causes of corneal vascularization: a preliminary report. Science 103: 194–196

Totter JR, Day PL (1942) Cataract and other ocular changes resulting from tryptophane deficiency. J Nutr 24: 159–166

von Sallmann L, Reid ME, Grimes PA, Collins EM (1959) Tryptophan-deficiency cataract in guinea pigs. Arch Ophthalmol 62: 662–672

Induced Cataracts, Lens, Rat

James A. Render and William W. Carlton

Gross Appearance

Exposure of animals to certain drugs and chemicals can result in a variety of gross lenticular alterations. The alterations may be transient or permanent, progressive or nonprogressive, and may locate in various regions of the lens. The opacities may appear as granular deposits on the anterior surface of the lenticular capsule, as scattered subcapsular gray dots, as fine striations, or as superficial vacuoles. Eventually, with long periods of exposure to some compounds, the entire anterior and posterior cortex becomes opaque.

Cataracts are seen in association with ocular anomalies, corneal changes, or inflammatory lesions. Ocular anomalies including open eye, exophthalmos, anophthalmia, microphthalmia, and corneal opacity are produced in fetal rats by administration of cyclophosphamide during 12–16 days of gestation (Hall, 1953; Singh and Sanyal 1976; Singh 1971). Sulfonyl urea hypoglycemic drugs, such as carbutamide, tolbutamide, and chlorpropamide, produce corneal opacities in addition to lenticular opacities after chronic administration (Wright 1963).

Different types of drugs and chemicals will produce different types of lenticular opacities. The lenticular opacification in rats receiving intravenous injections of streptozotocin first appears as a faint, feathery, or net-shaped cloudiness under the anterior capsule (Sasaki et al. 1983). Rats given chloroquine and other anphophilic drugs have, biomicroscopically, prominent sutural opacities and diffuse subcapsular opacities which are most prominent in the anterior cortex (Drenckhahn 1978). The early lenticular alterations of Myleran (2,4-dimethanesulfonoxybutane) toxicosis appear as white dots in the posterior and anterior cortex (Von Sallmann 1957). Small punctate cortical opacities in the posterior subcapsular region may be observed in rats given alloxan. Punctate cortical opacification may become diffuse with increasing severity (Charalampous and Hegsted 1950; Janes et al. 1952; Kok-Van Alphen and Cohen 1950). The first change in the lenses of rats fed 0.05% oder 0.075% Diquat (9,10-dihydro-8a, 10a-diazoniaphen-anthrene dibromide a herbicide) for 4–8 months is a regular "lacework" type of opacity immediately under the posterior lenticular capsule (Pirie et al. 1970). The cataracts produced by Diquat administration begin at the posterior pole of the lens; vacuoles appear in the cortex and progress to involve the entire lens (Conning et al. 1969).

The time of onset of cataractous change after administration of a drug or chemical may vary and the lenticular changes may be progressive. Weanling rats suddenly develop complete bilateral lenticular opacities about 2 weeks after the addition of N^2-phenyl-β-hydrazinopropionitrile to their diets at concentrations of 0.10%–0.25% (Dasler and Wang 1972; Dasler et al. 1970; Patterson and Heath 1967). Adult rats fed the compound develop cataracts that are mature in 6–8 weeks.

Thallium salts produce cataracts in young rats after about 6 weeks of exposure; these cataracts begin as striations in the anterior cortex between the suture and equator (Bellows 1944). With further development, a concentric opaque zone occurs between one clear equatorial area and the lenticular nucleus. The nucleus remains intact even in the mature cataract.

The course of development of lens opacification in rats may occur in stages such as described in streptozotocin toxicosis (Sasaki et al. 1983). Initially, the lenticular opacification appears as small vacuoles or short radial opacities in the equatorial regions or only as cloudiness. The vacuolation spreads near the mid-periphery from the equator toward the superficial cortex, and some vacuoles increase in size. The vacuoles disappear as a diffuse cloudiness develops in the anterior deep cortex. The cloudiness in the anterior deep cortex progresses into the deeper layers, which are distinguished from the superficial cortex by a complex irregular boundary. Opalescent changes become visible near the nucleus of the lens and spread into the surrounding cortex. Eventually, the whole lens is transformed into an opalescent body with only a thin relatively transparent layer just beneath the capsule.

Some of the lenticular opacities produced by specific compounds are confined to the lenticular sutures. For example, intraperitoneal injections of methionine sulfoximine in rats fed a diet low in protein cause accentuation of the suture lines and mature cataracts within 6–9 weeks of feeding (Bagchi 1959).

Cataracts may be localized to particular regions of the lens. For example, perinuclear cataracts are produced by several chemicals including naphthalene, bleomycin, and selenium. Fischer 344 rat given bleomycin beginning at 3 days of age develop bilateral perinuclear and nuclear lenticular opacities at the age of 14–16 days (Edwards et al. 1975). Selenium produces perinuclear and nuclear cataracts when injections are made into suckling rats. The nuclear cataracts are bilateral and develop within 3 days; the nucleus is opaque and a zone of diffuse cloudiness occurs around the nucleus (Bhuyan et al. 1981a, b; Ostadalova et al. 1978). Selenium-induced cataracts are shown to begin with the formation of a posterior equatorial subcapsular opacity which progresses in development to become a prominent "washer"-shaped opacity in the cortex. With time, bilateral dense central nuclear cataracts develop.

Selenite administration may cause both cortical and nuclear cataracts which progress from equatorial vacuolation to cortical and nuclear opacification (Anderson et al. 1986). Subcutaneous injection of sodium selenite in rats produces a 100% incidence of cataracts when administered between the 9th and 14th days after birth (Bunce and Hess 1981). The lens has a normal appearance for 2 days, but a well-formed central opacity is observed on the 3rd day postinjection. Injections at day 15 cause opacities in 80% of the lenses within 3–5 days, but administration at day 16 results in only a mild transient haziness or a more well defined opacification.

Administration of some compounds may result in a color change in the lens. Administration of naphthalene may cause the lens and intraocular fluids to become yellow or brown (Adams 1930). Naphthalene-induced cataracts are characterized by changes that begin with fiber swelling. This lenticular change is followed by development of cortical clefts and vacuoles that radiate from the cortex into the nucleus of the lens (Adams 1930; van Heyningen 1976, 1979;

van Heyningen and Pirie 1967; Koch and Doldi 1975; Pirie 1968). Changes observed by a slit lamp consisted of a supranuclear haziness and circular opacity (Adams 1930). Eventually, the cortex liquefies, but the nucleus remains intact.
Not all lenticular opacities are permanent. A rapid opacification of the lens has been reported in rats given opiates, opioids, or phenothiazine-based tranquilizers (Grant 1974). These substances given systemically produce an opacification of the anterior cortex of the lens within 1–2 h. This opacification is spontaneously reversible within another few hours.

Microscopic Features

Microscopic lenticular alterations may involve the lenticular epithelium or lenticular fibers or both; such alterations include cellular proliferation, migration, disorganization, degeneration, and necrosis. For example, the early changes in the lens due to mimosine administration occur in both the lenticular epithelium and lenticular fibers (Von Sallman et al. 1959 a). The epithelial cells of the equatorial region increase in size. Cellular hypertrophy combines with cellular proliferation. At the equator, large vesicular cells and nucleated cells form a broad zone about the lenticular nucleus posteriorly with loss of normal architecture of the nuclear bow.
Granular debris replaces the fibers in the anterior cortex. Superficial parts of the lenticular nucleus are broken up and become disorganzid. Clefts filled with granular material are formed.
Other examples of lenticular epithelial cell migration as the result of drug administration include bleomycin and naphthalene toxicosis. Epithelial cell migration along the posterior capsule has also been described as one of the histopathologic changes of the advanced cataract of bleomycin (Edwards et al. 1975).
The naphthalene-induced cataract has been characterized as having a lenticular epithelium that is several layers thick early in cataract development (Adams 1930; van Heyningen 1976, 1979; van Heyningen and Pirie 1967, 1976; Koch and Doldi 1975). Thirty days later, when the cataract is mature, the entire capsule is lined by epithelium and the cortex is liquefied.
Fiber swelling is a frequently reported alteration in the development of cataracts. A variety of compounds produce this change; the list includes methionine sulfoximine, mimosine, Mirex, and triparanol. The first changes of cataract development in rats given methionine sulfoximine are those of swelling of the lenticular fibers and disorientation of the nuclei in the equatorial region (Bagchi 1959). Histopathologic alterations in the mimosine-induced cataract includes degeneration of nuclei and hydropic swelling of the anterior cortical fibers (Von Sallman et al. 1959 a).
The earliest histologic change in the Mirex-induced cataracts at neonatal day 7 is slight swelling of individual cortical fibers followed at day 9 by more extensive swelling of intact fibers and, at days 11 and 13, by extensive degeneration and necrosis throughout the lenticular cortex. These changes are followed by only a slight proliferation of the anterior lenticular epithelium (Scotti et al. 1981).
Another frequently reported degenerative lenticular change is vacuolation. This alteration is reported in the lenses of rats given large doses of sugars and such compounds as alkylating agents, Myleran, selenium, and sulfonyl urea (Grant 1974). The cataract produced by alkylating agents is characterized by a granular cortex and vacuoles in the cortical regions of the anterior and posterior poles (Soloman et al. 1955; Light et al. 1956; Light 1967). The lesions of Myleran cataract include vacuolation in the anterior subcapsular region, suppression of mitosis, and a high incidence of nuclear fragmentation (Hamming et al. 1976). Extensive vacuolation of the lenticular cortical fibers is the principal change in the lenses of rats given excess selenium (Shearer et al. 1980). The lenticular lesions in rats given sulfonyl urea hypoglycemic drugs (carbutamide, tolbutamide, chlorpromide) include lenticular fragmentation, vacuolation, and globule formation (Wright 1963).
Suckling rats develop cataracts after a single subcutaneous injection of sodium selenite (Anderson et al. 1986). The first observable change in the lenses of rats given selenite is vacuolation, which starts at the lenticular bow and spreads throughout the posterior subcapsular region (Shearer and Anderson 1985). In the lenses of these young animals, mitosis is suppressed and karyorrhexis is observed in the nuclear bow region. Lesions of the lenticular epithelium include vacuolation and loss of normal epithelial morphology and are followed by clearing of the cortical opacity.
The lenses from rats given triparanol have small sudanophilic vesicles in the lenticular fibers, and larger complexes between fibers are formed by coalescence of the smaller vesicles. The lipid

material is probably composed of phospholipids, cholesterol, and cholesterol esters (Bellows 1963; Von Sallmann et al. 1963a, b).

In the cataract produced by chloroquine and other amphophilic drugs, lamellated inclusions accumulate in the lenticular epithelial cells and cortical fibers (Drenckhahn 1978). These lamellated inclusions are composed of lipids accumulated as a result of the impaired lipid catabolism. Numerous dense bodies and small vacuoles are present in the lenticular epithelium and in cortical lenticular fibers, especially the elongating fibers of the equator.

Ultrastructure

Ultrastructural lenticular alterations are not frequently reported but may involve the mitochondria endoplasmic reticulum, and other components of the cell. Changes in the mimosine cataract include swelling and distortion of the mitochondria and distention of the cisternae of the hyperplastic rough endoplasmic reticulum (von Sallmann et al. 1959a). Alterations due to the administration of chloroquine or other amphophilic drugs include accumulation of lipids with the formation of membrane-bound, lamellated, and crystalloid inclusions (Drenckhahn 1978). The lens of rats with galactose-induced cataracts have ultrastructural alterations of edematous, swollen, liquefied fibers and cellular cysts. Malaligned fibers are displaced by randomly distributed, variable-sized membrane-bound vesicles.

The cytoplasm is coarse and contains scattered electron-dense aggregates in the cytoplasm and adjacent to the cellular membrane. With increase in severity of the lenticular lesions, large intercellular spaces are found and the boundaries between fibers are ill defined (Unaker et al. 1978; Kuwabara et al. 1969). In the nuclear cataract induced by selenite, the lacy honeycomb appearance seen by light microscopy is ultrastructurally an aggregation or precipitation of cytoplasmic material (Russell et al. 1984).

Differential Diagnosis

Experimental cataracts are produced by the administration of chemical agents, by nutritional deficiencies, and by exposure to radiation. Toxic cataracts are caused by a variety of chemical agents (Gehring 1971) such as illustrated above. A deficiency of tryptophan and riboflavin and a severe protein deficiency combined with an imbalance in sulfur-containing amino acids results in the formation of cataracts (Koch et al. 1982; McAvoy et al. 1979; Ohrloff et al. 1978; Trotter and Day 1942; von Sallmann et al. 1959b). Cataracts induced by some chemicals seem to be analogous to those developing after exposure to X-rays or ionizing radiation (Grant 1974). Hereditary cataract may be induced by X-irradiation of young rats (Gorthy 1979; Leonard and Maisin 1965).

Biologic Features

The biologic activities of compounds which cause cataracts are numerous (Table 6). Alkylating agents are cytotoxic and attack molecules containing nucleophilic groups such as proteins, amino acids, and nucleic acids causing suppression of DNA synthesis and mitosis and interference with cellular proliferation (von Sallmann 1965).

Methionine sulfoximine, an antimetabolite of methionine, when given every other day by intraperitoneal injections, produces cataracts in rats fed a low-protein diet (Bagchi 1959). The cataract is considered the result of protein deficiency due to interference with protein synthesis by methionine sulfoximine.

Sulfhydryl content, especially glutathione, of the lenses, decreases prior to the observation of cataract.

Myleran (1,4-dimethanesulfonoxybutane), an anticancer drug, produces cataracts in rats (Grimes et al. 1964; Grimes and Von Sallmann 1966; Kandori and Kurimoto 1960; Light 1967; Von Sallmann 1957; Soloman et al. 1955). It acts on the relatively long Gl period, allowing normal DNA synthesis, but preventing miotic division (Grimes et al. 1964). Depression of miotic activity of the epithelial cells may be the direct cause of the lenticular opacification (Grimes and Von Sallmann 1966).

Naphthalene is metabolized to the unstable 1,2-dihydroxynaphthalene (van Heyningen and Pirie 1967), which is rapidly autoxidized to 1,2-naphthaquinone. This compound causes catalytic oxidation of ascorbic acid to hydrogen peroxide and dehydroascorbic acid. The lens may be vulnerable to naphthalene toxicosis because of its high concentration of ascorbic acid and low oxygen supply. The naphthaquinone-catalyzed reaction diminishes the already low oxygen sup-

Table 6. Biologic features of compounds causing cataract in rats

Compound	Biologic feature	Reference
Amphiphilic compounds (chloroquine, chlorphentermine, iprindole)	Intralysosomal drug-lipid complexes	Drenckhahn 1978
Diquat	Formation of free radicals and loss of lenticular ascorbic acid	Pirie et al. 1970; Pirie and Rees 1970
Methionine sulfoximine	Interference with protein synthesis	Bagchi 1959
Morphine, morphine-like compounds	Cataracts prevented by simultaneous administration of nalorphine	Weinstock and Stewart 1961
Myleran	Prevents lenticular epithelial cell division	Grimes et al. 1964; Grimes and Von Sallmann 1966
Naphthalene	More consistent, earlier, and severe cataracts in pigmented rats; changes due to a toxic metabolite, 1,2-dihydroxynaphthalene, which is metabolized to 1,2-naphthaquinone and hydrogen peroxide, diminishing the lenticular oxygen and ascorbic acid supply	van Heyningen and Pirie 1967
N^2-Phenyl-β-hydrazinopionnitriles	Decreased lenticular ATP concentrations	Patterson and Heath 1967; Dasler et al. 1970; Dasler and Wang 1972
Selenium	Decreased lenticular concentrations of sulfhydryl groups and glutathione, increased lenticular concentrations of insoluble protein, increased amount of lenticular water, interference with glutathione metabolism	Bhuyan et al. 1981 a, b; Bunce and Hess 1981; Bunce et al. 1984
Streptozotocin	Cataract due to hyperglycemia of diabetes resulting in lenticular osmotic changes from increased concentrations of sorbitol, glucose, and fructose	Arison et al. 1967; Von Sallmann and Grimes 1971; White and Cinotti 1972; Kojima et al. 1972
Triparanol	Inhibition of cholesterol biosynthesis with reduction of lenticular sulfhydryl content, accumulation of sudanophilic material causing uptake of water and sodium leading to swelling and disruption	Bellows 1963; Harris and Gruber 1973; Rathbun et al. 1973; Von Sallmann et al. 1963 a, b
Galactose	Lenticular accumulation of dulcitol resulting in an osmotic accumulation of water in the lens, decrease in lenticular glutathione concentrations, failure of cationic pump, decreased glycolysis, decreased concentrations of ATP	Bannon and Kaan 1939; Bannon et al. 1945; Bettman et al. 1964; Cotlier 1962; Dvornik et al. 1973; Kador et al. 1979; Keiding and Mellengaard 1972; Korc 1961; Lerman et al. 1961; Mitchell and Cook 1938; Segal and Bernstein 1963; Sippel 1966; Srivastava and Beuther 1972; Unaker et al. 1978

Diquat, 9,10-dihydro-8a, 10a-diazoniaphen-anthrene dibromide.

ply of the lens and produces toxic amounts of hydrogen peroxide. The highly reacitive 1,2-naphthaquinone combines with several constituents of the lens such as cysteine, other amino acids, glutathione, and proteins. Ocular pigmentation is significant in the development of naphthalene cataract in the rat. Rats of pigmented strains develop cataract more consistently with a shorter induction time and have more severe lenticular alterations than nonpigmented strains (van Heyningen and Pirie 1976). The susceptibility of pigmented strains may result from the activity of the polyphenol oxidase in the pigmented iris with the formation of the toxic 1,2-naphthaquinone.

Galactose feeding is an effective method for the experimental production of lenticular opacification (Bannon and Kaan 1939; Bannon et al. 1945; Bettman et al. 1964; Cotlier 1962; Dvornik et al. 1973; Kador et al. 1979; Korc 1961; Lerman et al. 1961; Mitchell and Cook 1938; Segal and Bernstein 1963; Sippel 1966; Srivastava and Beuther 1972). There is a great deal of uniformity in the appearance of the various stages from the initial peripheral striations to the final central cataract. In galactose-induced cataracts, the accumulated dulcitol, a metabolic product which is not further metabolized, results in an osmotic effect with accumulation of water. Initially, the dulcitol does not penetrate the lenticular membranes and becomes trapped within the cells with the highest concentration in the cells of the equatorial region. This accumulation draws water into the cells to maintain an osmotic balance, producing osmotic swelling and hydropic changes in the lenticular fibers.

During the early stages of galactose feeding an almost immediate and precipitous decrease in the glutathione concentration and a failure of the cation pump results in progressive decrease in the uptake of tracer potassium and the extrusion of sodium. Glycolysis is decreased to about 75% of normal and is even lower when the cataract matures. This depression in metabolism is reflected in a corresponding decrease in the concentration of ATP. Another result of galactose feeding is to reduce the concentration of free amino acids in the lens.

The formation of a mature sugar cataract may not be directly associated with purely osmotic effects. A dense nuclear opacity forms rapidly and the chemical changes include a marked reduction in cation pump efficiency and failure to maintain intracellular potassium and to extrude sodium. A failure of membrane function follows and even dulcitol is lost from the lens as well as increased amounts of glutathione associated with a further loss of the capacity to generate ATP. The net loss of potassium and protein from the lens is overcompensated for by an increase in sodium ions so that even more water is drawn osmotically into the lens.

Rats made severely diabetic by the administration of alloxan or streptozotocin develop cataractogenic changes, noted at 1 month, and are completely opaque at 6 months (Arison et al. 1967; Bounds et al. 1955; Janes et al. 1952; Kojima et al. 1972; Kok-van Alphen and Cohen 1950; Von Sallmann and Grimes 1971; White and Cinotti 1972). In spontaneous or experimental diabetes, concentrations of sorbitol, glucose, and fructose are elevated in the lens. The hyperglycemia of diabetes appears to be the initial factor for the lens as the accumulated glucose results in changes in osmotic characteristics of the lens. Lowering of the blood glucose increases the time required for the induction of cataracts. A potent aldose reductase inhibitor is effective in preventing the development of cataracts in rats made diabetic by streptozotocin.

Subcutaneous injection of sodium selenite into 9-day-old male or female Sprague-Dawley rats causes development of large nuclear cataracts within 72 h (Bunce and Hess 1981) accompanied by a three times increase in the lenticular calcium and a two times increase in inorganic phosphate (Bunce et al. 1984). The selenium interferes with glutathione metabolism in the lens with the early changes in the fibers at or near the lenticular bow with eventual formation of nuclear cataract (Shearer and Anderson 1985). Biochemical changes in the lens associated with the administration of excess selenium include decreased concentrations of sulfhydryl groups and glutathione and increased concentrations of insoluble proteins and water (Bhuyan et al. 1981a, b; Bunce and Hess 1981). Radioactive selenium accumulates in the soluble and insoluble proteins in the lens, but not in the nuclear cataract (Shearer et al. 1982, 1983). The simultaneous administration of mercury, silver, cyanide, arsenite, cadmium, and copper either reduces the incidence or prevents the induction of nuclear cataracts by excess selenium. Iron, zinc, lead, chromium, and tungsten are ineffective in preventing the selenium-induced cataract (Shearer et al. 1983a). The selenite cataract in neonatal rats is associated with an increase in calcium and proteolysis occurring specifically in the lenticular nucleus. The proteolysis appears to be activated by increased lenticular calcium (David and Shearer 1984).

Triparanol, a cholesterol-lowering drug, produces cataract in human patients and experimental animals (Bellows 1963; Harris and Gruber 1973; Rathbun et al. 1973; Von Sallmann et al. 1963a, b). The triparanol-induced cataract is reversible in many animals when the drug is discontinued. Soluble protein concentrations are greatly depressed in dense cataracts but increase as the cataract clears. Also, the sulfyhydryl content of the soluble protein is reduced in dense cataracts, but increases during the recovery phase. The development of opacity is accompanied by a marked increase in the water and sodium content of the lens, but with little change in the potassium content. Triparanol may produce cataract in rats by the inhibition of cholesterol synthesis in the lens, as in other tissues, leading to the accumulation of 2,4-dehydrocholesterol (Von Sallmann et al. 1963a). The accumulation of sudanophilic material may result in the uptake of water and sodium leading to swelling and eventual disruption of fibers.

The generation of toxic metabolites of oxygen is proposed as a mechanism of cataract formation via lipid peroxidation (Bhuyan and Bhuyan 1984). Hydrogen peroxide is increased in ocular fluids in several experimental cataracts and in ocular fluids in senile cataracts in humans. Also, some cataractogenic compounds increase hydrogen peroxide in ocular fluids prior to development of cataract. Malondialdehyde, a major breakdown product of lipid peroxides, is increased in experimental cataracts in rabbits and rats, in hereditary cataracts in mice, and in senile cataract in humans.

Comparison with Other Species

Many compounds are associated with the development of lenticular cataracts in rats and in other species such as chickens, cattle, cats, dogs, rabbits, guinea pigs, mice, monkeys, and humans (Table 7). Although many drugs and chemicals produce cataracts in rats and other species, some, such as lovastatin, produce cataracts in dogs but not in rats (MacDonald et al. 1988). Bethamethasone, a corticosteroid drug, produces cataract in some rabbits when used as an ointment or as drops (Bettman et al. 1968). Cataracts are produced in the lens of fetal mice from females given hydrocortisone during varying periods of gestation (Rogoyski and Trzcinska-Dabrowska 1969); lenticular alterations included swelling, vacuolation, and disintegration of swollen fibers. Posterior subcapsular cataracts are reported in human patients treated with moderately high doses of corticosteroids (Black et al. 1960a, b; Braver et al. 1967; Bihari and Grossman 1968). Initially, the cataracts consist of vacuoles centrally located immediately anterior to the posterior capsule. With time, small clusters of discrete opacities coalesce to eventually form a posterior cortical cataract (Crews 1963). Dogs and cats given a subcutaneous injection of deferoxamine mesylate (Desferal) at high doses (150–200 mg/kg daily

Table 7. Compounds causing cataracts in rats and other species

Compound	Species	Reference
Alkylating agents	Mouse	Christenberry et al. 1963
Corticosteroids	Human, chicken, rabbit, mouse fetus	Black et al. 1960b; Braver et al. 1967; Bihari and Grossman 1968; Crews 1963; Rogoyski and Trzcinska-Dabrowska 1969
Deferoxamine mesylate (Desferal)	Cat, dog	Bruckner et al. 1967
Diquat	Dog	Pirie et al. 1970; Ribelin et al. 1967
Methoxsalen	Guinea pig, mouse	Cloud et al. 1960, 1961; Freeman 1966
Mimosine	Cattle	Holmes et al. 1981
Morphine	Mouse, guinea pig	Weinstock and Stewart 1961
Naphthalene	Rabbit	van Heyningen and Pirie 1976; van Heyningen 1979; Ihimoto and Iwata 1978; Koch and Doldi 1975; Pirie 1968; Adams 1930
Selenium	Guinea pig, rabbit	Shearer et al. 1983a, b
Streptozotocin	Monkey	Howard and Peterson 1973; Howard 1972
Triparanol	Human, dog	Bellows 1963; Von Sallmann et al. 1963a, b; Kirby et al. 1962; Kirby 1967

Diquat, 9,10-dihydro-8a, 10a-diazoniaphen-anthrene dibromide.

for 13–89 days) develop irreversible opacities morphologically similar to those produced in rats (Bruckner et al. 1967).

Diquat administered to dogs at a dose of 15 mg/kg per day produces cataracts in 10 months. Dogs given daily oral doses of 30, 67, and 150 mg/kg develop cataracts by 14 weeks (Ribelin et al. 1967).

Methoxsalen, a methoxypsoralen derivative, produces cataracts in mice and guinea pigs as well as rats exposed to ultraviolet light (320°–400°C) (Cloud et al. 1960, 1961; Freeman 1966). The lenses of guinea pigs and mice develop multiple vacuoles; these lesions are reversible and disappear within 1 week after withdrawal of the compound. Methoxsalen found in the lenses of rats can lead to photosensitization enhancement of lenticular fluorescence (Koch et al. 1979; Wulf and Andreasen 1982). Photoaddition products are generated with certain amino acid residues in the lenticular proteins, which may result in permanent retention of the compound within the lens. This photosensitizing agent alters the effect of sunlight on the skin as well as causing lenticular changes. In guinea pigs, these changes are multiple punctate opacities in the anterior cortex. Daily injections of methoxsalen followed by exposure to sunlight or long-wave ultraviolet light result in mature cataracts (Cloud et al. 1961; Freeman 1966).

Cataracts, goiter, and infertility are observed in cattle grazing a legume that contains mimosine (Holmes et al. 1981). In the lens, severe vacuolation and disruption of lenticular fibers are accompanied by focal hyperplasia of the lenticular epithelium.

A reversible opacity is produced in mice and guinea pigs as well as rats by parenteral administration of morphine and morphine-like compounds (Weinstock and Stewart 1961).

Naphthalene produces cataract and retinal degeneration in rabbits and rats (van Heyningen and Pirie 1967, 1976; van Heyningen 1976, 1979; Ihimoto and Iwata 1978; Koch and Doldi 1975; Pirie 1968). The development of cataract is quite variable in the rabbit as severe lenticular changes appear after a few days in some animals, and in other rabbits no changes are produced after 1–2 weeks of dosing. In some animals only the lens is damaged and sometimes only the retina has lesions. In others both the lens and retina are damaged. In other rabbits the lens and retina have no lesion. In the rabbit, ocular pigmentation does not alter the response to naphthalene, and lenticular and retinal damage is similar in both albino and pigmented rabbits (van Heyningen and Pirie 1967, 1976).

Dogs given triparanol develop cataracts in 5–7 months when fed 40 mg/kg per day and cataracts develop in 50% of dogs when fed 10 mg/kg per day (Bellows 1963). Monkeys given similar doses of triparanol fail to develop cataracts. Triparanol-induced cataracts in humans are located in the posterior subcapsular region, with less severe changes in the anterior subcapsular region (Kirby 1967). The posterior opacity is usually gray and irregular, but is sometimes lacy. Vacuoles are often present in the opacity, and are usually noticeable in the periphery. These cataracts do not usually progress in severity.

Mongolian gerbils fed a 50% galactose diet develop cataracts similar to those produced in rats fed the same diet. The rate of occurrence of the cataract in the gerbil is about twice that in rats. Increased enzymic activity is associated with greater amounts of dulcitol in the gerbil lens during the early phase of cataractogenesis (El-Aguizy et al. 1983).

References

Adams DR (1930) The nature of the ocular lesions produced experimentally by naphthalene. Br J Ophthalmol 14: 49–60

Anderson RS, Shearer TR, Claycomb CK (1986) Selenite-induced epithelial damage and cortical cataract. Curr Eye Res 5: 53–61

Arison RN, Ciaccio EL, Glitzer MS, Cassaro JA, Pruss MP (1967) Light and electron microscopy of lesions in rats rendered diabetic with streptozotocin. Diabetes 16: 51–56

Bagchi K (1959) The effects of methionine sulphoximine induced by methionine deficiency on the crystalline lens of albino rats. Indian J Med Res 47: 437–447

Bannon SL, Kaan HW (1939) Normal development of the lens in the albino rat and the effect of a diet high in galactose. Anat Rec [Suppl] 73: 59

Bannon SL, Higginbottom RM, McConnell JM, Kaan HW (1945) Development of galactose cataract in the albino rat embryo. Arch Ophthalmol 33: 224–228

Bellows JG (1944) Cataract and anomalies of the lens. Mosly, St Louis

Bellows JG (1963) Lens opacities produced by cataractogenic agents. Am J Ophthalmol 55: 537–541

Bettman JW, Fung WE, Nayes PP (1964) Potential action of prednisone on galactose cataracts in rats. Invest Ophthalmol 3: 678–679

Bettman JW, Fung WE, Webster RG, Nayes PP, Vincent NL (1968) Cataractogenic effect of corticosteroids on animals. Am J Ophthalmol 65: 581–586

Bhuyan KC, Bhuyan DK (1984) Molecular mechanism of cataractogenesis: III. Toxic metabolites of oxygen as initiators of lipid peroxidation and cataract. Curr Eye Res 3: 67–81

Bhuyan KC, Bhuyan DK, Podos DM (1981 a) Selenium-induced cataract; biochemical mechanisms. In: Spallholz JE, Martin JL, Ganther HE (eds) Proceedings of the 2nd international symposium on selenium in biological medicine. AV I, Westport, pp 403–412

Bhuyan KC, Bhuyan DK, Podos SM (1981 b) Cataract induced by selenium in the rat. I. Effect on the lenticular protein and thiols. IRCS Med Sci Eye 9: 194–195

Bihari M, Grossman BJ (1968) Posterior subcapsular cataracts related to long-term corticosteroid treatment in children. Am J Dis Child 116: 604–608

Black RL, Oglesby RB, von Sallmann L, Bunim JJ (1960 a) The occurrence of posterior subcapsular cataracts induced in patients with rheumatoid arthritis treated with corticosteroids. Arthritis Rheum 3: 432–433

Black RL, Oglesby RB, von Sallmann L, Bunim JJ (1960 b) Posterior subcapsular cataracts induced by corticosteroids in patients in rheumatoid arthritis. JAMA 174: 166–171

Bounds GW Jr., Janes RG, Leinfelder PJ (1955) Cataracts induced by alloxan diabetes in rats and rabbits. Arch Ophthalmol 54: 564–572

Braver DA, Richards RD, Good TA (1967) Posterior subcapsular cataracts in steroid treated children. Arch Ophthalmol 77: 161–162

Bruckner R, Hess R, Keberle H, Pericin C, Tripod J (1967) Tierexperimentelle pathologische Linsenveränderungen nach langdauernder Verabreichung hoher Dosen von Desferal Hely. Physiol Pharmacol Acta 25: 62–77

Bunce GE, Hess JL (1981) Biochemical changes associated with selenite-induced cataract in the rat. Exp Eye Res 33: 505–514

Bunce GE, Hess JL, Batra R (1984) Lens calcium and selenite-induced cataract. Curr Eye Res 3: 315–320

Charalampous FC, Hegsted DM (1950) Effect of age and diet on the development of cataracts in the diabetic rat. Am J Physiol 161: 540–544

Christenberry KW, Conklin JW, Upton AC, Costrove GE (1963) Induction of cataracts in mice by 4-(*p*-dimethyl-aminostyryl) quinoline. Arch Ophthalmol 70: 250–252

Cloud TM, Hakim R, Griffin AC (1960) Photosensitization of the eye with methoxsalen. I. Acute effects. AMA Arch Ophthalmol 64: 346–351

Cloud TM, Hakim R, Griffin AC (1961) Photosensitization of the eye with methoxsalen. II. Chronic effects. Arch Ophthalmol 66: 689–694

Conning DM, Fletcher K, Swan AAB (1969) Paraquat and related bipyridyls. Br Med Bull 25: 245–249

Cotlier E (1962) Hypophysectomy effect on lens epithelium mitosis and galactose cataract development in rats. Arch Ophthalmol 67: 476–482

Crews SJ (1963) Posterior subcapsular lens opacities in patients on long-term corticosteroid therapy. Br Med J I (5346): 1644–1647

Dasler W, Wang HLS (1972) Studies on cataracts induced in rats by N^2-phenyl-hydrazinopropionitrile. Invest Ophthalmol 11: 236–240

Dasler W, Wang HL, Norton TB, McCoy FD (1970) Cataractogenic and lathyrogenic effects of *N*-phenylhydrazinopropionitriles and related compounds in rats. Proc Soc Exp Biol Med 135: 1–5

David LL, Shearer TR (1984) Calcium-activated proteolysis in the lens nucleus during selenite cataractogenesis. Invest Ophthalmol Vis Sci 25: 1275–1283

Drenckhahn D (1978) Anterior polar cataract and lysosomal alterations in the lens of rats treated with the amphophilic lipidosis-inducing drugs chloroquine and chlorphentermine. Virchows Arch Cell Pathol 27: 255–266

Dvornik D, Simard-Duquesne N, Krami M, Sestanj K, Gabbay KH, Kinoshita JH, Varma SD, Merola LO (1973) Polyol accumulation in galactosemic and diabetic rats: control by an aldose reductase inhibitor. Science 182: 1146–1148

Edwards GA, Bernardino VB Jr, Babcock VI, Southam CM (1975) Cataract in bleomycin-treated rats. Am J Ophthalmol 80 (2): 538–542

El-Aguizy HK, Richards RD, Varma SD (1983) Sugar cataracts in Mongolian gerbil *(Meriones unguiculatus)*. Exp Eye Res 36: 839–844

Freeman RG (1966) Morphologic changes resulting from photosensitization of the eye with 8-methoxypsoralen – a comparison with conventional ultraviolet injury. Tex Rep Biol Med 24: 588–596

Gehring PJ (1971) The cataractogenic activity of chemical agents. CRC Crit Rev Toxicol 1: 93–118

Gorthy WC (1979) Developmental ocular abnormalities in rats with x-ray-induced cataract mutation. Invest Ophthalmol Vis Sci 18: 936–946

Grant WM (1974) Toxicology of the eye: drugs, chemicals, plants, venoms, 2nd edn. Thomas, Springfield, pp 766–767

Grimes P, Von Sallmann L (1966) Interference with cell proliferation and induction of polyploidy in rat lens epithelium during prolonged myleran treatment. Exp Cell Res 42: 265–273

Grimes P, Von Sallmann L, Frichette A (1964) Influence of myleran on cell proliferation in the lens epithelium. Invest Ophthalmol 3: 566–576

Hall EK (1953) Development anomalies in the eye of the rat after various experimental procedures. Anat Rec 116: 383–393

Hamming NA, Apple DJ, Goldberg MF (1976) Histopathology and ultrastructure of busulfan-induced cataract. Graefes Arch Clin Exp Ophthalmol 200: 139–147

Harris JE, Gruber L (1973) The reversal of triparanol-induced cataracts in the rat. III. Amino acid content and update of AC-AIB in cataractous and clearing lenses. Invest Ophthalmol 12: 385–388

Holmes JHC, Humphrey JD, Walton EA, O'Shea JD (1981) Cataratcs, goiter and infertility in cattle grazed on an exclusive diet of *Leucaena leucocephala*. Aust Vet J 57: 257–261

Howard CF Jr (1972) Streptozotocin-induced diabetes mellitus by direct pancreatic infusion in *Macaca nemestrina*. Diabetes 21: 138–142

Howard CF Jr, Peterson LH (1973) Cataract development in streptozotocin-diabetic monkeys *(Macaca nemestrina.)* Lab Anim Sci 23: 366–369

Ihimoto F, Iwata S (1978) Sulfhydryl contents of soluble and insoluble lens protein in naphthalene and traumatic cataracts in rabbits. Ophthalmol Res 10: 194–201

Janes RG, Bounds GW Jr, Leinfelder PJ (1952) Ocular complications in the rat made diabetic with alloxan. Arch Ophthalmol 48: 414–419

Kador PF, Zigler JS, Kinoshita JH (1979) Alterations of lens protein synthesis in galactosemic rats. Invest Ophthalmol Vis Sci 18: 696–702

Kandori F, Kurimoto S (1960) An experimental study on the chronic toxicity of myleran and its influence upon the lens, endocrine glands and internal organs of rats. Acta Pathol Jpn 10: 35–45

Keiding S, Mellemgaard L (1972) Dose dependence of galactose cataract in the rat. Acta Ophthalmol 50: 174–182

Kirby TJ (1967) Cataracts produced by triparanol. Trans Am Ophthalmol Soc 65: 493–543

Kirby TJ Jr, Achor RW, Perry HO, Winkelmann RK (1962) Cataract formation after triparanol therapy. Arch Ophthalmol 68: 486–489

Koch HR, Doldi K (1975) Proceedings: naphthalene cataracts in rats of differently pigmented strains. Exp Eye Res 20: 180

Koch HR, Beitzen R, Kremer F, Lerman S (1979) Effect of 8-methoxypsoralen and long UV on the rat lens. Invest Ophthalmol Vis Sci [Suppl] 18: 218

Koch HR, Ohrloff C, Bours J, Riemann G, Dragonmirescu V, Hockwin O (1982) Separation of lens proteins in rats with tryptophan deficiency cataracts. Exp Eye Res 34: 479–486

Kojima K, Majima Y, Niimi Kajima K (1972) Light and electron microscopic studies on ocular tissues in streptozotocin-treated diabetic rats. Nippon Ganka Gakkai Zasshi (Acta Soc Ophthalmol) 76: 1001–1016

Kok-Van Alphen CC, Cohen EM (1950) The occurrence of cataract in alloxan diabetic rats. Acta Physiol Pharmacol Neerl 1: 400–407

Korc I (1961) Biochemical studies on cataracts in galactose-fed rats. Arch Biochim Biophys 94: 196–200

Kuwabara T, Kinoshita JH, Cogan DG (1969) Electron microscopic study of galactose-induced cataract. Invest Ophthalmol 8: 133–149

Leonard A, Maisin JR (1965) Hereditary cataract induced by x-irradiation of young rats. Nature 205: 615–616

Lerman S, Devi A, Hawes S (1961) The incorporation of labelled amino acids into lens proteins of normal, galactose, and xylose-fed rats. Am J Ophthalmol 51: 1012–1017

Light AE (1967) Additional observations on the effects of busulfan on cataract formation, duration of anesthesia and reproduction in rats. Toxicol Appl Pharmacol 10: 459–466

Light AE, Solomon C, DeBeer EJ (1956) Effects of dietary supplements in preventing or augmenting the production of cataracts in rats by 1,4-dimethanesulfonoxy-butane. J Nutr 60: 157–172

MacDonald JS, Gerson RJ, Kornburst DJ, Kloss MW, Prahalada S, Berry PH, Alberts AW, Bokelman DL (1988) Preclinical evaluation of lovastatin. Am J Cardiol 62: 16_j–27_j

McAvoy JW, Palfrey LJ, van Heyningen R (1979) A light microscopic study of the lens of the tryptophan deficient rat. Exp Eye Res 28: 533–538

Mitchell HS, Cook GM (1938) Galactose cataract in rats. Factors influencing progressive and regressive changes. Arch Ophthalmol 19: 22–33

Ohrloff C, Stoffel C, Koch HR, Wefers U, Bours J, Hockwin O (1978) Experimental cataracts in rats due to tryptophan-free diet. Graefes Arch Clin Exp Ophthalmol 205: 73–79

Ostadalova I, Babicky A, Obenberger J (1978) Cataract induced by administration of a single dose of sodium selenite to suckling rats. Experientia 34: 222–223

Patterson RA, Heath H (1967) Chemical changes in human diabetic, cataractous and B,B-iminodipropionitrile-treated rat lens capsules. Exp Eye Res 6: 233–238

Pirie A (1968) Pathology in the eye of the naphthalene-fed rabbit. Exp Eye Res 7: 354–357

Pirie A, Rees JR (1970) Diquat cataract in the rat. Exp Eye Res 9: 198–203

Pirie A, Rees JR, Holmberg NJ (1970) Diquat cataract: formation of the free radical and its reaction with constituents of the eye. Exp Eye Res 9: 204–218

Rathbun WB, Harris JE, Vagstad G, Gruber L (1973) The reversal of triparanol-induced cataracts in the rat. IV. Reduced sulfyldryl groups in soluble protein and glutathione. Invest Ophthalmol 12: 388–390

Ribelin WE, Owen G, Rubin LF, Levinskas GJ, Agersborg HPK (1967) Development of cataracts in dogs and rats from prolonged feeding of sulfaethoxypyridazine. Toxicol Appl Pharmacol 10: 557–564

Rogoyski A, Trzcinska-Dabrowska Z (1969) Corticosteroid-induced cataract and palatoschisis in the mouse fetus. Am J Ophthalmol 68: 128–133

Russell NJ, Royland JE, McCawley EL, Shearer TR (1984) Ultrastructural study of selenite-induced nuclear cataracts. Invest Ophthalmol Vis Sci 15: 751–757

Sasaki K, Kuriyama H, Yeh LI, Fukuda M (1983) Studies on diabetic cataract in rats induced by streptozotocin I. Photodocumentation of lens opacification. Ophthalmic Res 15: 185–190

Scotti TM, Chernoff N, Linder R, McElroy WK (1981) Histopathologic lens changes in mirex-exposed rats. Toxicol Lett 9: 289–294

Segal S, Bernstein H (1963) Observations on cataract formation in the newborn offspring of rats fed a high-galactose diet. J Pediatr 62: 363–370

Shearer TR, Anderson RS (1985) Histologic changes during selenite cataractogenesis: a light microscopy study. Exp Eye Res 40: 557–565

Shearer TR, McCormack DW, De Sart DJ, Britton JL, Lopez MT (1980) Histological evaluation of selenium-induced cataracts. Exp Eye Res 31: 327–333

Shearer TR, Anderson RS, Britton JL (1982/83) Uptake and distribution of radioacitve selenium in cataractous rat. Curr Eye Res 2: 561–564

Shearer TR, Anderson RS, Britton JL (1983a) Influence of selenite and fourteen trace elements on cataractogenesis in the rat. Invest Ophthalmol Vis Sci 24: 417–423

Shearer TR, Anderson RS, Britton JL, Palmer EA (1983b) Early development of selenium-induced cataract: slit lamp evaluation. Exp Eye Res 36: 781–788

Singh S (1971) The teratogenicity of cyclophosphamide in rats. Indian J Med Res 58: 1128–1135

Singh S, Sanyal AK (1976) Eye anomalies induced by cyclophosphamide in fetuses. Acta Anat 94: 490–496
Sippel TO (1966) Energy metabolism in the lens during development of galactose cataract in rats. Invest Ophthalmol 5: 576–582
Solomon C, Light AE, De Beer EJ (1955) Cataracts produced in rats by 1,4-dimethanesulfonoxybutane (Myleran). Arch Ophthalmol 54: 850–852
Srivastava SK, Beutler E (1972) Galactose cataract in riboflavin deficient rats. Biochem Med Metab Biol 6: 372–379
Trotter JR, Day PL (1942) Cataract and other ocular changes resulting from tryptophane deficiency. J Nutr 24: 159–166
Unaker NJ, Genyea C, Reddan JR, Reddy VN (1978) Ultrastructural changes during the development and reversal of galactose cataracts. Exp Eye Res 26: 123–133
van Heyningen R (1976) Experimental studies on cataract. Am J Med Sci 272: 15: 685–697
van Heyningen R (1979) Naphthalene cataract in rats and rabbits: a resumé. Exp Eye Res 28: 435–439
van Heyningen R, Pirie A (1967) The metabolism of naphthalene and its toxic effect on the eye. Biochem J 102: 842–852
van Heyningen R, Pirie A (1976) Naphthalene cataract in pigmented and albino rabbits. Exp Eye Res 22: 393–394
Von Sallmann L (1957) The lens epithelium in the pathogenesis of cataract. Am J Ophthalmol 44: 159–170
Von Sallmann L (1965) Cytologic studies on lens epithelium. A comparison of effects of x-rays, Myleran, and TEM. Invest Ophthalmol 4: 471–479
Von Sallmann L, Grimes P (1971) Eye changes in streptozotocin diabetes in rats. Am J Ophthalmol 71: 312–319
Von Sallmann L, Grimes P, Collins E (1959a) Mimosine cataract. Am J Ophthalmol 47: 107–117
Von Sallmann L, Reid ME, Grimes PA, Collins EM (1959b) Tryptophan-deficiency cataract in guinea pigs. AMA Arch Ophthalmol 62: 662–672
Von Sallmann L, Grimes P, Collins E (1963a) Triparanol-induced cataract in rats. Trans Am Ophthalmol Soc 61: 49–58
Von Sallmann L, Grimes P, Collins E (1963b) Triparanol-induced cataract in rats. Arch Ophthalmol 70: 522–529
Weinstock M, Stewart HC (1961) Occurrence in rodents of reversible drug-induced opacities of the lens. Br J Ophthalmol 45: 408–414
White JH, Cinotti AA (1972) Streptozotocin-produced cataracts in rats. Invest Ophthalmol 11: 56–57
Wright HN (1963) Corneal and lenticular opacities in the eyes of rats following long-term administration of sulfonylurea derivatives. A preliminary report. Diabetes 12: 550–554
Wulf HC, Andreasen MP (1982) Concentration of 3H-8-methoxysoralen and its metabolites in the rat lens and eye after a single oral administration. Invest Ophthalmol Vis Sci 22: 32–36

Radiation-Induced Cataracts, Mouse and Rat

Robert L. Peiffer, Jr.

Synonyms. Radiation cataracts. The lens is susceptible to a broad range of radiant energy from diathermy (wavelength, 1010 nm), microwave and infrared sources through the visible spectrum to ultraviolet, and X-, and gamma-radiation; this discussion is limited to cataracts associated with exposure to X- and gamma-radiation (101–104 nm). Terminology should distinguish these cataracts from radiation-induced mutant strains with inherited cataracts.

Gross Appearance

Cataracts in general, including radiation cataracts, are difficult to diagnose grossly in fixed specimens due to inability to distinguish lesions from lens fixation artifact. With intumescent cataracts the lens will be swollen; with hypermature cataracts the lens will be shrunken with capsular wrinkling. Calcification and fibrous metaplasia will appear as localized white densities.

In general, all forms of ionizing radiation give rise to cataracts that are similar in appearance, both clinically (as viewed with the slit-lamp biomicroscope) and histologically.

Initially, radiation cataracts appear as fine dot-like subcapsular opacities in the anterior cortex, with granular and vacuolar subcapsular opacities in the posterior and equatorial cortex (Fig. 59). Increasing severity results in increased involvement of the peripheral posterior cortex, progressing to complete opacification (Fig. 60). Radiation applied to portions of the lens may result in localized opacification (Table 8).

Table 8. Clinical (slit-lamp) appearance of cataracts in Fischer rats exposed to divided doses of 333 rads three times a week from a ^{60}Co source. (From Pfeiffer et al. 1981)

	At 30 days after initial exposure		At about 120 days after initial exposure	
Group (exposure dose)	No. of eyes affected/ total No.	Changes (No. of eyes)	No. of eyes affected/ total No.	Changes (No. of eyes)
A (control)	0/20	None	0/20	None
B (2000 rads)	0/20	None	5/20	Anterior cortical vacuoles and/or granules (4) and radiating anterior cortical fiber opacities (1)
C (3000 rads)	13/20	Anterior cortical vacuoles and/or granules (9/–), equatorial vacuoles (1), and posterior cortical vacuoles (1)	20/20	Anterior cortical vacuoles and/or granules (13), equatorial vacuoles (5), and posterior cortical vacuoles (4)
D (4000 rads)	20/20	Anterior cortical vacuoles and/or granules (15), equatorial vacuoles (3), posterior cortical vacuoles (19), and cuneiform cortical opacity (1)	20/20	Anterior cortical vacuoles and/or granules (8), equatorial vacuoles (2), posterior cortical vacuoles (13), "snowflake" opacity of posterior capsule (2), clefting of posterior cortical fibers (1), and 1 in ear fiber opacities (2)
E (6000 rads)	20/20	Anterior cortical vacuoles and/or granules (2), posterior cortical vacuoles (5), anterior cortical clefting (3), diffuse mature cataracts (4)	20/20	Posterior cortical vacuoles (5), anterior cortical fiber opacities (3), diffuse nuclear opacity (14), and diffuse mature cataracts (4)

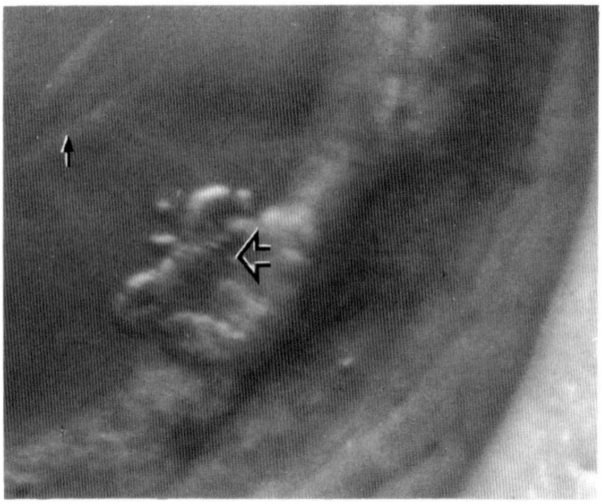

Fig. 59. Rat lens, 120 days after 4000 rads. A cluster of equatorial vacuoles *(open arrow)* and linear fiber opacities *(arrow)*. (From Peiffer 1981)

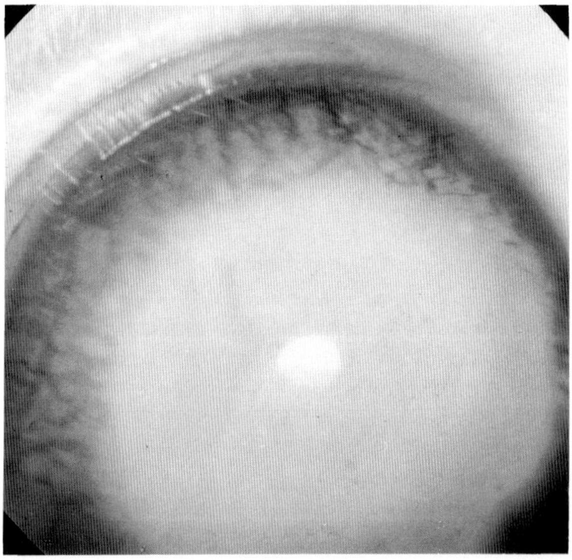

Fig. 60. Rat lens, 120 days following 6000 rads. A dense nuclear opacity and less dense cortical change are evident with clefting of the fibers along the anterior "Y" suture lines. (From Peiffer 1981)

Table 9. Histopathologic changes in eyes of Fischer rats exposed to divided doses of 333 rads three times a week from a ^{60}Co source. (From Pfeiffer et al. 1981)

Group (exposure dose)	No. of eyes	Mean postirradiation survival in days (range)	Histopathologic changes
A (control)	10		None
B (2000 rads)	10	182 (144–233)	Epithelial layer intact, lens bow migration of nuclei into cortex, small intercellular vacuoles anterior and at equator, and a few migratory subcapsular epithelial cells in anterior cortex
C (3000 rads)	10	173 (141–240)	Epithelial layer intact, lens bow migration of nuclei into cortex, small intercellular vacuoles anteriorly, intraccllular vacuoles posteriorly subcapsular, small focal areas of Morgagni's globules, and posterior and anterior subcapsular migration of epithelial cells into cortex
D (4000 rads)	10	166 (145–202)	Epithelial layer markedly reduced with foamy cells, pyknotic nuclei, karyolysis, occasional "bladder" cells at equator, marked liquefactive degeneration of cortex, numerous vacuoles at anterior equator, Morgagni's globules in subcapsular cortex, and subcapsular epithelium, bladder cells posteriorly
E (6000 rads)	16	143 (96–205)	Epithelium sparse and vacuolated, lens bow ranged from nearly acellular mass of liquefactive debris to focal areas of massive epithelial cell proliferation, large confluent areas of cortical vacuoles, reticular cortical debris, total cortical degeneration, sparse subcapsular epithelium posteriorly with areas of large clumps of bladder cells, mononuclear inflammatory cells lining anterior capsule in single layer – occasionally on posterior capsule – and posterior synechiae

Microscopic Features

In the rat, the earliest slit-lamp changes occur about 3 weeks following exposure to 440 rad X-ray and consist of narrow anterior cortical clefts and scattered opacities that follow the course of the subepithelial lens fibers; these changes are correlated with the swelling of the cortical fibers and the appearance of interfibrilliary spaces (Figs. 61–63). The second stage of posterior subcapsular opacities consists of lens epithelial cells that have failed to elongate and differentiate into normal lens fibers; as the lens grows, these cells are pushed to the posterior subcapsular region and swell to transform into bladder or Wedl cells. At about 4 weeks following irradiation, a rather well-circumscribed white granular opacity becomes apparent in the region of the posterior subcapsular lens suture and increases in size to cover the entire posterior pole of the lens. This lesion comprises swollen and ruptured lens fibers, cellular debris, and bladder cells. Fibrous metaplasia of lens epithelial cells may occur (Figs. 64, 65) (Friedenwald and Rytel 1955; Von Sallmann 1959; Evans et al. 1960; Pfeiffer et al. 1981) (Table 9).

Further progression is dependent on the reparative ability of the lens which is related to radiation exposure dose and age of the animal. Recovery with the formation of new healthy lens fibers will be accompanied by central condensation of the opaque area, which histologically will be surrounded by normal lens fibers. If the lens is unable to repair itself, progression to complete opacification can occur rapidly, as a result of alteration of osmotic balance and acute swelling of cortical fibers.

Ultrastructure

Following exposure of 4-week-old Columbia-Sherman rats to 2400 rad, lens epithelial cell nuclear membranes are disrupted and the nuclear shape is distorted 4.5 h postirradiation, followed by membrane breakdown and condensation of nucleoplasm (Broglio and Worgul 1982). In Sprague-Dawley rats exposed to 1500 rad X-rays, visualization of epithelial cells may be noted 3 days postirradiation, with subsequent progressive edema and shrinkage. Lens fibers are swollen and vacuolated (Figs. 66–69) (Palva and Palkama 1978).

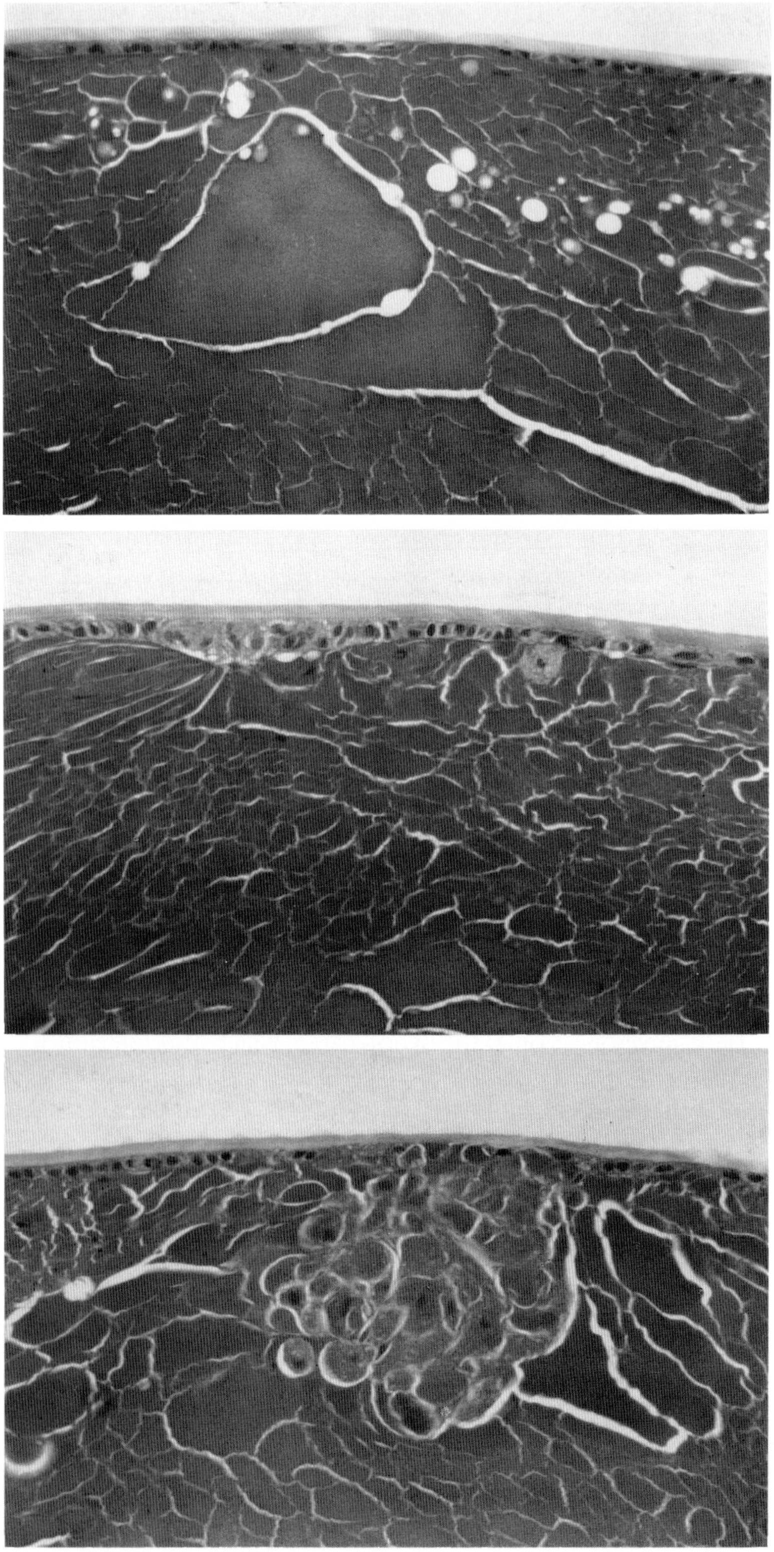

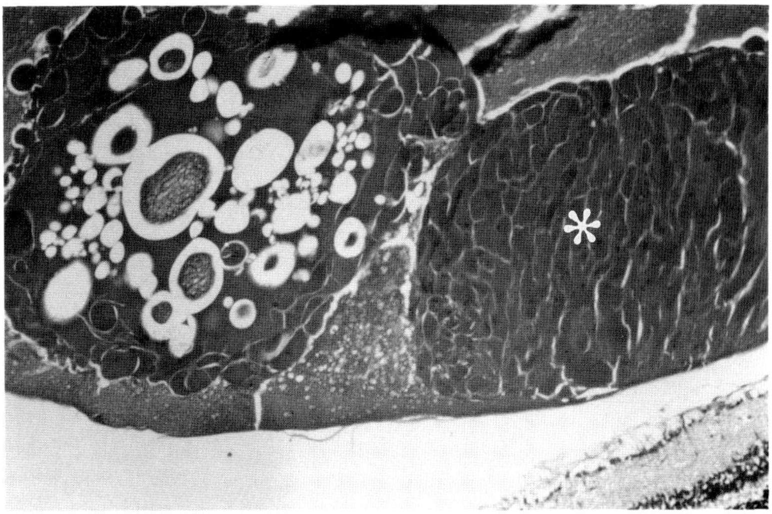

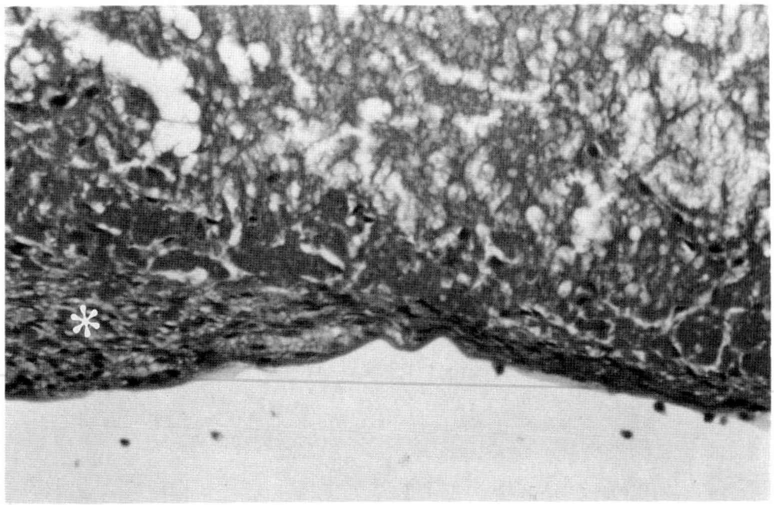

◂**Fig. 61** *(above)*. Rat lens, 141 days after 3000 rads. Anterior lenticular changes with sparse subcapsular epithelial cells (many with pyknotic nuclei), large intercellular vacuoles, and cortical degeneration with liquefaction. (From Peiffer et al. 1981) H & E, ×310

Fig. 62 *(middle)*. Rat lens, 233 days, 2000 rads. Anterior pole of lens, with minimal cataractous changes with disruption of the normal monolayer of the anterior subcapsular epithelium, enlarged foamy epithelial bladder cells, and disruption of the normal cortical architecture. (From Peiffer et al. 1981) H & E, ×310

Fig. 63 *(below)*. Rat lens, 145 days following 4000 rads. Anterior pole of lens with abnormal and typical focal area of epithelial proliferation resulting in foamy swollen bladder cells surrounded by degenerated cortex. (From Peiffer et al. 1981) H & E, ×310

Fig. 64 *(above)*. Rat lens, 116 days following 6000 rads. Posterior equatorial cataractous changes showing focal region of epithelial proliferation (*) adjacent to an area with a lacunar pattern of proteinaceous matrix containing moderate to large vacuoles filled with debris. (From Peiffer et al. 1981) H & E, ×310

Fig. 65 *(below)*. Rat lens, 114 days following 6000 rads. Focal posterior subcapsular epithelial cell fibrous metaplasia (*), showing totally liquefactive cortex with an intact posterior capsule and retrolental mononuclear inflammatory cells. (From Peiffer et al. 1981) H & E, ×310

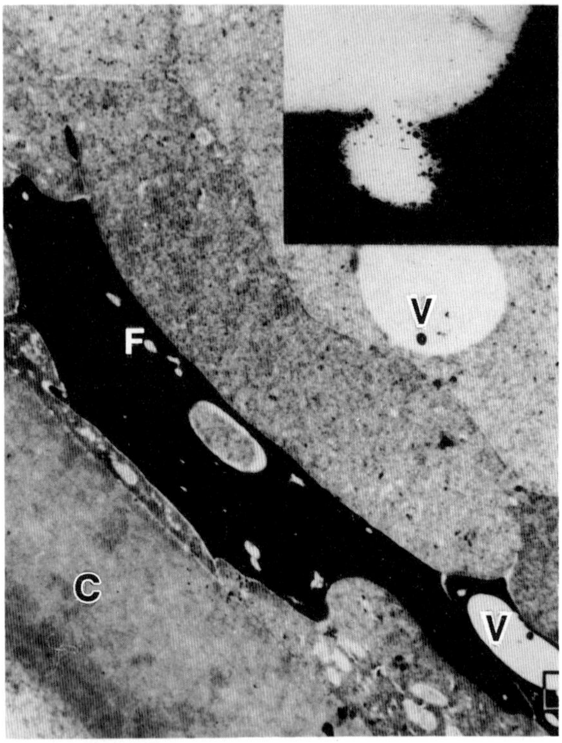

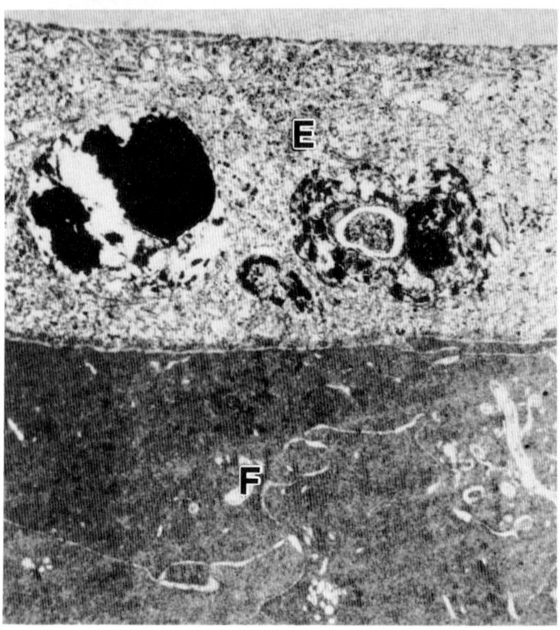

Fig. 66 *(upper left).* Rat lens, 7 days after 1500 rads. The posterior subcapsular region contains electron-dense fibers *(F)* and intracytoplasmic vacuoles *(V).* These seem to be formed by the coalescence of smaller vacuoles *(insert).* (From Palva and Palkama 1978) TEM, ×2850, *insert,* ×55350

Fig. 67 *(lower left).* Rat lens, 1 month following 1500 rads. At this stage occasional nuclei of the epithelial cells *(E)* have undergone severe degenerative changes. (From Palva and Palkama 1978) TEM, ×4600

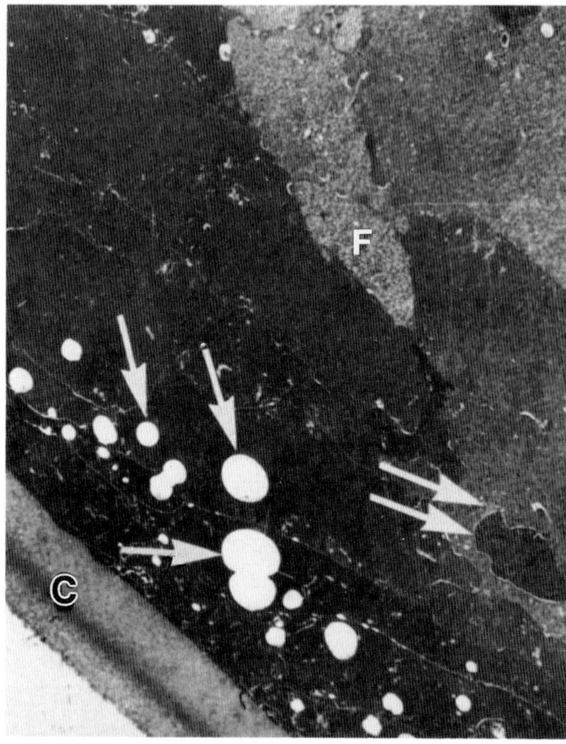

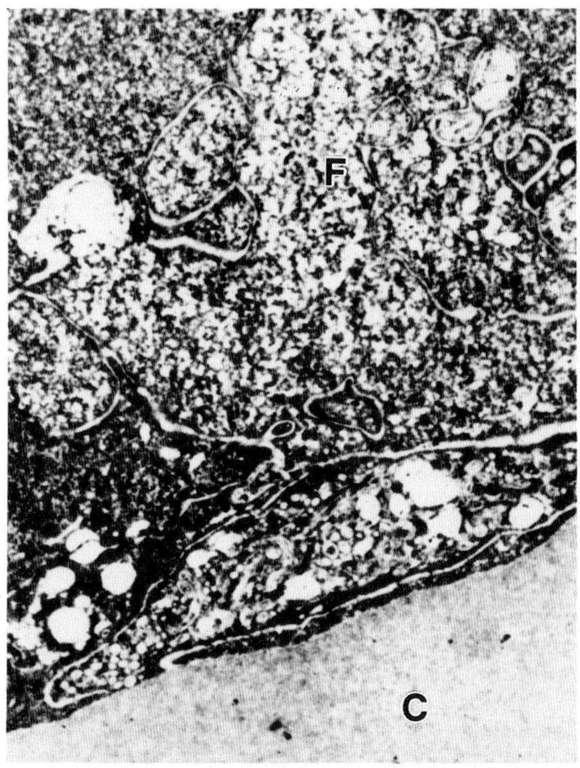

Fig. 68 *(upper right).* Rat lens, 2 months following 1500 rads. The lens fibers *(F)* below the intact posterior capsule *(C)* are arranged irregularly and are heavily deformed due to swelling. Intracytoplasmic vacuoles *(arrows)* are visible. At this stage a nucleus of "pseudoepithelium" *(double arrow)* can also be noted. (From Palva and Palkama 1978) TEM, ×4950

Vacuolization, hydration, and swelling of lens fibers with intracellular cysts and fiber disorganization were shown in RF mice at variable periods following exposure to 1000 r X-rays using scanning electron microscopy (Kodama et al. 1983), and similar techniques were utilized to study, from 12 h to 1 year postirradiation, lens fiber changes in young Columbia-Sherman albino rats exposed to 600–1800 r X-rays (Rini et al. 1986). In early stage and low dosage, damage was limited to the equatorial and posterior subcapsular regions. Cataracts in late stage, following high doses, were associated with clusters of 4- to 10-μm globules at the poles subcapsularly, massive disruption of the equatorial region, and formation of a granular matrix that extended to the posterior pole. Ultrastructural changes were also noted in the superficial cortical region, while the nucleus and remainder of the cortex were unchanged.

Differential Diagnosis

The histopathology of cataract is nonspecific, representing a common tissue response to a variety of insults. Clinical history, latency, location, and cytopathologic features may be suggestive but rarely diagnostic of a particular type of cataract.

Biologic Features

Natural History

Latency between exposure and appearance of cataract will vary depending on dose and age of the animal, with the younger and more actively growing lens being more susceptible to high levels of ionizing radiation. Depending on dose and reparative capabilities of the lens (greater in the young eye), the cataracts may or may not progress to total lens opacification (Merriam and Szechter 1973, 1975).

◂ **Fig. 69** *(lower right)*. Rat lens, 3 months after 1500 rads. At this stage the posterior lens fibers *(F)* are markedly destroyed. The fibers are heavily vacuolized and the intercellular spaces are dilated. The capsule *(C)* is still intact. (From Palva and Palkama 1978) TEM, ×4600

Etiopathogenesis

Minimal cataractogenic dose is dependent on the nature of the radiation, species, and method of exposure. Heavy-charged particles and neutrons have a greater effect when compared with X- and gamma-rays. Critical dose levels for man are about 200 rads for X- and gamma-rays and 75–80 rads for neutrons (Merriam et al. 1972). Dividing the doses increases threshold values for radiation cataractogenesis (Focht et al. 1966).

Radiation cataracts are the consequence of altered fibrogenesis with the epithelial cell, the primary cell of involvement. The anterior epithelium is divided into four regions, from axial to peripheral: central, germinative, pre-equatorial, and equatorial. The cells with the highest mitotic index and lowest turnover time are located in the germinative zone, and these cells are the initial as well as primary sites of radiation damage (Riley and Devi 1965). Microscopically apparent damage precedes the development of clinically visible changes by days or weeks, with mitotic arrest occurring within 30 min postirradiation and subsequent nuclear fragmentation, degeneration, and extrusion of chromatin material from these cells. Mitotic activity recovers after 4 days followed by a phase of abnormal mitoses and cytopathologic effects including vacuolated and multinucleated cells. Changes become evident in the lens fibers located in the nuclear bow region, with misalignment or displacement of the nuclei in this region, probably an expression of defective differentiation of epithelial cells into lens fibers (Von Sallmann 1950, 1951, 1952, 1957; Von Sallmann et al. 1955, 1957; Wanko et al. 1959). Radiation damage proceeds in two stages, with an initial direct effect on the DNA of lens epithelium and a second stage of lens fiber damage that may or may not be a delayed manifestation of the first. Exposure to radiation causes acute loss of integrity of the blood aqueous barrier (Worgul et al. 1977); however, this is likely insignificant in terms of radiation cataractogenesis. Biochemical changes that have been charted include progressive decrease in glutathione (Hockwin 1962b) related to both radiation-induced generation of free radicals and impaired glutathione synthesis (Pirie 1956). Permeability of cell membranes is altered (Von Sallmann and Locke 1951; Lambert and Kinoshita 1967), and changes in enzyme activity have been noted prior to the clinical appearance of radiation cataracts (Lerman 1965; Koch et al. 1976). It has been suggested that these and other biochemical processes that accompany irradiation of the lens (alterations in carbohydrate metabolism, increase in relative concentration of insoluble protein, and decrease in synthesis of soluble lens protein) (Pirie et al. 1953; Pirie 1956; Hockwin 1962a; Orekhovich et al. 1962; Lerman 1965; Liem-The et al. 1975; 1978; Giblin et al. 1978) are analogous to the aging process in this tissue. It would seem that these biochemical changes are most likely the result of ionizing radiation on lens nucleic acid components rather than of primary influence on cataract formation.

As with other tissues, there is an oxygen enhancement effect of radiation on the lens (Howard-Flanders and Pirie 1957); ligation of the carotid artery has a similar effect (Koch et al. 1974, 1977). A synergistic association between radiation and galactose (Hockwin et al. 1968) and naphthalene cataractogenesis has been demonstrated (Hockwin 1962b).

Frequency

Incidence is predictable, related to dose. In Table 8 it can be seen that all rats receiving 3000 rads or greater in divided doses develop cataracts 4 months following exposure.

Comparison with Other Species

The lens is perhaps the most radiosensitive tissue in the body; however, significant species variation exists in sensitivity of the lens to ionizing radiation. The latency period is longer in dogs and monkeys than in rabbits, mice, rats, guinea pigs, and cats (Upton et al. 1956). This is most likely related to species differences in lens mitotic activity (Von Sallmann 1957). The avian lens is extremely resistant, probably resulting from slow lens epithelial turnover at the lens pad and/or extremely slow fiber maturation (Pirie 1959; Hanna and O'Brien 1961; Hanna and Keatts 1966).

References

Broglio TM, Worgul BV (1982) The lens epithelium and radiation cataract. IV. Ultrastructural studies of interphase death in the meridional rows. Virchows Arch [Cell Pathol] 39: 49–57

Evans TC, Richards RD, Riley EF (1960) Histologic studies of neutron- and x-irradiated mouse lenses. Radiat Res 13: 737 –50

Focht EF, Merriam GR Jr, Schwartz M, Velasquez V, McNeill D (1966) A method of radiation cataract analysis and its uses in experimental fractionation studies. Radiology 87: 465–74

Friedenwald JS, Rytel D (1955) Contribution to the histopathology of cataract. Arch Ophthalmol 53: 825–31

Giblin FJ, Chakrapani B, Reddy VN (1978) High molecular weight protein aggregates in x-ray cataract. Exp Eye Res 26: 507–519

Hanna C, Keatts HC (1966) Chicken lens development: epithelial cell production and migration. Exp Eye Res 5: 111–115

Hanna C, O'Brien JE (1961) Cell production and migration in the epithelial layer of the lens. Arch Ophthalmol 66: 103–107

Hockwin O (1962a) Experimenteller Beitrag zur Wirkung von Röntgenstrahlen auf Stoffwechselabläufe der Augenlinse in Abhängigkeit vom Lebensalter. Fortschr Med 80: 659–666

Hockwin O (1962b) Early changes of lens metabolism after x-irradiation. Exp Eye Res 1: 422–426

Hockwin O, Bergeder HD, Kaiser L (1968) Über die Galactose-Katarakt junger Ratten nach Ganzkörper-Röntgenbestrahlung. Berl Dtsch Ophthalmol Ges 68: 135–139

Howard-Flanders P, Pirie A (1957) The effect of breathing oxygen on the radiosensitivity of the rabbit lens and the use of oxygen in x-ray therapy. Radiat Res 7: 357–364

Koch HR, Kremer F, Linner E, Hockwin O, Kaufmann H, Breuli W, Dahners HW (1974) On the influence of a monolateral carotid ligation upon the formation of radiation cataracts in rats. Ophthalmic Res 6: 175–182

Koch HR, Hockwin O, Kremer F (1976) Changes of several enzyme activities in the course of x-ray cataract development in rats. Exp Eye Res 22: 294

Koch HR, Kremer F, Hockwin O, Kaufmann H (1977) Formation of radiation cataracts in rats after monolateral carotid ligature. Biochemical results. Ophthalmic Res 9: 31–37

Kodama T, Reddy VN, Giblin F, Kinoshita JH, Harding C (1983) Scanning electron microscopy of x-ray induced cataract in mice on normal and galactose diet. Ophthalmic Res 15: 324–333

Lambert BW, Kinoshjta JH (1967) The effects of ionizing irradiation of lens cation permeability, transport and hydration. Invest Ophthalmol 6: 624–633

Lerman S (1965) Metabolic pathways in experimental sugar and radiation cataract. Physiol Rev 45: 98–122

Liem-The KN, Stols AL, Jap PH, Hoenders HJ (1975) X-ray induced cataract in rabbit lens. Exp Eye Res 20: 317–328

Liem-The KN, Ringens PJ, Holtslag JC, Hoenders HJ (1978) Changes in the proportion and composition of structural proteins during the development of x-ray cataract in rabbit lens. In: Hockwin O (ed) Lens ageing and development of senile cataracts. Karger, Basel

Merriam GR, Szechter A (1973) The effect of age on the radiosensitivity of rat lenses. Trans Am Ophthalmol Soc 71: 88–110

Merriam GR, Szechter A (1975) The relative radiosensitivity of rat lenses as a function of age. Radiat Res 62: 488–497

Merriam GR Jr, Szechter A, Focht EF (1972) The effects of ionizing radiation on the eye. Radiat Ther Oncol 6: 346–362

Orekhovich VN, Firfarova KF, Kedrova EM, Levdikova GA (1962) Studies of lens proteins in x-ray cataracts. Exp Eye Res 1: 324–329

Palva M, Palkama A (1978) Ultrastructural lens changes in x-ray induced cataract of the rat. Acta Ophthalmol 56: 587–598

Pfeiffer RL, Wright W, Steinbok P, Mahaley MS (1981) Long-term study of the ocular effects of orthovoltage irradiation in rats. Am J Vet Res 42: 1598–1605

Pirie A (1956) Biochemical changes in radiation cataract. Trans Ophthalmol Soc UK 76: 461–475

Pirie A (1959) The effects of x-radiation of the lens of the embryo and the adult hen. Radiat Res 11: 260–270

Pirie A, Van Heyningen R, Boag JW (1953) Changes in lens during the formation of x-ray cataracts in rabbits. Biochem J 54: 682–688

Riley EF, Devi SK (1965) Characteristics of cell populations in the rat lens epithelium after x-irradiation of half or all of the eye. Radiat Res 25: 232–233 (abstract)

Rini FJ, Worgul BV, Merriam GR Jr (1986) Radiation cataractogenesis in rat lenses. Bull NY Acad Med 62: 744–753

Upton AC, Christenberry KW, Melville GS, Furth J, Hurst GS (1956) The relative biological effectiveness of neutrons, x-rays, and gamma rays for the production of lens opacities. Observations on mice, rats, guinea-pigs and rabbits. Radiology 67: 686–696

Von Sallmann L (1950) Experimental studies on early lens changes after x-ray irradiation. Trans Am Ophthalmol Soc 48: 228–242

Von Sallmann L (1951) Experimental studies on early lens changes after roentgen irradiation. I: morphological and cytochemical changes. Arch Ophthalmol 45: 149–164

Von Sallmann L (1952) Experimental studies on early lens changes after roentgen irradiation. III. Effect of x-radiation on mitotic activity and nuclear fragmentation of lens epithelium in normal and cysteine treated rabbits. Arch Ophthalmol 47: 305–320

Von Sallmann L (1957) The lens epithelium in the pathogenesis of cataract. Am J Ophthalmol 44: 159–170

Von Sallmann L (1959) Symposium: ocular effects of ionizing radiation and radiotherapy. Early lenticular lesions resulting from ionizing radiation. Trans Am Acad Ophthalmol 63: 439–448

Von Sallmann L, Locke BD (1951) Experimental studies on early lens changes after roentgen irradiation. II. Exchange and penetration of radioactive indicators (Na 24, K 42, I 131, P 32) in normal and irradiated lenses of rabbits. Arch Ophthalmol 45: 431–444

Von Sallmann L, Tobias CA, Anger HO, Welch C, Kimura SF, Munoz CM, Drungis A (1955) Effects of high energy particles, x-rays, and aging on lens epithelium. Arch Ophthalmol 54: 489–514

Von Sallmann L, Caravaggio L, Munoz CM, Drungis A (1957) Species differences in the radiosensitivity of the lens. Am J Ophthalmol 43: 693–704

Wanko T, Von Sallmann L, Gavin MA (1959) Early changes in the lens epithelium after roentgen irradiation. Arch Ophthalmol 62: 977–984

Worgul BV, Bito LZ, Merriam GR Jr (1977) Intraocular inflammation produced by x-irradiation of the rabbit eye. Exp Eye Res 25: 53–61

Light-Induced Retinal Degeneration, Rat

Robert L. Peiffer, Jr. and Dean P. Porter

Gross Appearance

This condition has not been well described in terms of gross appearance; generally, the process diffusely involves the fundus with retinal thinning with or without alteration of the underlying retinal pigment epithelium (more obvious in pigmented animals) and as such will appear as total or geographic areas of change in intensity of coloration.

Microscopic Features

Light microscopic findings vary with the severity of retinal damage, which in turn is related to variables of light exposure. O'Steen and Lytle (1971) performed a study in which albino rats were exposed to 18 ftc (1.67 lx) of continuous light at 25°C for periods of 20 h to 16 days. The first change, noted at 28 h, was a stratified appearance of the photoreceptor outer segments, with a dark inner band and an outer lighter band. After several days, phagocytes were seen within the fragmented photoreceptor layer and the outer plexiform layer. Subsequently, pyknosis of the photoreceptor nuclei occurred and the outer plexiform layer narrowed. Maximal effects were noted at 16 days of exposure, when the photoreceptor and outer plexiform layers had disappeared, with few photoreceptor nuclei remaining. No changes were noted in inner retinal layers, although discontinuity of the retinal pigment epithelium occurred after 4 days (Figs. 70–72).

With increased illumination and elevated body temperature, Noell et al. (1966) noted similar changes over 4–48 h, as well as damage to the retinal pigment epithelium; at 4 h this epithelium was swollen, with increased nuclear size. After ½ day, the nuclei had vanished, with subsequent disappearance of the cells.

In a study over 4–6 months, nuclei of bipolar cells were displaced from the outer nuclear layer to the inner ganglion layer along retinal blood vessels (O'Steen et al. 1972).

Ultrastructure

Kuwabara and Gorn (1968) exposed albino rats to 750 ft c (69.58 lx) of continuous light at room temperature from 1 h to several weeks. Photoreceptor changes noted within 24 h included swelling and disruption of the lamellae, with disk membrane thinning, separation, and formation of tubules and vesicles. Pyknosis of photoreceptor nuclei was observed. Within ½ week, the outer segments transformed into large round or pear-shaped bodies; the swollen outer segments separated from the photoreceptor inner segments and were broken into smaller fragments. Atrophic changes of the photoreceptor nuclei were seen. The microvilli of the retinal pigmented epithelium (which began to contact Müller cell microvilli) became elongated and the epithelial cells were increased in height. Glial cells contained lysosomes and cellular debris. After ½ week, disappearance of photoreceptors was noted. The microvilli of the retinal pigment epithelium and Müller cells interdigitated and adhered to each other. This process continued over a period of ½ month (Fig. 73).

Other studies have identified different patterns of degeneration. Grignolo et al. (1969) exposed albino rats to 1500–2000 lux at 38°–39°C for periods of 8–100 h; in contrast to Kuwabara (1970), they noticed complete degeneration of the retinal pigment epithelium at 80–100 h.

Hansson (1970) exposed albino rats at 39°C to "intense" light for two 30-min periods separated by 2 h of darkness. The first structural change noted was an increase in space between the basal processes of the retinal pigment epithelium and Bruch's membrane, as well as vesicula-

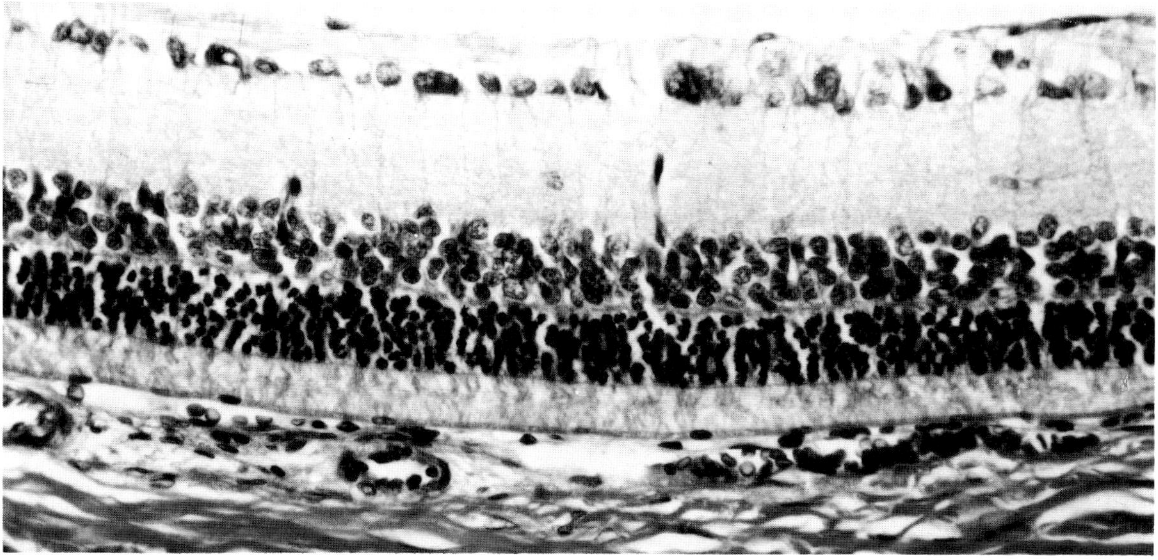

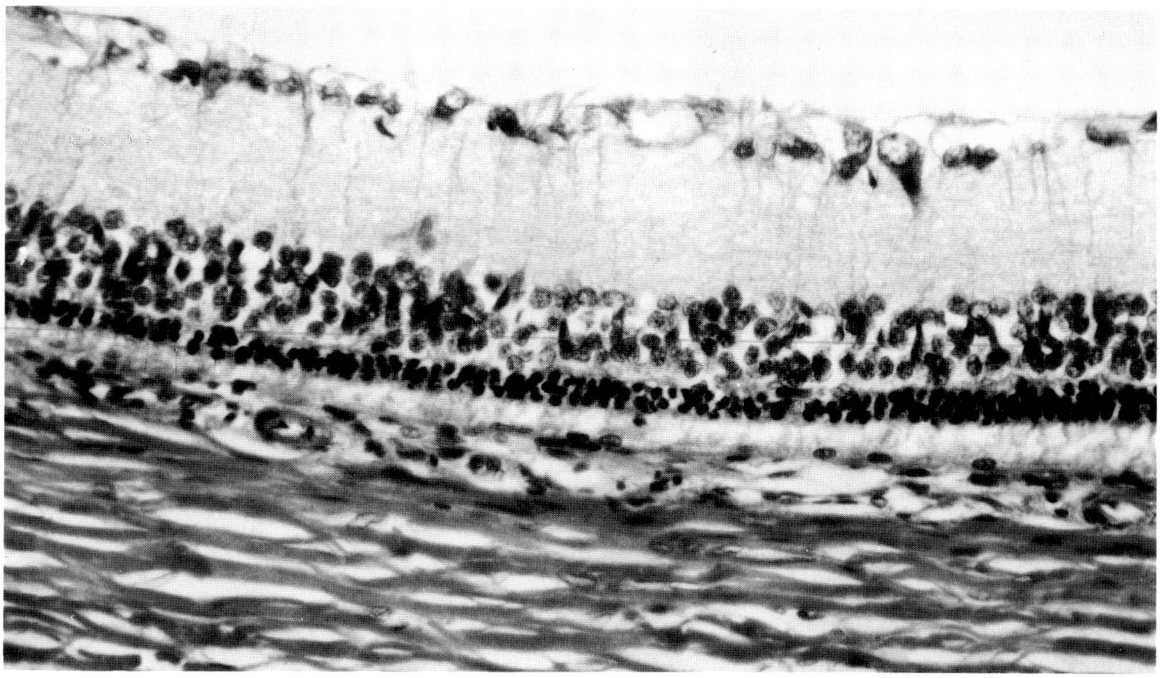

Fig. 70 *(above).* Mild light-induced retinal degeneration in an albino rat exposed to a fluorescent source. The outer plexiform and outer nuclear layers of the central retina are thinner than normal. (From Saunders 1975)

Fig. 71 *(below).* Moderate light-induced retinal degeneration in an albino rat. The outer plexiform layer is thinned, the inner nuclear layer is reduced to two to three nuclei in thickness, and the outer segments are compressed and disorganized. The RPE is unaffected. (From Saunders 1975)

tion of the smooth endoplasmic reticulum and increase in number of lysosomes in the cells of the retinal pigmented epithelium. Complete disintegration of the epithelial cells occurred within 3 days. One other difference was a proliferation of Müller cells, which segregated the damaged outer half of the retina from the undamaged inner half. A study by O'Steen et al. (1972) in which albino rats were exposed for 4–6 months was remarkable because of the extension of bipolar cells through the inner plexiform layer to the ganglion cell layer.

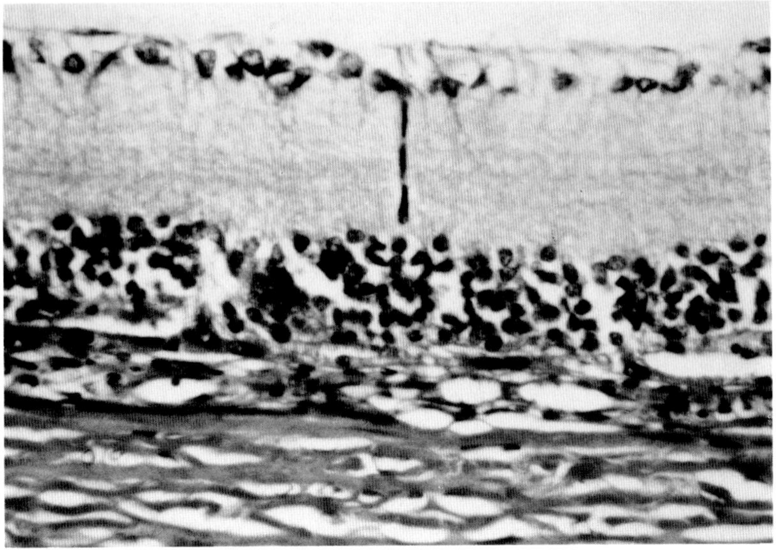

▲ **Fig. 72.** Advanced light-induced retinal degeneration in albino rat. The photoreceptors have disappeared entirely and there is pyknosis of inner nuclear layer nuclei. RPE is preserved but appears discontinuous. (From Saunders 1975)

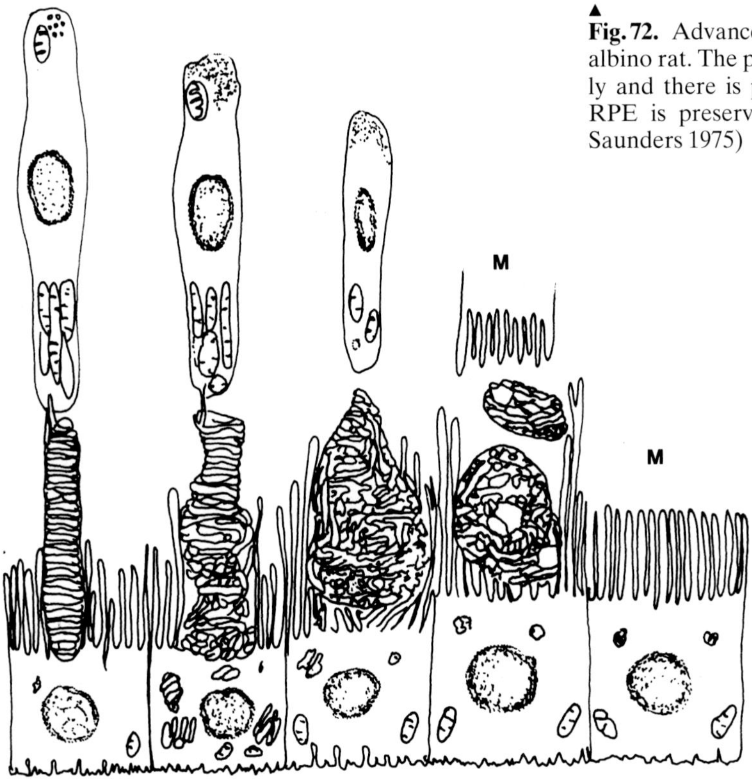

Fig. 73. A typical course of retinal damage by light exposure is shown schematically. With a 3-h exposure, only the outermost tip of the photoreceptor contains vacuoles. At 24 h, the photoreceptor outer segment is tortuous and swollen. Myelin membranes separate from each other and form vesicular and tubular structures, and the synaptic end of the photoreceptor undergoes pathologic changes. Pigment epithelium has a conspicuous increase in myeloid bodies. At 3–5 days, damaged outer segment is isolated from inner segment and becomes a large round or pear-shaped body filled with tubular material, followed by cellular degeneration at 2–3 weeks with complete adhesion of pigment epithelium and Müller cells *(M)* in 1 month. (Kuwabara and Gorn 1968)

Differential Diagnosis

Light-induced retinal damage must be differentiated from several conditions. In a study by Dowling et al. (1961), chronic vitamin A deficiency presented many of the same changes noted with light-induced retinal degeneration. These were first noted at 2 months when swelling and fragmentation of the photoreceptor outer segment occurred with vesicle and tubule formation. The outer segments eventually disappeared. The inner segments and nuclei were depleted in number by 50% at 6 months. At 10 months, only a single row of photoreceptor nuclei remained. Other layers of the retina remained healthy. These changes occurred over a greater period than required for light-induced damage and were reversible by administration of vitamin A, administration as long as the inner segments and nuclei were present. Regeneration was complete in 14 days.

Inherited retinal dystrophy of rats is also characterized by retinal degeneration. Initial changes occur at several weeks (Dowling and Sidman 1962) to 12 months of age (Frank and Mancini 1986) depending on the strain. Dowling and Sidman (1962) described an initial accumulation of extracellular lamellar material between the photoreceptor outer segments and retinal pigment epithelium. Degeneration of the photoreceptor subsequently occurred, and, by 60 days of age, inner segments and photoreceptor nuclei had disappeared entirely. The outer segment and extracellular material was gradually absorbed over 6 months or more. Changes in retinal pigment epithelium occurred after 40 days with separation and migration into the inner retinal layers. Rats in the dark underwent slower degeneration, but arrest of the process was not possible.

Other mechanisms of retinal degeneration have been noted in mammalian species. These include X-irradiation (Noell 1962), hyperoxia (Noell 1962), iodate, and iodoacetate (Noell 1955).

Biologic Features

Natural History

The natural history of light-induced retinal degeneration parallels microscopic findings. In general, early effects are noticed within several days as the photoreceptor outer segments lose their lamellar structure, separate from the photoreceptor inner segments, and eventually disappear. Concomitantly, the inner segments shrink and the nuclei become pyknotic. Over a period of days to weeks the photoreceptors vanish completely. The response of the retinal pigment epithelium is variable, in both extent and relative time course of injury. Disappearance of the epithelium has been noted at high light intensities and with elevated body temperature (Noell et al. 1966; Grignolo et al. 1969; Hansson 1970). Hansson (1970) observed changes in the retinal pigment epithelium to be the first evident in the retina, but other observers noticed changes accompanying or following damage to the photoreceptor cells (Noell et al. 1966; Grignolo et al. 1969).

The reversibility of damage to the retina depends on the extent of damage. Kuwabara (1970) investigated recovery in rats exposed to fluorescent or incandescent light. Recovery was observed in both treatments, and was closely related to photoreceptor and pigment epithelial damage. Mild damage was reversed including thinning and separation of the photoreceptor outer segment lamellae as well as inclusion bodies and edema in the retinal pigmented epithelium following incandescent exposure. Recovery started in the retinal pigmented epithelium at 2 days postexposure, with return to normal morphology by 5 days. The outer segments recovered more slowly, with structural irregularities still visible at 1 month despite a return of normal electroretinogram recordings at 10 days. Moderate damage, consisting of outer segment lamellar degeneration as well as vacuolization of cells in the pigmented epithelium and damage to microorganelles, was similarly reversible. Recovery started in the retinal pigment epithelium with a return to normal appearance within 1 week. Recovery of the outer segments was slow, with new lamellae formation, but the irregular appearance continued even after several months. Recovery in the electroretinogram was noted in 6–8 weeks. No morphologic or functional recovery was noted after advanced damage, characterized by loss of photoreceptor cells or retinal pigment epithelium.

Etiopathogenesis

Mechanisms of retinal damage produced by light remain speculative. Damage is produced independent of thermal means, and is associated with the effect of light on rhodopsin (Noell 1980). Noell (1980) has proposed that there are two types of light damage, primarily differing in whether there is damage to the retinal pigment epithelium. Several mechanisms have been hypothesized, including photooxidation, induced membranolysis of the retina, and rhodopsin-mediated physiologic responses (Noell 1980).

Frequency

The frequency of light-induced damage is not well documented; however, Kuwabara and Gorn (1968) studied 300 rats and noted that all exposed animals exhibited some effects. These varied in accordance with age (younger animals with less damage) and location in the retina (posterior retina more susceptible to damage than the anterior retina). Several variables influence the extent of retinal degeneration. Increasing intensity of light has been shown to increase retinal damage (Noell et al. 1966). The rate, extent, and involvement of retinal pigment epithelium in the degenerative process are all greater with increasing light intensity (Noell et al. 1966). The location within the retina may vary, the superior hemisphere being most sensitive (Rapp and Williams 1980). Duration of exposure is linked to retinal degeneration (Noell et al. 1966) in a nonlinear manner (Lawwill 1973). Degeneration is dependent on wavelength, the most damaging wavelengths being those that cause efficient bleaching of rhodopsin (Noell et al. 1966; Williams and Howell 1983). Elevated body temperature (Noell et al. 1966), aging (O'Steen et al. 1974), lack of eye pigmentation (Rapp and Williams 1980; LaVail 1980), decreased prior daily light exposure ("light history") (Penn et al. 1985; Noell 1979), and changes in the light/dark cycle length (Noell et al. 1966; O'Steen 1970) have been associated with increased retinal damage. Removal of the pituitary (O'Steen and Kraeer 1977), ovary (O'Steen 1977), and pineal gland (O'Steen 1980) have all been associated with decreased susceptibility to light-induced damage. Vitamin A deficiency is also decreased in severity by obliteration of these organs (Noell 1979). Strain differences noted in respect to susceptibility to light-induced retinal degeneration suggest a genetic factor (LaVail et al. 1987; O'Steen and Donnelly 1982).

Comparison with Other Species

Light damage has been extensively studied in the rat, and has been noticed in other species as well. Pigeons (Marshall et al. 1972), rabbits (Lawwill 1973), hamsters (Noell and Albrecht 1971), and monkeys have all been used in studies involving constant light exposure. Fish are also susceptible (B.P. Wilcock 1988, personal communication). As the rat retina is predominantly composed of rods (Noell 1980), other animals have been used to study degeneration of cones. Rats have the advantage of a low threshold for light-induced damage relative to many other species (Noell and Albrecht 1971; Lawwill 1973).

The pattern of light-induced degeneration in mice proceeds differently than in the rat, without formation of large, membranous outer segment packets and with relatively rapid outer segment degeneration (LaVail et al. 1987).

Knowledge of human light-induced retinal degeneration is largely based on indirect evidence. Several studies have documented temporary elevation of dark adaptation threshold (Clark et al. 1946; Hecht et al. 1948; Dawson and Herron 1970). Radnot et al. (1969) have demonstrated ultrastructural changes in photoreceptor in rods and cones following exposure to incandescent light. These changes are similar to those observed in animals.

References

Clark B, Johnson ML, Dreher RE (1946) The effect of sunlight on dark adaptation. Am J Ophthalmol 29: 828–836

Dawson WW, Herron WL (1970) Retinal illumination during indirect ophthalmoscopy: subsequent dark adaptation. Invest Ophthalmol Vis Sci 9: 89–96

Dowling JE, Sidman RL (1962) Inherited retinal dystrophy in the rat. J Cell Biol 14: 73–109

Dowling JE, Gibbons IR, Smelser GK (1961) The effect of vitamin A deficiency on the fine structure of the retina. In: Smelser GK (ed) The structure of the eye. Academic, New York, pp 85–99

Frank RN, Mancini MA (1986) Presumed retinovitreal neovascularization in dystrophic retinas of spontaneously hypertensive rats. Invest Ophthalmol Vis Sci 27: 346–355

Grignolo A, Orzalesi N, Castellazzo R, Vittone P (1969) Retinal damage by visible light in albino rats: an electron microscope study. Ophthalmologica 157: 43–59

Hansson HA (1970) Ultrastructural studies on rat retina damaged by visible light. Virchows Arch [B] 6: 247–262

Hecht S, Hendley CD, Ross S, Richmond PN (1948) The effect of exposure to sunlight on night vision. Am J Ophthalmol 31: 1573–1580
Kuwabara T (1970) Retinal recovery from exposure to light. Am J Ophthalmol 70: 187–198
Kuwabara T, Gorn RA (1968) Retinal damage by visible light: an electron microscope study. Arch Ophthalmol 79: 69–78
Lawwill T (1973) Effects of prolonged exposure of rabbit retina to low intensity light. Invest Ophthalmol Vis Sci 12: 45–51
LaVail MM (1980) Eye pigmentation and constant light damage in the rat retina. In: Williams TP, Baker BN (eds) The effects of constant light on visual processes. Plenum, New York, pp 357–387
LaVail MM, Gorrin GM, Repaci MA, Yasumura D (1987) Light induced retinal degeneration in albino mice and rats: strain and species differences. In: Prog Clin Biol Res 247: 439–454
Marshall J, Mellerio J, Palmer DA (1972) Damage to pigeon retinae by moderate illumination from fluorescent lamps. Exp Eye Res 14: 164–169
Noell WK (1955) Metabolic injuries of the visual cell. Am J Ophthalmol 40: 60–68
Noell WK (1962) X-irradiation studies on mammalian retina. In: Haley TJ, Snider RS (eds) Response of the nervous system to ionizing radiation. Academic, New York, pp 543–559
Noell WK (1979) Effects of environmental lighting and dietary vitamin A on the vulnerability of the retina to light damage. Photochem Photobiol 29: 717–723
Noell WK (1980) Possible mechanisms of photoreceptor damage by light in mammalian eyes. Vision Res 20: 1163–1171
Noell WK, Albrecht R (1971) Irreversible effects of visible light on the retina: role of vitamin A. Science 172: 76–80
Noell WK, Walker VS, Kang BS, Berman S (1966) Retinal damage by light in rats. Invest Ophthalmol Vis Sci 5: 450–473
O'Steen WK (1970) Retinal and optic nerve serotonin and retinal degeneration as influenced by photoperiod. Exp Neurol 27: 194–205
O'Steen WK (1977) Ovarian steroid effects on light induced retinal photoreceptor damage. Exp Eye Res 25: 361–369
O'Steen WK (1980) Hormonal influences on retinal photodamage. In: Williams TP, Baker BN (eds) The effects of constant light on visual processes. Plenum, New York, p 29
O'Steen WK, Donnelly JE (1982) Chronologic analysis of variations in retinal damage in two strains of rats after short-term illumination. Invest Ophthalmol Vis Sci 22: 252–255
O'Steen WK, Kraeer SL (1977) Effects of hypophysectomy, pituitary gland homogenates and transplants, and prolactin on photoreceptor destruction. Invest Ophthalmol Vis Sci 16: 940
O'Steen WK, Lytle RB (1971) Early cellular disruption and phagocytosis in photically-induced retinal degeneration. Am J Anat 130: 227–234
O'Steen WK, Shear CR, Anderson KV (1972) Retinal damage after prolonged exposure to visible light: a light and electron microscope study. Am J Anat 139: 5–22
O'Steen WK, Anderson KV, Shear CR (1974) Photoreceptor degeneration in albino rats: dependency on age. Invest Ophthalmol Vis Sci 13: 334–339
Penn JS, Howard AG, Williams TP (1985) Light damage as a function of "light history" in the albino rat. In: LaVail MM, Hollyfield JG, Anderson RE (eds) Retinal degeneration: experimental and clinical studies. Liss, New York, pp 439–447
Radnot M, Jabbágy P, Heszberger I, Lovas B (1969) Les donées à l'ultrastructure de la rétine humanine sous l'effet de la lumière. Ophthalmologica 159: 460–471
Rapp LM, Williams TP (1980) A parametric study of retinal light damage in albino and pigmented rats. In: Williams TP, Baker BN (eds) The effects of constant light on visual processes. Plenum, New York, pp 135–159
Saunders LZ (1975) Ophthalmic pathology of animals. Karger, Basel
Williams TP, Howell WL (1983) Action spectrum of retinal light damage in albino rats. Invest Ophthalmol Vis Sci 24: 285–287

Lipidosis of the Retina Due to Cationic Amphiphilic Drugs, Rat

Renate Lüllman-Rauch

Synonyms. Drug-induced retinal lipidosis, drug-induced lysosomal storage of polar lipids resulting from impaired degradation.

Gross Appearance

Drug-induced lipidosis in the retina of rats is not recognizable by the naked eye.

Microscopic Features

The unequivocal diagnosis of this lysosomal storage disease can be made on the basis of ultrastructural observations only. Paraffin sections are entirely unsuitable; the light microscopic examination of semithin plastic sections (Figs. 74, 75) from glutaraldehyde-fixed, osmicated tissues may yield indirect indications of

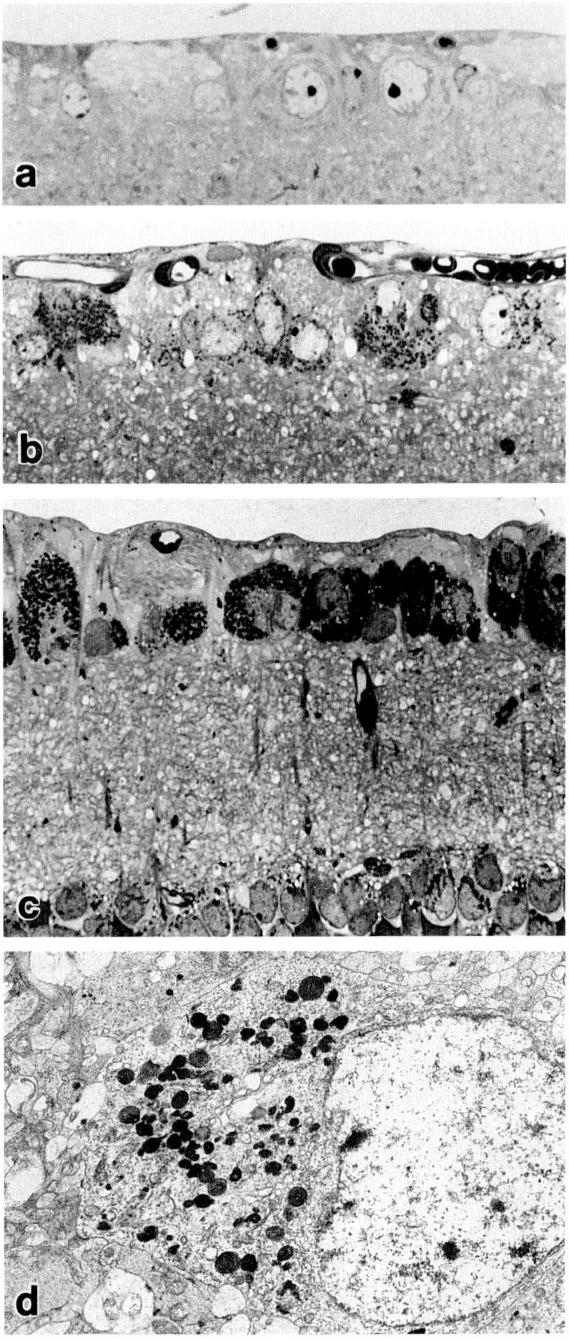

Fig. 74a–d. Drug-induced lipidosis in retinal ganglion cells, rat. **a** Untreated control; **b, d** chlorphentermine, 60 mg/kg per os, 4 weeks; **c** chloroquine 75 mg/kg per os, 13 weeks. Dense cytoplasmic inclusions are seen in the ganglion cells of the drug-treated rats. **a–c** are semithin plastic sections (1 μm) stained with alkaline toluidine blue, ×560. **d** TEM, ×3600

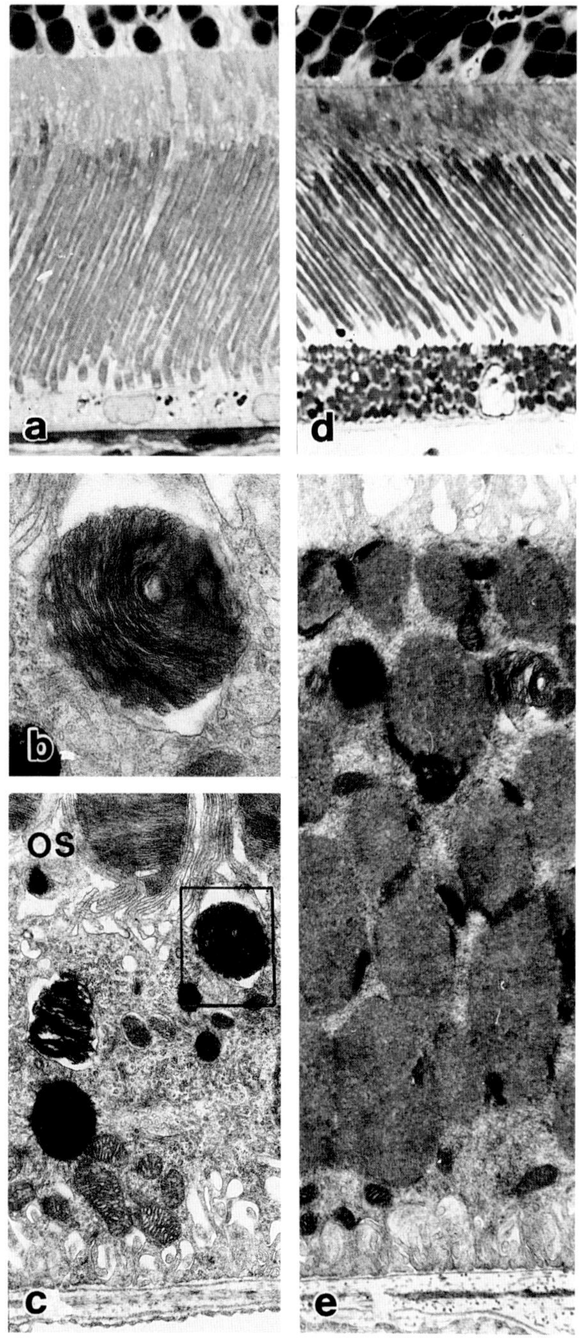

Fig. 75a–e. Drug-induced lipidosis in retinal pigment epithelium, rat. **a–c** Untreated control; **d, e** 1-chloroamitriptyline 120 mg/kg per os, 10 weeks. The epithelial cells of the drug-treated rat contain numerous cytoplasmic inclusions and are increased in height. In the epithelium of the control rat, partially degraded fragments of rod outer segments are seen, one of which is shown at higher magnification in **b**. *OS*, rod outer segment. **a, d** semithin sections, ×900. **c, e** TEM ×10000; **b** TEM ×25000

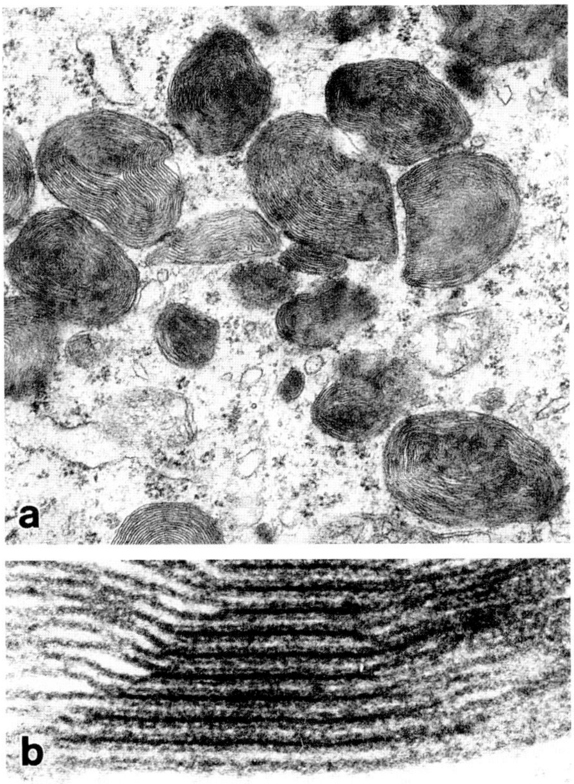

Fig. 76 a, b. Drug-induced lipidosis, retinal ganglion cell, rat (chlorphentermine 60 mg/kg per os, 4 weeks). The lamellated inclusions are membrane limited. At high magnification (**b**), the lamellar material is seen to have a periodic pattern. TEM, **a** ×30600; **b** ×200000

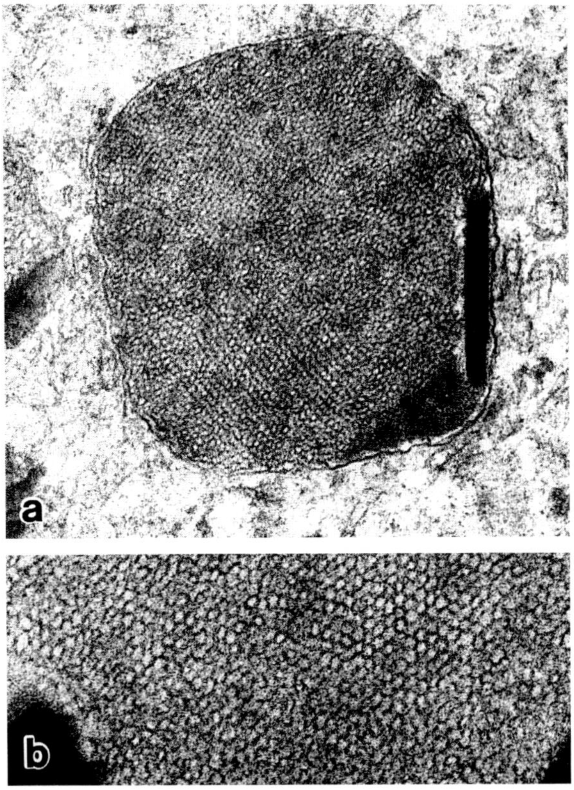

Fig. 77 a, b. Drug-induced lipidosis, retinal pigment epithelium, rat (triparanol 60 mg/kg per os, 2 weeks). An inclusion with a crystalline internal pattern is shown. TEM. **a** ×61500, **b** ×100000

the lysosomal storage. When retinal lipidosis is fully developed, abnormal dense cytoplasmic inclusions can be seen in the retinal ganglion cells, in neurons of the inner nuclear layer, in Müller cell processes, and in the pigment epithelium. In the latter, the storage may lead to a significant increase of the height of the epithelial cells (Fig. 74 a, d); the cytoplasmic inclusions can be packed so densely that they are barely discerned as solitary inclusion bodies and may thus escape detection by light microscopy. The frequency of abnormal inclusions is quite homogeneous throughout the pigment epithelium of the pars optica retinae, but decreases abruptly with the beginning of the pars caeca retinae (Lüllmann-Rauch 1979, 1981). This correlates with the fact that the pigment epithelium in the pars optica phagocytizes phospholipid-rich membranes of the rod outer segments while the pigment epithelium in the pars caeca does not.

Ultrastructure

Drug-induced lipidosis is characterized by the transformation of normal lysosomes into enlarged storage organelles which can have two distinct ultrastructural patterns (Lüllmann-Rauch 1976, 1981). (1) The more frequently occurring type (Fig. 76) consists of concentrically arranged lamellae. At high resolution, the lamellated material has a periodic pattern of alternating dense and lucent bands. (2) In the second type of inclusion (Fig. 77), the storage material has crystalline or reticular patterns. This type is most often seen in the retinal pigment epithelium but may also occur in retinal neurons. Transitions between the lamellated and reticular patterns are observed in the inclusions of retinal neurons.

By the freeze-fracture technique, the lamellated inclusions have been shown to contain the polar lipids aggregated in the lamellar phase, while in the inclusions with crystalline or reticular pat-

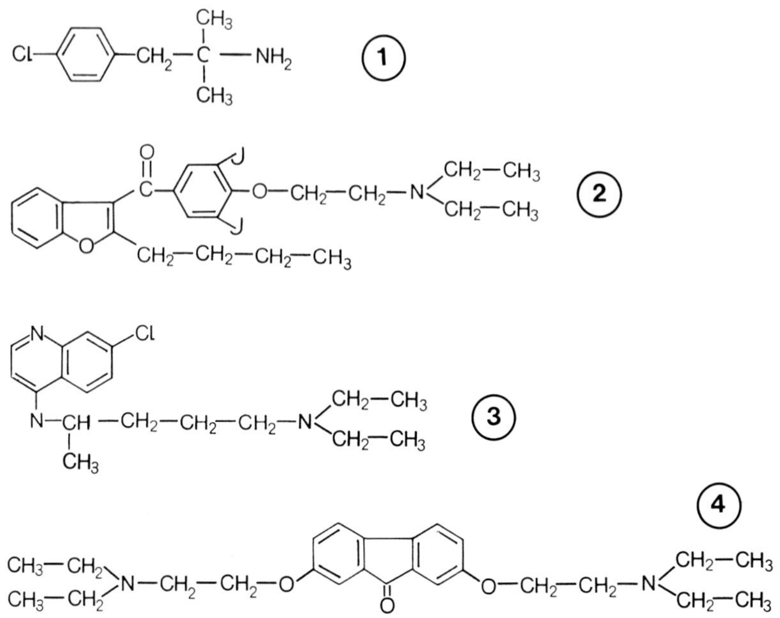

Fig. 78. Lipidosis-inducing drugs, selected examples. All compounds consist of an apolar portion (aromatic ring system) and one or two polar side chains carrying a protonizable nitrogen. *1*, chlorphentermine (anorectic); *2*, amiodarone (antianginal); *3*, chloroquine (antimalarial, antirheumatic); *4*, tilorone (experimental immunostimulatory agent). The latter three drugs have been reported to induce lipidosis also in human patients

terns the polar lipids were aggregated in a hexagonal phase (Buchheim et al. 1979). The degree of lipid storage in the neuroretina as compared with that in the pigment epithelium may vary greatly depending on the amphiphilic cationic drug under study.

Differential Diagnosis

In rats, no other conditions are known to be associated with the retinal lesions described above. In untreated control rats, the lysosomes of the retinal ganglion cells may occasionally have a few dense lines in the lysosomal matrix, but lamellated structures such as described above do not occur. The pigment epithelium of the pars optica retinae in control rats (Fig. 75b, c) regularly contains some phagosomes, i.e., freshly engulfed fragments of rod outer segments (Young 1976), and some lamellated inclusion bodies. The latter represent partially degraded phagosomes and must not be confused with the drug-induced abnormal inclusions described above.

Biologic Features

Retinal lipidosis is part of a generalized storage disease inducible by various drugs (Lüllmann et al. 1978; Lüllmann-Rauch 1979). The essential feature in the molecular structure common to all lipidosis-inducing compounds is that they consist of an apolar ring (system) and a short polar side chain which carries a protonizable nitrogen. Thus lipidosis-inducing drugs can be grouped by their amphiphilic, cationic character rather than by their therapeutic actions, which differ greatly (anorectics, tricyclic antidepressants, antimalarials, antianginal agents, antihistaminics, hypocholesterolemic agents, immunostimulants, etc.). The molecular structures of selected examples are shown in Fig. 78. Drug treatment with high doses for several weeks is required to induce lipidosis in the retina of rats.

Pathogenesis

The lysosomal storage of polar lipids results from impaired degradation. This can be explained in the simplest way by the following hypothesis (Lüllmann et al. 1978): The drugs are accumulated within the acid lysosomal compartment, due to the affinity of the cationic amphiphilic drugs toward polar lipids (phospholipids, gangliosides). The drugs form complexes with polar lipids and thereby impair the digestibility of the lipids. Another assumption is that drug-enzyme interaction inhibits the lipid-degrading enzymes (Kubo and Hostetler 1987). Lipidosis is slowly reversible (within weeks) after drug treatment is discontinued. It is noteworthy that not every cationic compound with marked amphiphilic features induces lipidosis in intact animals. When a drug (e.g., chlorpromazine) is rapidly metabolized, giving rise to less amphiphilic metabolites, generalized lipidosis will not occur.

With respect to the resulting cytologic alterations, drug-induced lipidosis is an imitation of the inherited lipidoses, which are due to a genetically determined deficiency, usually affecting one particular lysosomal enzyme (Berman 1982). However, drug-induced lipidosis is not a suitable model for the pathogenesis and the qualitative biochemical alterations (spectrum of stored lipids) of inherited lipidoses.

The retina of rats is fairly susceptible to drug-induced lipidosis when compared with other parts of the nervous system. For example, 24 h after a single oral dose of the anorectic agent chlorphentermine (40 mg/kg) or of the tricyclic antidepressant iprindole (100 mg/kg), the first abnormal inclusions with a crystalline pattern are seen in the pigment epithelium (Lüllmann-Rauch 1976). Twenty-four hours after a single oral dose of chloroquine (100 mg/kg) the first lamellar bodies are found in the retinal ganglion cells (R. Lüllmann-Rauch, unpublished).

The distribution of lipidosis-related lesions throughout the retinal layers may vary with the drug (Drenckhahn and Lüllmann-Rauch 1978). For example, chloroquine and tilorone affect the neuroretina mainly, whereas the pigment epithelium is barely changed. In contrast, the hypocholesterolemic drug triparanol causes severe lipidosis in the pigment epithelium, while the neuroretina is unaffected. Most lipidosis-inducing drugs, however, affect either part of the retina. The reasons for the diversities are not clear. Differences in drug distribution might account for the absence of lesions from the neuroretina. Qualitative differences concerning the affinities toward the various species of polar lipids may be responsible for the finding that some drugs have little effect on the pigment epithelium: these cells apparently store mostly the phospholipids that originate from the phagocytized rod outer segment membranes (Daemen 1973). Drugs which have relatively low affinities to these particular phospholipids (e.g., chloroquine) will not impair the degradation and thus not cause significant lipid storage in the pigment epithelium. The high affinity of chloroquine toward gangliosides (Lüllmann and Wehling 1979) may explain why the retinal neurons undergo severe lipidosis after chronic treatment with this drug.

Two drugs (chloroquine and the immunomodulatory agent tilorone) were found to induce irreversible photoreceptor cell degeneration in albino rats treated for many weeks (Gregory et al. 1970; Ivanina et al. 1983; Lüllmann-Rauch and Lüpkes 1987). The histologic lesions correspond to those of the chloroquine-induced retinopathy known to occur in patients (Bernstein and Ginsberg 1964; Wetterholm and Winter 1964). Tilorone has also induced a retinopathy in human patients; histologic data have not been reported (Weiss et al. 1980). At present, an explanation of the pathogenic mechanisms is not available. It is not clear (1) whether or not there is any pathogenic relationship between retinal lipidosis and photoreceptor degeneration and (2) what are the essential molecular features responsible for the drugs' potencies to induce photoreceptor destruction.

Comparison with Other Species

Drug-induced lipidosis as a generalized disease has been shown to occur in several other animal species and in man. Retinal lipidosis in particular has been described in rabbits (Ramsey and Fine 1972), mice, cats, dogs (Gregory et al. 1970), pigs (Gleiser et al. 1969), monkeys (Rosenthal et al. 1978), and minipigs (Klinghardt et al. 1981) treated long-term with chloroquine. The latter study contains a biochemical determination of the accumulated lipids.

References

Bernstein HN, Ginsberg J (1964) The pathology of chloroquine retinopathy. Arch Ophthalmol 71: 238–245

Berman ER (1982) Sphingolipidoses and neuronal ceroidlipofuscinosis. In: Garner A, Klintworth GK (eds) Pathobiology of ocular disease, part. B. Dekker, New York, pp 897–929

Buchheim W, Drenckhahn D, Lüllmann-Rauch R (1979) Freeze-fracture studies of cytoplasmic inclusions occurring in experimental lipidosis as induced by amphiphilic cationic drugs. Biochim Biophys Acta 575: 71–80

Daemen FJM (1973) Vertebrate rot outer segment membranes. Biochim Biophys Acta 300: 255–288
Drenckhahn D, Lüllmann-Rauch R (1978) Drug-induced retinal lipidosis: differential susceptibilities of pigment epithelium and neuroretina toward several amphiphilic cationic drugs. Exp Mol Pathol 28: 360–371
Gleiser CA, Dukes TW, Lawwill T, Read WK, Bay WW, Brown RS (1969) Ocular changes in swine associated with chloroquine toxicity. Am J Ophthalmol 67: 399–405
Gregory MH, Rutty DA, Wood RD (1970) Differences in the retinotoxic action of chloroquine and phenothiazine derivatives. J Pathol 102: 139–150
Ivanina TA, Zueva MV, Lebedeva MN, Bogoslovsky AI, Bunin AJ (1983) Ultrastructural alterations in rat and cat retina and pigment epithelium induced by chloroquine. Graefes Arch Clin Exp Ophthalmol 220: 32–38
Klinghardt GW, Fredman P, Svennerholm L (1981) Chloroquine intoxication induces ganglioside storage in nervous tissue: a chemical and histophatological study of brain, spinal cord, dorsal root ganglia, and retina in the miniature pig. J Neurochem 37: 897–908
Kubo M, Hostetler KY (1987) Diethylaminoethoxyhexestrol inhibition of purified rat liver lysosomal phospholipase A_1: role of drug binding to substrate. J Pharmacol Exp Ther 240: 88–92
Lüllmann H, Wehling M (1979) The binding of drugs to different polar lipids in vitro. Biochem Pharmacol 28: 3409–3415
Lüllmann H, Lüllmann-Rauch R, Wassermann O (1978) Lipidosis induced by amphiphilic cationic drugs. Biochem Pharmacol 27: 1103–1108
Lüllmann-Rauch R (1976) Retinal lipidosis in albino rats treated with chlorphentermine and with tricyclic antidepressants. Acta Neuropathol 35: 55–67
Lüllmann-Rauch R (1979) Drug-induced lysosomal storage disorders. In: Dingle JT, Jacques PJ, Shaw IH (eds) Lysosomes in applied biology and therapeutics, vol 6. North Holland, Amsterdam, pp 49–130
Lüllmann-Rauch R (1981) Experimentally induced lipidosis in rat retinal pigment epithelium. Greafes Arch Clin Exp Ophthalmol 215: 297–303
Lüllmann-Rauch R, Lüpkes S (1987) Drug-induced degeneration of photoreceptor cells. Adv Biosci 62: 471–476
Ramsey MS, Fine BS (1972) Chloroquine toxicity in the human eye. Histopathologic observations by electron microscopy. Am J Ophthalmol 73: 229–235
Rosenthal AR, Kolb H, Bergsma D, Huxsoll D, Hopkins JL (1978) Chloroquine retinopathy in the rhesus monkey. Invest Ophthalmol 17: 1158–1175
Weiss JN, Ochs AL, Abedi S, Selhorst JB (1980) Retinopathy after tilorone hydrochloride. Am J Ophthalmol 90: 846–853
Wetterholm DH, Winter FC (1964) Histopathology of chloroquine retinal toxicity. Arch Ophthalmol 71: 82–87
Young RW (1976) Visual cells and the concept of renewal. Invest Ophthalmol 15: 700–725

Inherited Retinal Degeneration, RCS Rat

Yousef Matuk

Synonyms. Royal College of Surgeons rat, RCS rat, dystrophic rat.

Gross Appearance

There are four congenic strains of RCS rats, which differ from one another only in melanin pigmentation. When present, this pigmentation appears on the face and head and runs as a stripe along the back (Fig. 79). Thc cycs may also be pigmented. The four strains of RCS rat are: (1) the pink-eyed tan-hooded Royal College of Surgeons (RCS) strain, which is the descendent of the strain studied by Bourne et al. in 1938 and is homozygous for the pink-eye dilution gene *(p/p);* (2) The pink-eyed albino strain, designated RCS-*c* (LaVail et al. 1975); and (3) two black-eyed black-hooded strains: (a) the RCS-

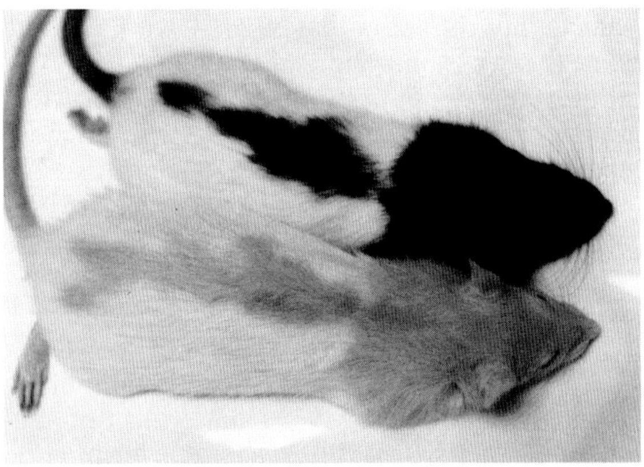

Fig. 79. RCS (tan-hooded, *below*) and RCS-p + (black-hooded, *above*) rats. Note pigmentation on head and along the back

p/+ strain, whose progeny are approximately 50% black-eyed (*p*/+) and 50% pink-eyed, tan-hooded *(p/p)* and (b) the RCS-*p*+ strain, whose progeny are 100% black-eyed (*p*+) (LaVail 1981).
Congenic, tan-hooded, pink-eyed (RCS-*rdy*+) and black-hooded, black-eyed (RCS-*rdy*+*p*+) rats which are homozygous wild type (+/+) at the retinal dystrophy genetic locus are available as controls for the RCS and the RCS-*p*+ strains respectively (LaVail 1981).

Fundoscopy (Herron et al. 1974)

Ophthalmoscopic examination of the 3- to 4½-week-old fundus of a normal pigmented rat shows the gray color of the pigment epithelium and the red blood vessels of the choroid (Fig. 80a). Scanning ophthalmoscopy shows fundoscopic changes in the pigmented dystrophic rat at about 3 weeks of age. At this stage the normal red reflex of the fundus becomes almost white. This abnormality can be used to detect dystrophic rats in a mixed population. Careful ophthalmoscopic examination reveals a slight lightening of the gray background color of the fundus. This change begins to shroud the choroidal vessels. Between 3 and 4½ weeks of age, the intensity of the whitish reflex is sufficient to mask the choroidal vessels and the details of the retina (Fig. 80b). The whitish reflex dissipates from the posterior of the eye by about 6 or 7 weeks of age, revealing the choroidal vessels and a granular retina (Fig. 80c).
The blood vessels in the posterior retina, especially the arteries, are now quite thin. At this time the peripheral retina is still masked by the whitish reflex.
Further pigment granulation of the fundus and thinning of the blood vessels occur with increasing age.

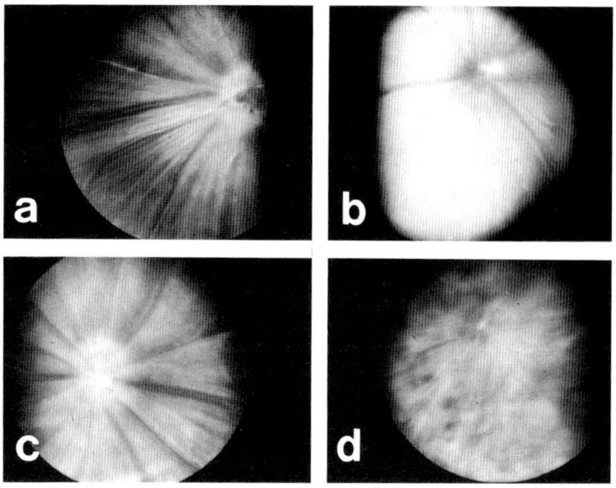

Fig. 80a–d. Fundi of pigmented normal and dystrophic rats. **a** Normal rat aged 3–4 weeks: the choroidal vessels and the gray background of the pigment epithelium are visible. **b** Dystrophic rat aged 3–4 weeks: whitish reflection obscures the pigment epithelium and choroidal vessels. **c** Normal rat aged 6 weeks: gray background of pigment epithelium and the choroidal vessels can be seen. **d** Dystrophic rat aged 6 weeks: clumped pigment, thinned retina, and narrowed blood vessels are visible at this time. (From Herron et al. 1974)

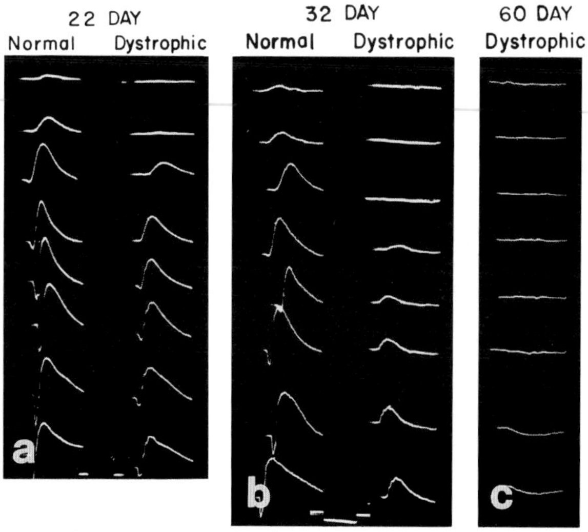

Fig. 81a–c. Electroretinograms of control and RCS rats. **a** Twenty-two-day-old rat: compared with the normal retina, the stimulus response of the dystrophic retina increased by about 1.5 log units and the a- and b-waves were reduced. **b** Thirty-two-day-old rat: in the RCS retina, the a-wave has disappeared and the b-wave is elicited only at high levels of light intensity. **c** Sixty-day-old RCS rat: the b-wave is extinguished and an electroretinogram cannot be elicited at any light intensity. Electroretinograms were elicited with 1/50-s flashes of white light over an intensity range of 7 log units. A 200-μV calibration signal is shown *at the bottom* of each set of results. The duration of the oscilloscope time was 0.5 s. (From Dowling and Sidman 1962)

Electroretinography
(Dowling and Sidman 1962)

A significant increase above normal levels in the stimulus threshold of the dystrophic retina may be observed at the age of 18 days. Otherwise the electroretinogram of the RCS rat develops normally until about the age of 22 days. At this time the stimulus response is increased by about 1.5 log units above the normal levels. In addition the a-wave and the b-wave of the electroretino-

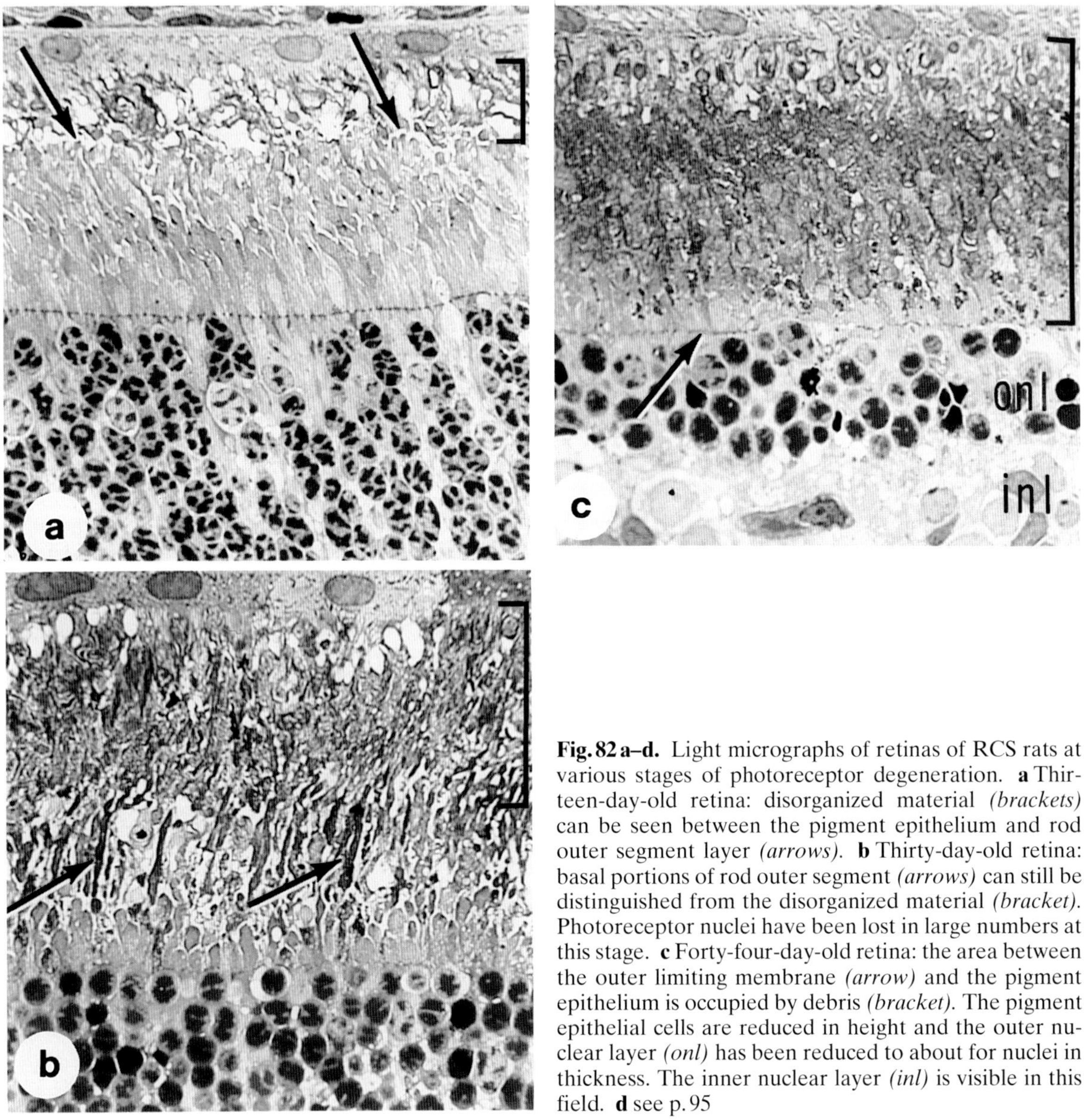

Fig. 82 a–d. Light micrographs of retinas of RCS rats at various stages of photoreceptor degeneration. **a** Thirteen-day-old retina: disorganized material *(brackets)* can be seen between the pigment epithelium and rod outer segment layer *(arrows)*. **b** Thirty-day-old retina: basal portions of rod outer segment *(arrows)* can still be distinguished from the disorganized material *(bracket)*. Photoreceptor nuclei have been lost in large numbers at this stage. **c** Forty-four-day-old retina: the area between the outer limiting membrane *(arrow)* and the pigment epithelium is occupied by debris *(bracket)*. The pigment epithelial cells are reduced in height and the outer nuclear layer *(onl)* has been reduced to about for nuclei in thickness. The inner nuclear layer *(inl)* is visible in this field. **d** see p. 95

gram are decreased at the lower levels of light stimulation (Fig. 81 a). The levels of the a-wave and the b-wave continue to decrease with age. The a-wave disappears at about the age of 32 days (Fig. 81 b) and the b-wave is no longer observed at the age of 60 days (Fig. 81 c).

Microscopic Features
(Dowling and Sidman 1962; Bok and Hall 1971)

The first indication of abnormality in the RCS retina is observed at about the age of 12–13 days. At this age a distinct zone of disorganized material is seen between the retinal pigment epithelial cells and the layer of photoreceptor outer segments (Fig. 82 a). The zone of disorganized debris continues to increase in width without any indication of histologic changes in the retinal cells until about the age of 21 – 22 days, when pyknotic nuclei and swollen inner segments start to appear in the photoreceptor layer. Degenerative changes in the apical ends of rod outer segments are not evident until about 27 – 28 days of age. The degenerative changes in the outer segents progress rapidly. By 30 days of age only a few basal outer segments can be recognized in the zone of rod outer segments. At this stage the

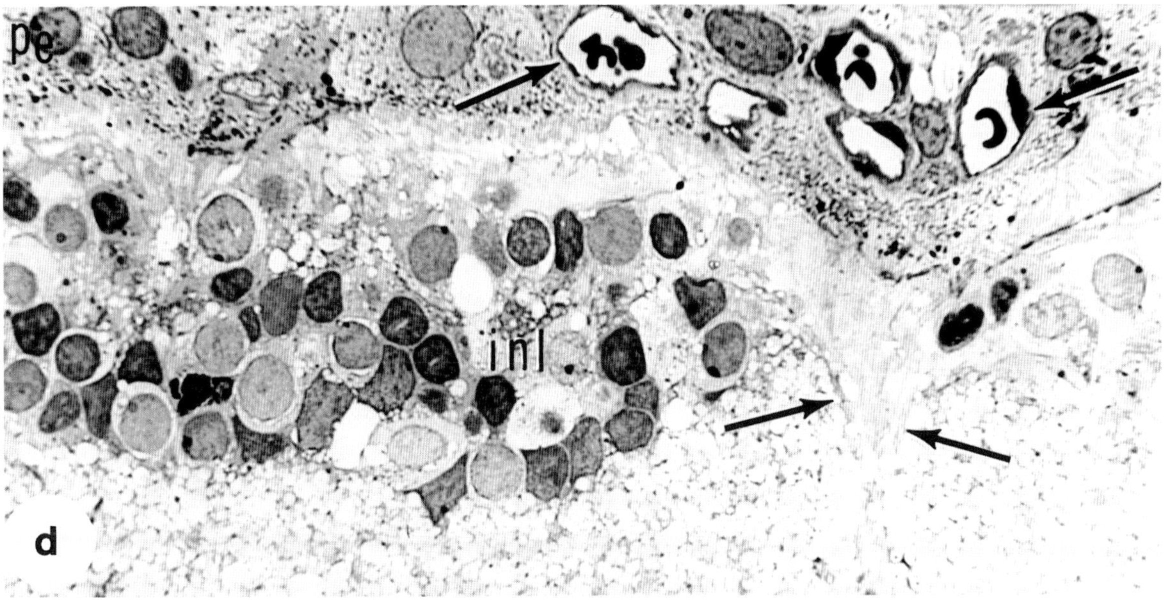

Fig. 82 d. Seven-month-old retina: the photoreceptor layer and the rod outer segment debris have disappeared and the retinal pigment epithelium has been invaded by capillaries *(upper arrows)*. The inner nuclear layer *(inl)* is now adjacent to the pigment epithelium and is interrupted in places *(lower arrows)* by aggregates of Müller cell fibers (gliosis). 0.5-μm epoxy resin (Araldite) sections. (From Bok and Hall 1971) Toluidine blue stain, ×800

inner segment layer has become much thinner and a significant number of photoreceptor nuclei have been lost (Fig. 82b).

Between the ages of 40 and 44 days the outer nuclear layer has been reduced from the normal 11–13 to 2–4 nuclei in width. The rod inner segment layer has disappeared and distinct inner and outer photoreceptor segments can no longer be recognized. The thickness of the zone of disorganized materials is reduced and the area adjacent to the pigment epithelium is virtually unstainable with periodic acid Schiff reagent. In addition, abnormal changes in the retinal pigment epithelium become apparent at this stage. These cells lose their characteristic cuboidal arrangement along Bruch's membrane and become flattened. Both their cytoplasm and nuclei appear irregular in shape and larger in volume than those of normal retinal pigment epithelial cells. Cells of unknown origin may now be seen scattered in the area of the disorganized material (Fig. 82c). The vestiges of the photoreceptor cell continue to disappear with age. By 7 months the debris has disappeared and the inner nuclear layer rests against the pigment epithelium, which now appears thicker than at earlier stages of the disease. The pigment epithelium is invaded by capillaries and evidence for gliosis is observed (Fig. 82d).

Cationic stains selectively stain the normal interphotoreceptor matrix in the areas around the rod outer segment-pigment epithelial cell interface, and around the junction of the inner and the outer segments (LaVail et al. 1981). Less intense staining is seen in the interstices between the rod outer segments (Fig. 83a).

The first signs of abnormal staining in the RCS retina appear at 12 days of age. At this time the intensity of the apical band of stain in the interphotoreceptor matrix of the posterior retina is less pronounced than in the normal retina of the same age. This differences becomes progressively more apparent. By 16 days of age, the stain at the apical pigment epithelial cell surface of the RCS retina appears patchy (Fig. 83b). The stain is virtually absent from the dystrophic interphotoreceptor matrix by the age of 24 – 26 days (Fig. 83c). At this stage the highest density of reaction product is found among the basal area of the dystrophic rod outer segments (Fig. 83c). This frequently appears more dense than in the same area of the normal retina.

In the peripheral retina, near the ora serrata, the intensity of stain at the surface of the pigment epithelial cells is substantially greater than in the posterior retinas of both control and dystrophic rat. In this area the density of the stain at the apical surface of the pigment epithelium of control

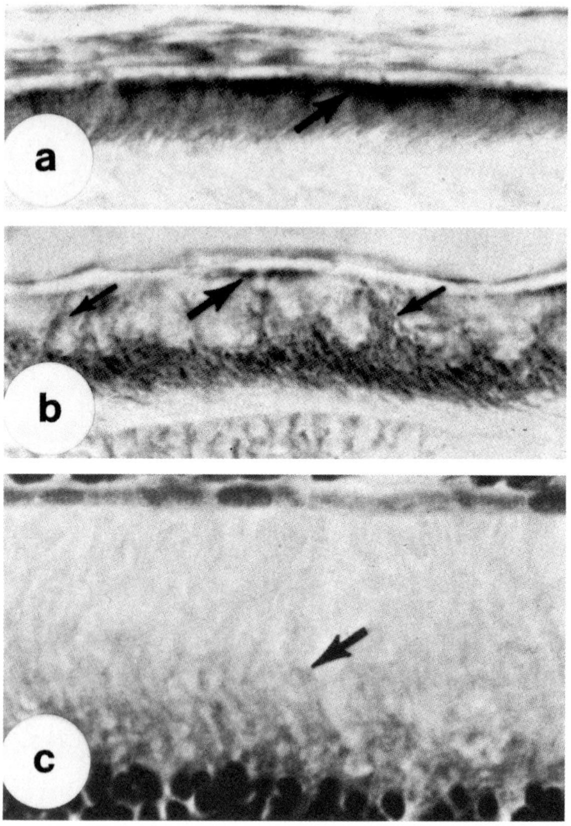

Fig. 83 a–c. Interphotoreceptor matrix of control (RCS-rdy +) and dystrophic (RCS) rat retinas. **a** Twelve-day-old normal retina: a prominent band of reaction product *(arrow)* lies at the interface of the rod outer segments and the retinal pigment epithelial cells *(top)*. A similar band of reaction product appears in this region of older normal rats and, with a slightly reduced intensity, in the 12-day-old interphotoreceptor matrix of the RCS retina. **b** Sixteen-day-old RCS retina: the intense band of reaction product which appears at the surface of the retinal pigment epithelium of the 12-day-old RCS rat has now been reduced to small patches *(large arrows)*. Some strands of interphotoreceptor matrix are seen extending from the outer segment layer through the debris to the pigment epithelial cell layer *(small arrow)*. **c** Twenty-six-day-old RCS retina: the reaction product is now mainly absent from the regions of the retinal pigment epithelium and the rod outer segment debris. Some reaction product is still, however, observed in the basal area of the outer segments *(arrow)*. Ten-micrometer sections of polyester wax-embedded eyes were stained with colloidal iron, **a** and **b**, or toluidine blue (**c**). (From LaVail et al. 1981) ×740

retinas aged 12 days and older does not vary. In the mutant retina a slight change in the density of the stain of the peripheral interphotoreceptor matrix may be observed at the age of 29 days. The stain disappears rapidly from this region of the RCS retina between the ages of 30 and 40 days.

Ultrastructure (Dowling and Sidman 1962)

Low magnification by transmission electron microscopy reveals that the disorganized material which accumulates between the outer segment layer and the retinal pigment epithelium consists of membranes which may be arranged in elongated bundles or in sheets parallel to or closely associated with the processes of the pigment epithelium. They may be large lamellar structures arranged in whorls between the rod outer segments and the retinal pigment epithelium. The double membrane structure, dimensions, and density of the lamellae are similar to those of the normal rod outer segment disk

Fig. 84 *(upper left)*. Disorganized material from the retina of an 18-day-old rat. Lamellar extracellular double membranes *(EL)* are in close contact with apical processes of the pigment epithelial cells *(PE)*. The lamellae have similar dimensions and density to the disks of the rod outer segments *(arrows)*. The ROS disks differ from the lamellar membranes in that they are enclosed within a surface membrane *(left arrow)*. (From Dowling and Sidman 1962) TEM, ×6600 ▶

Fig. 85 *(below)*. Section taken about the middle of the outer segment layer of the retina of a 27-day-old RCS rat. Extracellular and rod outer segment material are now mixed together. Some lamellae of each show vesiculation, indicating early degeneration. (From Dowling and Sidman 1962) TEM, ×8300

Fig. 86 *(upper right)*. Retina of a 40-day-old RCS rat. Two relatively normal photoreceptor nuclei *(N)* are seen at the top of the micrograph, but the other photoreceptor nuclei have undergone various degrees of degeneration. The synaptic zone *(S)* is thinner than normal, but some synapses still appear relatively intact. The nucleus at the bottom of the micrograph belongs to a bipolar cell *(B)*; the large nucleus to its left may be either a Müller or a horizontal cell nucleus. (From Dowling and Sidman 1962) TEM, ×3360

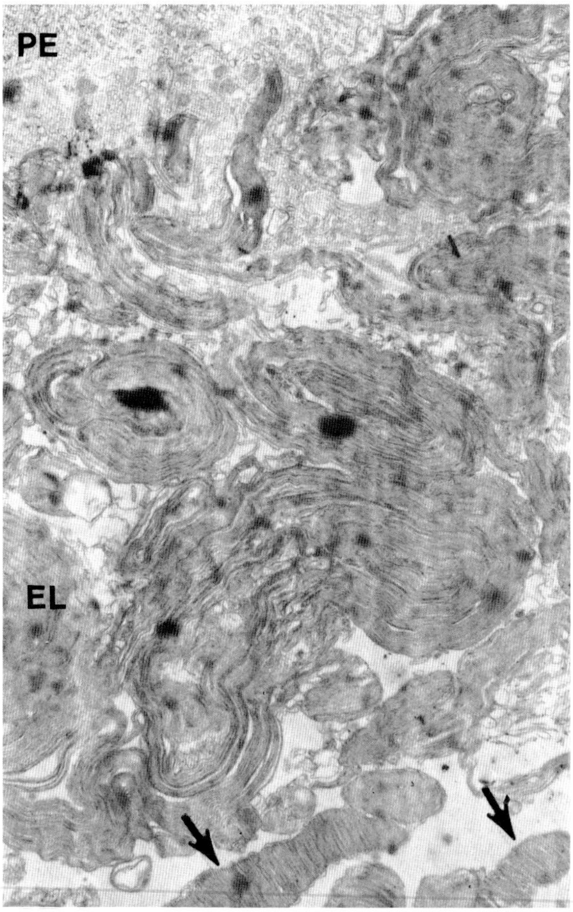
PE
EL

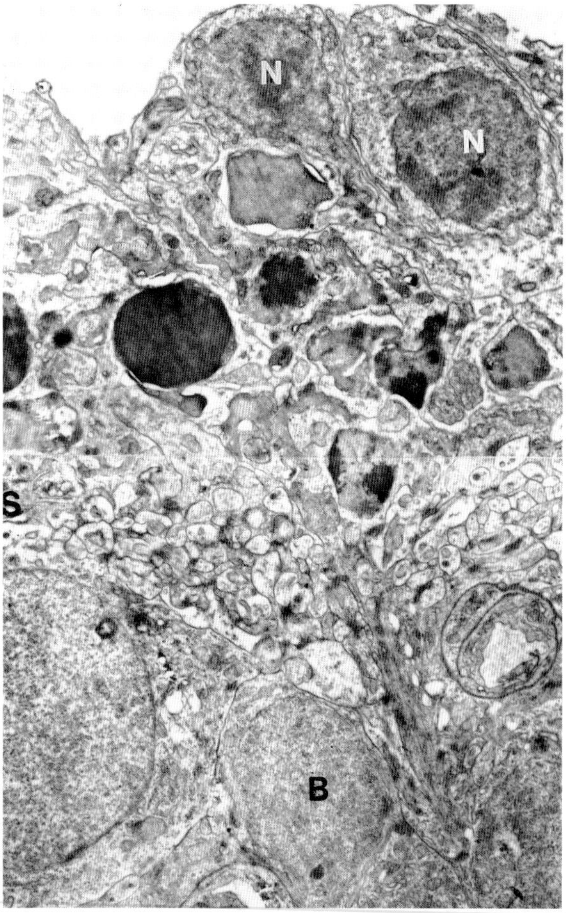
N
N
S
B

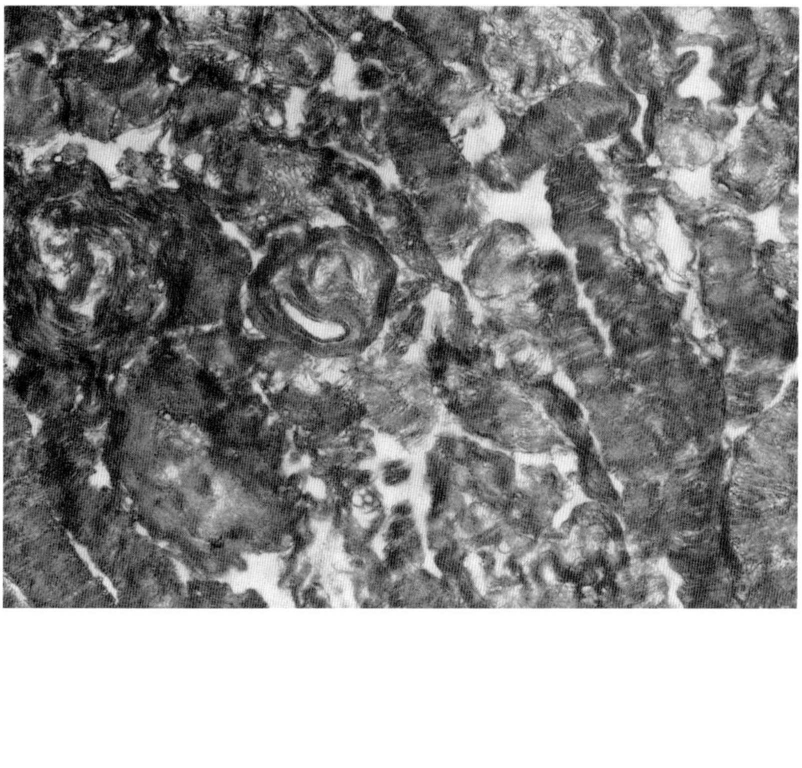

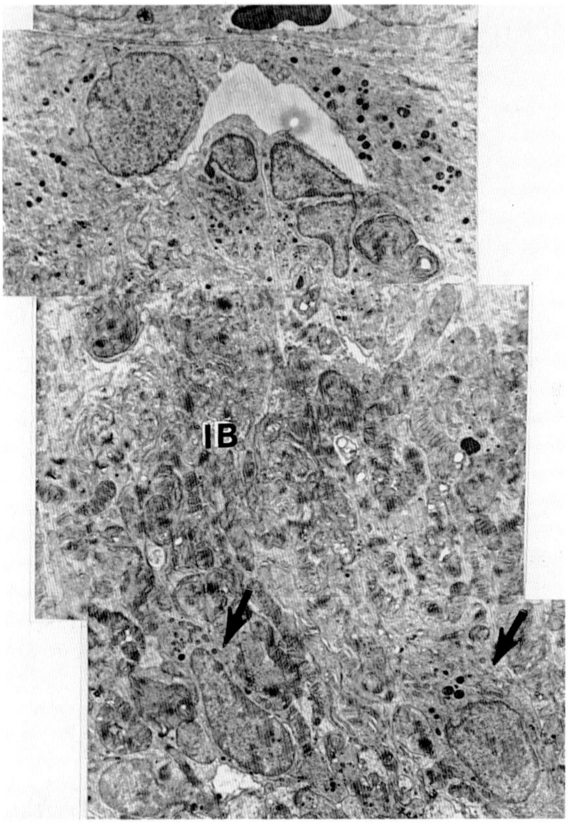

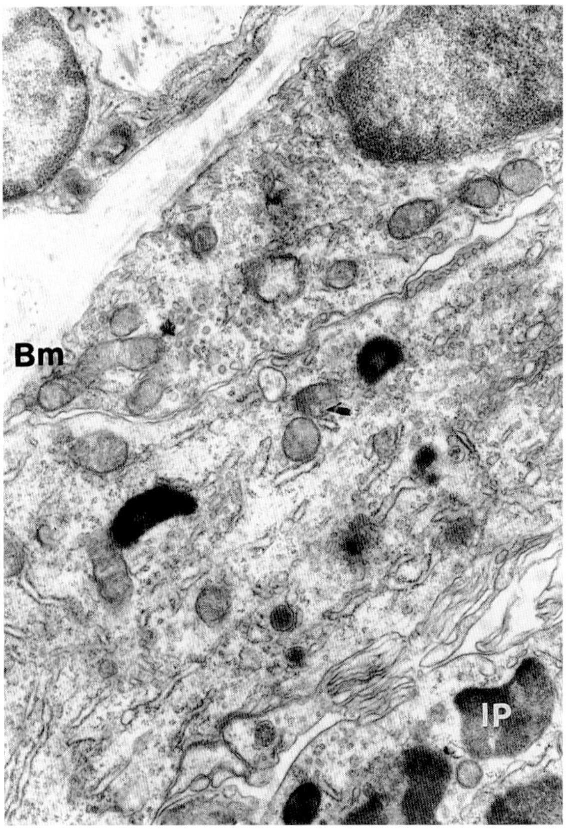

membranes (Fig. 84) and have been shown to contain rhodopsin (Dowling and Sidman 1962). Autoradiography indicates that the lamellar membranes originate from the rod outer segment disks (Herron et al. 1969; Bok and Hall 1971).

By age 27 days, degenerating rod outer segments and some extracellular lamellae contain disks which have swollen into vacuoles and tubules (Fig. 85). The vesiculation becomes quite prominent at the age of 32 days. At this time the nuclei are also rapidly degenerating and by 40 days very few nuclei are left. Normally, the photoreceptor cell nuclei are finely grained, uniform in size, with low contrast in electron micrographs. The degenerating photoreceptor cell nuclei of the dystrophic retina are dense in appearance and varied in size (Fig. 86). Some of these nuclei are quite large.

At 40 days, the rod outer segment layer contains a few intact outer segments and the zone of debris appears less electron dense than at earlier stages of the disease. The space between the remaining outer segments and debris is filled with cytoplasmic processes emanating from pigment epithelial cells which have migrated from Bruch's membrane (Fig. 87).

At the age of 60 days, the pigment epithelial cells, which normally have straight lateral borders at right angles to Bruch's membrane and never overlap, are now elongated, lie parallel to Bruch's membrane, and usually overlap each

◂**Fig. 87** *(above)*. Montage of electron micrographs from retina of a 40-day-old RCS rat. *At the top of the micrograph* two cells appear to be breaking away from the pigment epithelial cell layer. Two other cells are seen at the bottom of the micrograph. The interstices between outer segments or pieces of debris are filled with processes of pigment epithelial cells, many containing inclusion bodies *(IB)*. (From Dowling and Sidman 1962) TEM, ×2500

Fig. 88 *(below)*. Parts of three pigment epithelial cells in the retina of a 60-day-old rat. The cells appear to have differentiated to some extent: the endoplasmic reticulum is less dense than normal and often tubular in form, the cell surface bordering Bruch's membrane *(Bm)* is no longer extensively infolded, and the cells have changed in shape and overlap one another. The area of pigment cell cytoplasm which occupies the lower right corner of the micrograph contains typical granular inclusion particles *(IP)* found in rat pigment epithelial cells. (From Dowling and Sidman 1962) TEM, ×24200 other. More changes in the dystrophic pigment epithelium can be seen under higher electron microscopic magnification (Fig. 88). The normally dense vesicular cytoplasm is now frequently observed in the form of long tubules. The extensive infolding of the basement membrane along Bruch's membrane and the characteristic alignment of mitochondria in this region is no longer observed. In addition, the number of apical processes that normally extend among the outer segments from the cells of the pigment epithelium is reduced.

Differential Diagnosis

Two features characterize retinal degeneration in the RCS rat: (1) the accumulation of rod outer sement debris between the outer segment layer and the retinal pigment epithelium in young (12- to 20-day-old) RCS rats, without apparent changes in the photoreceptor cells, and (2) the virtual absence of phagocytic activity by the dystrophic retinal pigment epithelium. These characteristics distinguish retinal degeneration in the RCS rat from (1) generalized retinal degeneration caused by light and (2) photoreceptor degeneration observed in vitamin-A-deficient animals.

Biologic Features

Autoradiographic evidence (Heron et al. 1969; Bok and Hall 1971) and rhodopsin content (Dowling and Sidman 1962) indicate that the disorganized material which accumulates between the retinal pigment epithelium and the rod outer segment layer consists of rod outer segment disk debris. The appearance of fundoscopic, electroretinographic, and histologic changes about 10 days after the detection of the disorganized material suggests that retinal degeneration in the RCS rat is secondary to the accumulation of the debris.

The pathologic changes described above are for animals maintained under controlled laboratory cyclic light-dark illumination. The rate of retinal degeneration is significantly reduced in rats with pigmented eyes and in those maintained in the dark, suggesting a role for light in the retinal degeneration of the dystrophic rat.

Etiology and Frequency

The glycoproteins of the rod outer segment disks are synthesized in the photoreceptor inner segments and exported to the outer segments, where they are laid into disks at the proximal end of the structure. The older disks are pushed apically, where they are eventually shed and phagocytized by the retinal pigment epithelial cells (Young 1976). Available evidence indicates that retinal degeneration in the RCS rat is due to the failure of the retinal pigment epithelium to phagocytize the shed rod outer segment disks (Herron et al. 1969; Bok and Hall 1971; Mullen and LaVail 1976). Chaitin and Hall (1983) demonstrated that, although the retinal pigment epithelial cells of the dystrophic rat bind rod outer segments, they do not internalize them. The molecular basis of the defect in phagocytosis is, however, not clear. Several investigators have shown that simple sugars interfere with the process of shedding and phagocytosis of the rod outer segment disks. This suggests a role for the oligosaccharides of the disk membrane glycoproteins in this process. Recent evidence indicates that there is a deficiency in the transfer of galactose to endogenous glycoproteins in the mutant rod outer segments (Mok and Matuk 1987). It is not clear whether this defect is involved in the retinal degeneration of the RCS rat.

Retinal degeneration in the RCS rat is a strictly autosomal recessive disorder in which the recessive retinal degeneration gene *(rdy/rdy)* is homozygous. The progeny of the RCS, RCS-*c*, and RCS-*p* + rats are 100% dystrophic and have the same pigmentation as their parents. On the other hand, the progeny of the RCS-*p*/ + strain are 100% dystrophic but approximately 50% black-eyed *(p/ +*) and 50% pink-eyed *(p/p)* (LaVail 1981).

Comparison with Other Species

The RCS rat, particularly the tan-hooded strain, is one of the most extensively studied animal models of the human retinal degenerative group of diseases, retinitis pigmentosa. There are, however, significant differences between the human and rat diseases. The human disease is inherited as an autosomal dominant, an autosomal recessive, or an X-linked trait. Many cases are sporadic, with no known genetic links. Light microscope and ultrastructural studies of advanced cases of the human disease do not show accumulations of rod outer segment debris between the rod outer segment layer and the retinal pigment epithelium. The time of onset of the human disease and the rate of retinal degeneration is related to the mode of inheritance of the disorder.

Retinal degeneration in the RCS rat also differs from that observed in other animals. As in the RCS rat, rod outer segments appear to develop normally in the early stages of retinal degeneration in the miniature poodle dog. However, no accumulation of debris is seen between the rod outer segment layer and the retinal pigment epithelium. Moreover, phagocytosis by the retinal pigment epithelium of the miniature poodle appears to be normal. In the *rd* mouse and the Irish setter dog, the lesion is expressed at the time of photoreceptor cell differentiation as an abnormal development of rod outer segments. In the *rd* mouse, photoreceptors do not develop outer segments and the cells degenerate at about the age of 20 days. On the other hand, the photoreceptors of the Irish setter dog develop disorganized outer segments which degenerate within 18–24 weeks of age. The inner segments of these photoreceptors degenerate over a period of 9–12 months. Biochemically, the degeneration of the photoreceptor cells in the mouse and the Irish setter dog has been shown to be related to abnormalities in the metabolism of cyclic guanosine-3′,5′-monophosphate (see Matuk 1984 for references).

Acknowledgments. The preparation of this manuscript was supported by grants from the Eye Research Committee, Independent Order of Odd Fellows and Rebekahs, Ontario Lodge, and the RP Eye Research Foundation. The author wishes to thank Dr. Ching Mok for assistance in preparing the illustrations.

References

Bok D, Hall MO (1971) The role of the pigment epithelium in the etiology of inherited retinal dystrophy in the rat. J Cell Biol 49: 664–682

Bourne MC, Campbell DA, Tansley K (1938) Hereditary degeneration of the rat retina. Br J Ophthalmol 22: 613–623

Chaitin MH, Hall MO (1983) Defective ingestion of rod outer segments by cultured dystrophic rat pigment epithelial cells. Invest Ophthalmol Vis Sci 24: 812–820

Dowling JE, Sidman RL (1962) Inherited retinal dystrophy in the rat. J Cell Biol 14: 73–109

Herron WL Jr, Riegel BW, Myers OE, Rubin ML (1969) Retinal dystrophy in the rat – a pigment epithelial disease. Invest Ophthalmol 8: 595–604

Herron WL Jr, Riegel BW, Berman E, Rubin NL (1974) Retinal dystrophy in the pigmented rat. Invest Ophthalmol 13: 87–94

LaVail MM (1981) Photoreceptor characteristics in congenic strains of RCS rats. Invest Ophthalmol Vis Sci 20: 671–675

LaVail MM, Sidman RL, Gerhardt CO (1975) Congenic strains of RCS rats with inherited retinal dystrophy. J Hered 66: 242–244

LaVail MM, Pinto LH, Yasumura D (1981) The interphotoreceptor matrix in rats with inherited retinal dystrophy. Invest Ophthalmol Vis Sci 21: 658–668

Matuk Y (1984) Retinitis pigmentosa and retinal degeneration in animals: a review. Can J Biochem Cell Biol 62: 535–546

Mok C, Matuk Y (1987) Effect of light on the transfer of sugars from sugar nucleotides to rod outer segment membranes of control and dystrophic rats. Curr Eye Res 6: 1173–1180

Mullen RJ, LaVail MM (1976) Inherited retinal dystrophy: primary defect in pigment epithelium determined with experimental rat chimeras. Science 192: 799–801

Young RW (1976) Visual cells and the concept of renewal. Invest Ophthalmol 15: 700–725

Herpesvirus Infection, Experimental, Eye, Mouse

Sally S. Atherton, Herbert E. Whiteley, and John A. Shadduck

Synonyms. HSV-1 chorioretinitis, HSV-1 retinal necrosis.

Introduction

Following inoculation of herpes simplex virus, type 1, KOS strain (HSV-1), into the anterior chamber of one eye of a BALB/c mouse, an interesting pattern of bilateral ocular disease is observed. In the injected eye, there is massive inflammation of the anterior segment which results in the loss of the anterior chamber and destruction of the associated anterior segment structure (iris, ciliary body). The posterior segment of the inoculated eye remains relatively uninvolved in the inflammatory process and exhibits only mild inflammation of the vitreous chamber with preservation of the retinal architecture. In contrast, the uninoculated eye displays the opposite pattern of disease; the retina of this eye is destroyed while the anterior segment is preserved (Whittum et al. 1984). Two temporally distinct waves of virus are recovered from the uninoculated eye. An early low-titered wave, 10^2–10^3 plague-forming units (PFUs/ml) is present in the uninjected eye within 24 h of inoculation, and a later, high-titered wave ($>10^5$ PFUs/ml) is recovered from the uninoculated eye at day 10 postinoculation coincident with the destruction of the retina (Atherton and Streilein 1987b).

The spread of the second wave of virus into the uninjected fellow eye at the time of retinal destruction is via the optic nerve from the brain. The spread of virus from the injected eye to the central nervous system is also via one or several of the neural routes which connect the central nervous system and the eye (Atherton and Streilein 1987b; Whittum-Hudson and Pepose 1987; Olson et al. 1987). Following inoculation of HSV-1 (KOS) into one eye of a BALB/c mouse, the incidence of retinitis in the uninoculated contralateral eye is approximately 75%. BALB/c mice inoculated with the KOS strain of HSV-1 survive; infectious virus can no longer be recovered from any CNS structure or ocular tissue at 2 weeks after inoculation.

Gross Appearance

The eyes of mice inoculated with HSV-1 are most easily examined with the aid of a dissecting microscope or by the use of a slit-lamp biomicroscope. In the inoculated eye, the site of injection in the cornea becomes opaque. Within 5–7 days postinoculation, the lens of the injected eye becomes cataractous. The cornea of this eye becomes edematous and infiltrated with mononuclear inflammatory cells. Frequently, there is extensive corneal neovascularization. By 2 weeks, the injected eye undergoes phthisis. Occasionally, herpetic vesicles are observed on the lids and on the skin surrounding the orbit of the inoculated eye.

The uninoculated contralateral eye remains grossly normal until 6–7 days after inoculation, when dilatation of vessels of the iris becomes apparent. Pupillary dilatation and fixation accompany engorgement of the iris. Sometimes pupillary fixation is not uniform and an eccentric pupil results. Usually there are no external lesions observed on the cornea or on the adnexa of the contralateral eye (Whittum et al. 1984; Atherton and Streilein 1987b).

To monitor the progress of retinitis in the inoculated eye, the fundus of this eye may be examined (after pupillary dilatation with scopolamine) using a 28D lens and an indirect ophthalmoscope. The fundus of the uninoculated eye remains normal clinically until 6–7 days when subtle venous engorgement is noted. Vitreous opacities are often seen in the posterior vitreous overlying a swollen optic disk. The affected retina quickly begins to lose its transparency and its normal sheen and appears to become white. Between 8 and 10 days, the retinal veins become increasingly dilated and tortuous, and choroidal infiltrates are observed in the posterior pole. Tractional elevation of the retina occurs in many affected eyes; these areas of tractional elevation are associated with hemorrhage and inflammation. Multiple focal hemorrhages are observed along the retinal vessels. By day 10 or day 11, the entire retina of affected animals becomes opaque due to diffuse tractional elevation and progression of retinal inflammation. Opacification of the vitreous, presumably due to inflammatory cells and adhe-

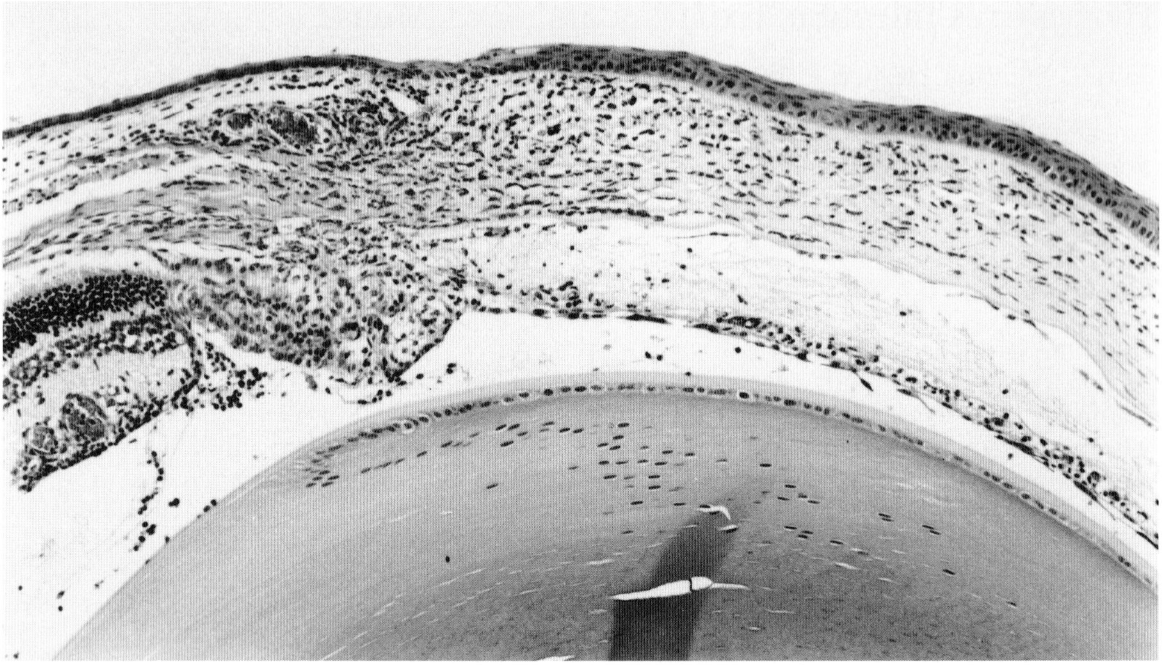

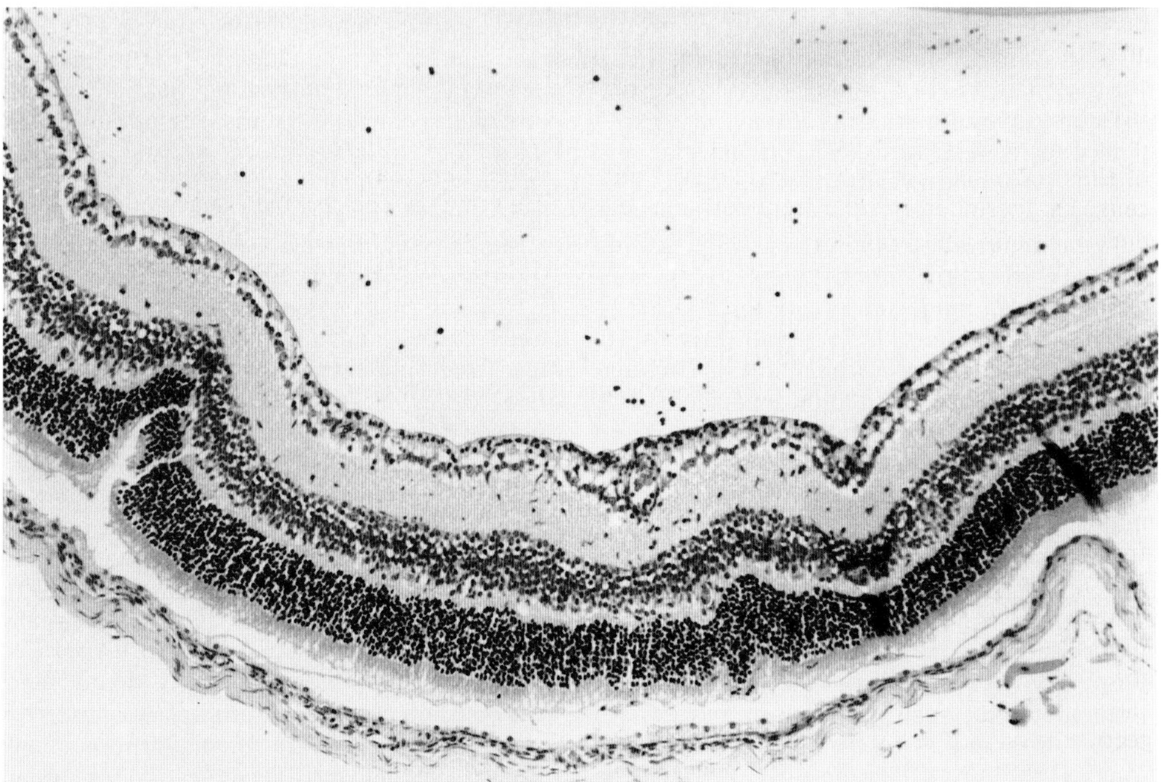

Fig. 89 *(above)*. Anterior segment, eye, BALB/c mouse. Three days after inoculation of (HSV-1) (KOS) into the anterior chamber. Note iridocyclitis and inflammatory cell infiltrate in the anterior chamber and mild inflammation of the nerve fiber and ganglion cell layers of the peripheral retina. H & E, ×140

Fig. 90 *(below)*. Retina, BALB/c mouse, 3 days following injection with HSV-1. Note mild vitreal inflammation and localized retinal folding with loss of the photoreceptor layer. The layered appearance of the retina is maintained. H & E, ×140 sion of the retina to the posterior surface of the lens, generally prohibits examination of the retina beyond this time. Because the lens of the injected eye becomes opaque and because of the massive inflammation in the anterior segment, the fundus of this eye cannot be examined clinically (Kielty et al. 1987).

Microscopic Findings

Inoculated Eye

Within 24 h of inoculation of HSV-1 into the anterior chamber, the anterior segment of the injected eye becomes markedly inflamed. Inflammation in the anterior chamber is accompanied by severe anterior uveitis, which results in the destruction of the iris and ciliary body of the injected eye (Fig. 89). Frequently, the iris becomes adherent to the posterior aspect of the cornea. The anterior chamber is obscured by the massive inflammatory process within 10–14 days after inoculation, and eventually the anterior chamber is replaced by fibrovascular scar tissue. In contrast to the massive inflammatory reaction in the anterior segment, the posterior segment of the inoculated eye remains relatively quiescent. The peripheral retina frequently has evidence of inflammation in all layers, but the spread of such inflammation to the central retina appears to be unusual. Mild inflammation of the vitreous and mild infiltration of the ganglion cells are also seen; the inflammatory infiltrate associated with the ganglion cells and the nerve fiber layer of the ipsilateral eye does not appear to be localized to any particular region of the retina (Whittum et al. 1984). Folds are observed in the outer nuclear layer which appear to result from the collapse of the subjacent photoreceptors (Fig. 90). These folds correlate with the changes in the electroretinogram that have been reported following inoculation of HSV-1 (Hamasaki et al. 1988). Although the retina is not physiologically normal, the layered retinal architecture is maintained in the inoculated eye.

Uninoculated Eye

The uninoculated eye remains normal microscopically until day 6 or day 7, when mild uveitis of the iris and ciliary body is observed. This anterior uveitis does not progress throughout the course of the disease (Fig. 91). In the posterior segment, the first histopathologic signs of retinitis are observed concomitant with development of the anterior uveitis and the first clinical signs of retinal involvement (vascular dilatation and tortuosity). The course of the disease in the contralateral eye may be divided into three stages, which frequently overlap with one another. Early retinitis (the *first stage*) is characterized by the presence of a mild inflammatory cell infiltrate in the nerve fiber and ganglion cell layers which is accompanied by a mild inflammation of the vitreous chamber. The *second stage* (retinal necrosis) begins around day 9 or day 10 and is characterized by disorganization of the retinal architecture and focal areas of choroidal infiltration by mononuclear cells (Fig. 92). Many eyes in the later part of stage two exhibit *schisis* of the retina, which involves separation of the nerve fiber layer from the underlying ganglion cell layer. This separation results in avulsion of the Müller cell footplates and retinal vessels, hemorrhage into the schisis cavity, and disruption of the underlying retinal architecture. Retinal *schisis* appears to contribute to the necrosis which follows the panretinal inflammation. Traction-induced avulsion of vessels also occurs which results in intraretinal hemorrhage. At this time (day 10–11) no normal retinal structure remains. The choroid is massively inflamed and papillitis is observed in association with cuffing of the major vessels as they exit the disk. Resolution, the *third stage* of the disease in the uninoculated eye, begins around day 15 and is characterized by attempts at repair which eventually result in formation of a hypertrophic scar (Whittum et al. 1984; Cousins et al. 1989).

Ultrastructure

In experiments in which outbred ICR mice were inoculated with the RE strain of HSV-1 via one anterior chamber, electron microscopic examination of the retinas of the uninoculated eyes revealed that virus particles were present in the inner nuclear and ganglion cell layers of the retina at the time when the retina was being destroyed. Virus particles were observed only rarely in the outer layers of the retina even though the outer layers of the retina become necrotic. Virus particles were also observed in the retinal pigment epithelium. No virus particles were observed in the structures comprising the anterior chamber (iris, ciliary body, cornea) in spite of the anterior uveitis which occurs in unin-

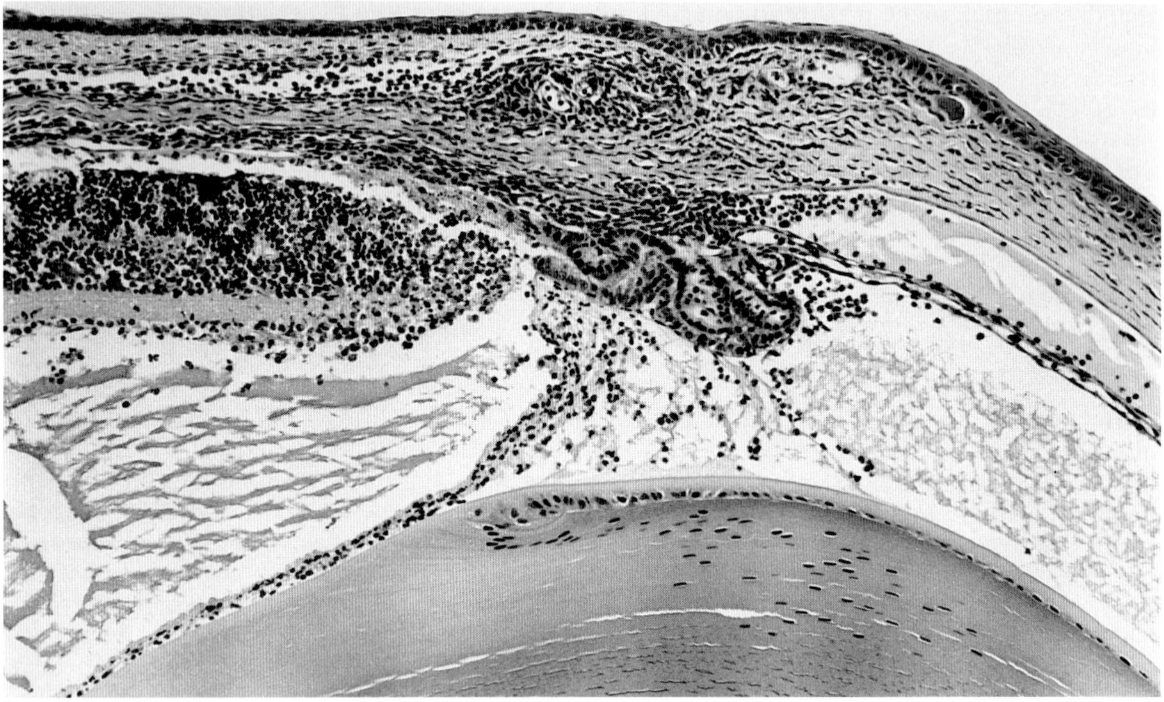

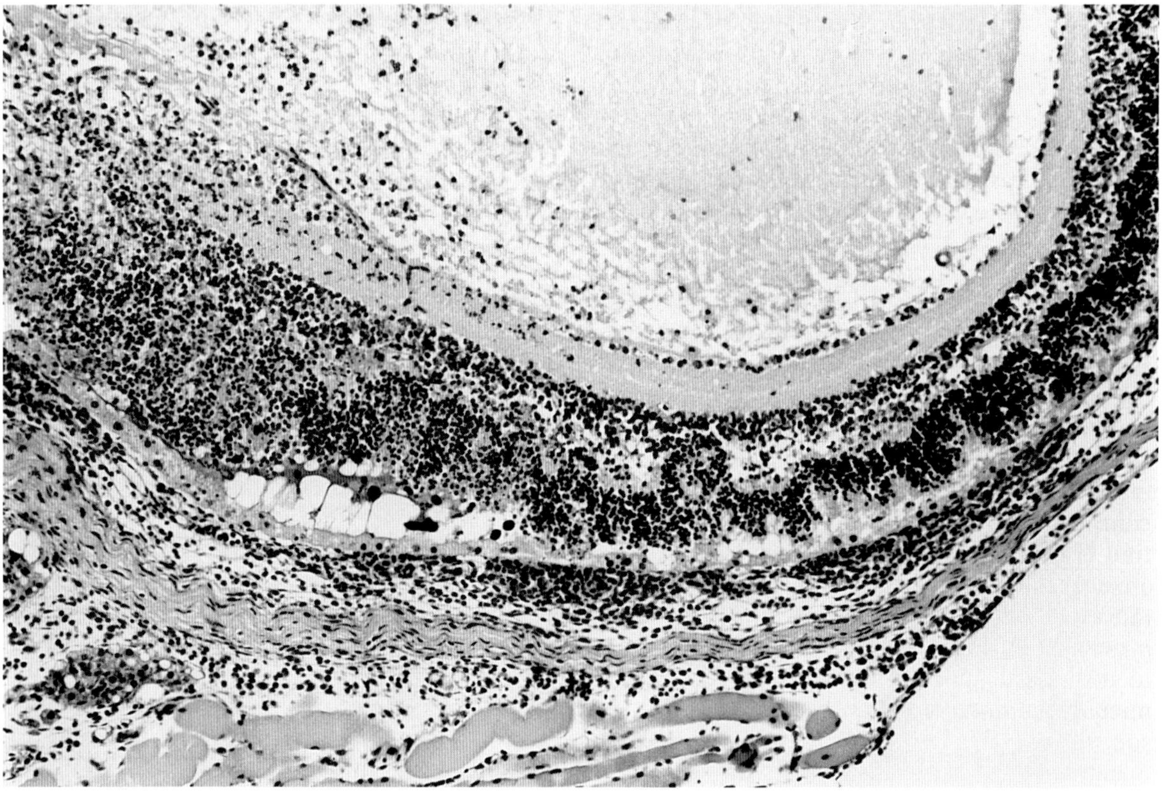

Fig. 91 *(above).* Anterior segment, uninoculated eye, BALB/c mouse 10 days after inoculation into opposite eye. Note: anterior uveitis and inflammatory cells in the anterior chamber. All layers of the peripheral retina are diffusely infiltrated. H & E, ×140

Fig. 92 *(below).* Retina of the uninoculated eye, BALB/c mouse 10 days after uniocular anterior chamber inoculation of HSV-1. Part of the retina is necrotic subjacent to an area of retinal schisis; the remaining retina is infiltrated in all layers. *Note:* karyorrhexis, loss of the photoreceptors, and massive choroiditis. H & E, ×140 jected eyes coincident with retinitis (Holland et al. 1987). These results support the hypothesis that retinitits results, at least in part, from the presence of virus in the uninoculated eye.

Biologic Features

The pathogenesis of retinitis observed in the uninjected eyes of micc aftcr uniocular antcrior chamber inoculation of the KOS strain of HSV-L results from the interplay of several variablcs: (1) the strain of HSV-L used for the experiments, (2) the titer of virus in the uninoculated eye, (3) the immune response of the host, (4) the innate susceptibility of the mouse strain to herpes simplex virus infection, and (5) additional factors related to the amount of posterior segment inflammation and to the integrity of the retinal architecture.

The pathogenesis of disease in the uninoculated eye is influenced by the strain of HSV-1 used for the anterior chamber inoculation. Unicameral anterior chamber injection of strains recently isolated from human patients with herpetic ocular and nonocular diseases and other more neurovirulent laboratory strains often does not produce the same bilateral pattern of ocular disease and may cause death of the mouse from encephalitis before the onset of retinal necrosis in the uninoculated eye. Live virus is required for production of disease in the uninoculated eye. On day 10 postinoculation (the time at which the maximum titer of virus is recovered from the uninoculated eye), virus titers from eyes of mice with clinical evidence of retinitis were compared with the titers of virus recovered from the contralateral eyes of BALB/c mice without retinitis. At this point, there was significantly more virus in the eyes of mice with retinitis than was recovered from the eyes of animals without clinical evidence of retinitis (5.57 +0.13 vs. 2.20 +0.36 log 10 PFUs/ml; $p < 0.001$) (Cousins et al. 1989). It is interesting to note that all uninoculated eyes of BALB/c mice contain virus at day 10; however, the reason why only 75% of the contralateral eyes have a high titer of virus and develop retinitis remains to be answered (Atherton and Streilein 1987 a, b).

The injection of ultraviolet-inactivated virus into one anterior chamber does not cause disease in either eye, a finding which confirms the requirement for infectious virus and which discounts the possibility that the retinal reaction in the contralateral eye is due merely to a sympathetic ophthalmia.

Both the ability of the animal to make an immune response to the virus and the type of immune response appear to be important in the pathogenesis of this disease. The host must be immunocompetent in order to clear infectious virus from the ocular and central nervous system structures. When HSV-1 is injected into one anterior chamber of BALB/c *nu/nu* (athymic) mice, retinitis is observed in both eyes, suggesting that protection of the ipsilateral retina of immunocompetent mice from total necrosis is immune mediated. Protection of the ipsilateral retina can be restored by adoptive transfer of T cells. Athymic BALB/c mice succumb to encephalitis in 10 – 14 days (Whittum-Hudson et al. 1985).

Injection of the KOS strain of HSV-1 into one eye of an immunocompetent euthymic BALB/c mouse induces *anterior chamber associated immune deviation,* the hallmarks of which are: (1) suppression of virus-specific delayed hypersensitivity responsiveness and (2) vigorous production of virus-specific neutralizing antibody (Whittum et al. 1983). The role of this phenomenon in the unique pattern of bilateral ocular disease which follows anterior chamber injection of HSV-1 may be to allow virus to replicate in the injected eye and to spread from there to the central nervous system and to the contralateral eye (Streilein et al. 1987). In this ocular system, the induction of anterior chamber associated immune deviation and the herpes virus resistance of the host mouse may be interconnected. By using other strains of mice, it has been demonstrated that mice from the HSV-1-susceptible strain DBA/2 develop both the immune deviation and contralateral retinitis following uninocular anterior chamber injection of HSV-1. Similar to HSV-1-inoculated BALB/c mice, DBA/2 mice that develop contralateral retinitis have high titers of virus in the uninoculated eye at day 10. In contrast, mice of the HSV-1-resistant strain C57BL/6 do not develop retinitis following uninocular anterior chamber injection of HSV-1 (Pepose and Whittum-Hudson 1987). C57BL/6 mice also develop vigorous virus-specific delayed hypersensitivity responsiveness following anterior chamber inoculation of HSV-1 (KOS). Mice of the strains resistant to HSV-1 have low titers of virus in the contralateral eye at day 10. These results suggest that the ability of the host to make a delayed hypersensitivity response to the virus after anterior chamber inoculation allows the animal to limit the replication of virus in the ipsilateral eye and brain and hence the amount of second-wave virus which reaches the contralateral eye (Kielty et al. 1987).

Infectious virus and viral antigens are present in the retina of the uninoculated eye at the time when retinitis occurs (Pepose and Whittum-Hudson 1987; Whittum-Hudson and Pepose 1987). Traction-induced schisis affects both the physical and physiologic integrity of the retina. However, it is still not clear how much of the damage to the retina of the uninoculated eye is due to the direct cytopathic effect of the virus; how much is due to virus-specific, host-mediated cytotoxicity toward virus-infected retinal cells; and how much is due to "innocent" bystander damage of uninfected retinal tissue caused by inflammation in the intraocular compartment of the uninoculated eye.

Comparison with Other Species

Some features of the model of herpes simplex virus type 1 retinitis resemble the human disease acute retinal necrosis. Both the mouse model of retinitis and the human disease are characterized by acute and rapidly progressive retinal inflammation. The human disease has been shown to be caused by several members of the herpesvirus family, varicella zoster virus, HSV-1, and HSV-2 (Culbertson et al. 1986; Freeman et al. 1986; Dix et al. 1988). Clinical features such as episcleritis, retinal vasculitis, and retinitis are similar between the human and the mouse disease. Papillitis, scleritis, granulomatous choroiditis, and migration of retinal pigment epithelium occur in both, and vitreous infiltration and traction are important features of both diseases. Several features, however, distinguish the two. Tractional schisis is not an important feature of acute retinal necrosis even though late retinal detachments do occur in these patients. The requirement for anterior chamber presentation of the virus probably does not have a direct human counterpart. However, since intracerebral inoculation of HSV-1 has been shown to produce a bilateral retinal necrosis in mice similar to that observed in the contralateral eye of a BALB/c mouse inoculated in one anterior chamber with HSV-1 (Pfeiffer et al. 1983); Anderson and Field 1984), it is possible that the brain of a patient with acute retinal necrosis could have a depot of latent virus which upon reactivation could be transported to the eye. This could occur via routes similar to those responsible for intraocular and central nervous system spread in the mouse.

References

Anderson JR, Field HJ (1984) An animal model of ocular herpes. Keratitis, retinitis and cataract in the mouse. Br J Exp Pathol 65: 283–297

Atherton SS, Streilein JW (1987a) Virus-specific DTH prevents contralateral retinitis following intracameral inoculation of HSV-2. Curr Eye Res 6: 133–139

Atherton SS, Streilein JW (1987b) Two waves of virus following anterior chamber inoculation of HSV-1. Invest Ophthalmol Vis Sci 28: 571–579

Cousins SW, Gonzalez A, Atherton SS (1989) Herpes simplex retinitis in the mouse: clinicopathologic correlations. Invest Ophthalmol Vis Sci 30: 1485–1494

Culbertson WW, Blumenkranz MS, Pepose JS, Stewart JA, Curtin VT (1986) Varicella zoster is a cause of the acute retinal necrosis syndrome. Ophthalmology 93: 559–569

Dix RD, Stewart RV, Culbertson W, Atherton SS, Vann V, Miller D, Lewis ML (1988) Clinical association of herpes simplex virus type I (HSV-1) with acute retinal necrosis. Invest Ophthalmol Vis Sci [Suppl] 29: 159

Freeman WR, Thomas EL, Rao NA, Pepose JS, Trousdale MD, Howes EL, Nadel AJ, Mines JA, Bowe B (1986) Demonstration of herpes group virus in active retinal necrosis syndrome. Am J Ophthalmol 102: 701–709

Hamasaki DI, Dix RD, Atherton SS (1988) Bilateral alterations of the ERG and retinal histology following unilateral HSV-L inoculation. Invest Ophthalmol Vis Sci 29: 1242–1254

Holland GN, Togni BI, Briones OC, Dawson CR (1987) A microscopic study of herpes simplex virus retinopathy in mice. Invest Ophthalmol Vis Sci 28: 1181–1190

Kielty D, Cousins SW, Atherton SS (1987) HSV-L retinitis and delayed hypersensitivity in DBA/2 and C57BL/6 mice. Invest Ophthalmol Vis Sci 28: 1994–1999

Olson RM, Holland GN, Goss SJ, Bowers WD, Meyers-Elliot RH (1987) Routes of viral spread in the von Szily model of herpes simplex virus retinopathy. Curr Eye Res 6: 59–62

Peiffer RL Jr, Dekker CD, Siegel FL (1983) Ocular lesions in mice following intracerebral injection of herpes simplex virus type 1. Invest Ophthalmol Vis Sci 24: 1070–1078

Pepose JS, Whittum-Hudson JA (1987) An immunogenetic analysis of resistance to herpes simplex versus retinitis in inbred strains of mice. Invest Ophthalmol Vis Sci 28: 1549–1552

Streilein JW, Atherton SS, Vann V (1987) A critical role for ACAID in the distinctive pattern of retinitis that follows anterior chamber inoculation of HSV-I. Curr Eye Res 6: 127–131

Whittum JA, Niederkorn JY, McCulley JP, Streilein JW (1983) Intracameral inoculation of herpes simplex

virus type 1 induces anterior chamber associated immune deviation. Curr Eye Res 2: 691–697
Whittum JA, McCulley JP, Niederkorn JY, Streilein JW (1984) Ocular disease induced in mice by anterior chamber inoculation of herpes simplex virus. Invest Ophthalmol Vis Sci 25: 1065–1073
Whittum-Hudson JA, Pepose JS (1987) Immunologic modulation of virus-induced pathology in a murine model of acute herpetic retinal necrosis. Invest Ophthalmol Vis Sci 28: 1541–1548
Whittum-Hudson JA, Farazdaghi M, Prendergast RA (1985) A role for T lymphocytes in preventing experimental herpes simplex virus type 1-induced retinitis. Invest Ophthalmol Vis Sci 26: 1524–1532

Lymphocytic Choriomeningitis Virus Infection, Experimental, Eye, Rat

Herbert E. Whiteley, Sally S. Atherton, and John A. Shadduck

Synonyms. None.

Gross Appearance

Most rats inoculated with lymphocytic choriomeningitis virus intracerebrally at birth do not develop external lesions, although in a few corneal leukoma may be seen 2 months after infection. Others develop iridocorneal adhesions within 10 months (del Cerro et al. 1982). Funduscopic examination reveals mottling of the retinal pigment epithelium, vascular attenuation, thinning of the retina, and retinal detachment with or without subretinal hemorrhage or exudate (del Cerro et al. 1982). Electroretinographic examination demonstrates a continual reduction in a- and b-wave response beginning by 2 months postinoculation and resulting in some eyes failing to respond by 10 months postinoculation (del Cerro et al. 1982).

Microscopic Features

The initial lesion identified at 2 months after intracerebral inoculation of neonatal rats is an inflammatory cell infiltrate consisting of macrophages in the subretinal space (Fig. 93) (del Cerro et al. 1984). This cellular infiltrate is associated with areas of retinal detachment and focal loss of inner and outer segments. Smaller numbers of macrophages are also found within the vitreous along the internal limiting membrane (Fig. 94). Dysplastic rosettes composed of photoreceptor cells (Fig. 95) and intraretinal cysts are also found. Retinal destruction continues with time; lymphocytes and plasma cells are mixed with macrophages. Complete destruction of all retinal layers can occur with replacement by fibrovascular tissue and proliferating pigment epithelial cells (Fig. 96) (del Cerro et al. 1982). The inflammatory response affects principally the retina, does not have a significant neutrophilic component, and does not involve the uvea.

Ultrastructure

Initial changes in the loss of photoreceptor cells are characterized by outer segment disorganization with subsequent involvement of inner segments and cell bodies. These cells become necrotic in situ or are extruded into the subretinal space (del Cerro et al. 1982). Macrophages in the lumina of dysplastic rosettes contain ingested fragments of outer segments. In addition, macrophages mixed with fibrin are present along the vitreal surface of the retina.

As retinal degeneration progresses, the associated retinal pigment epithelial cells develop hyperplastic apical microvilli, microvilli on the lateral surface, and numerous intracellular phagosomes. Retinal pigment epithelium (RPE) may also become hyperplastic and vascularized (del Cerro et al. 1982).

Differential Diagnosis

Spontaneous retinitis and uveitis are rare in mice and rats. Immunohistochemical techniques should reveal the presence of LCM virus, at

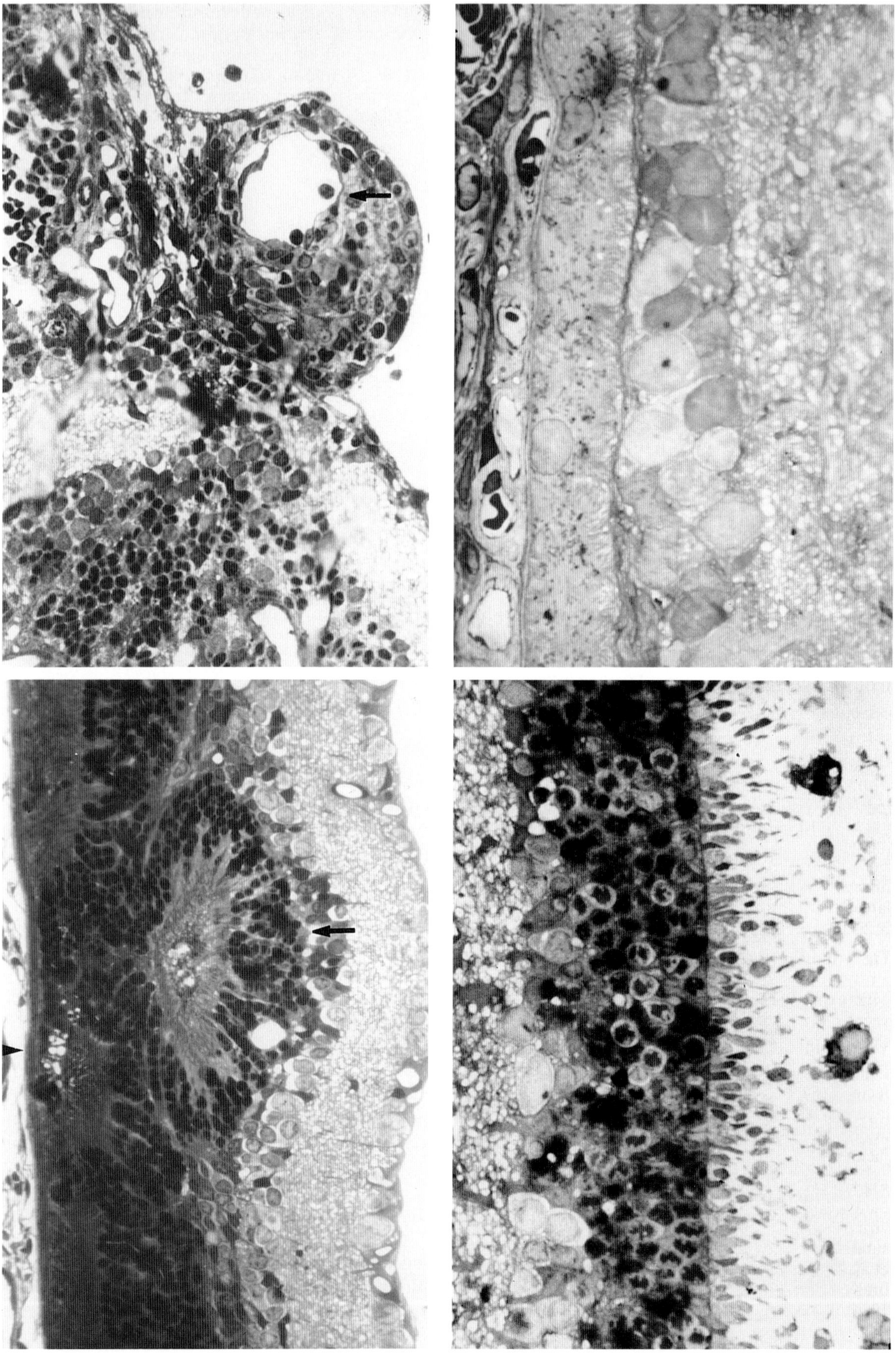

least in the early stages, and thus permit the diagnosis of spontaneously occurring LCM infections which might occur in control animals.

Biologic Features

The features of newborn rats inoculated intracerebrally with lymphocytic choriomeningitis virus are consistent with a rapidly progressing immune-mediated retinitis with persistence of viral antigen in the specifically affected tissues (Silverstein et al. 1976). Even after viral antigens have disappeared, the retinitis continues, suggesting it could be, at least in part, a chronic response to release of sequestered retinal antigens (del Cerro et al. 1982). The lesion process can be abrogated by neonatal thymectomy or significantly reduced by treatment with antilymphoid serum (Monjan and Hogan 1979). Less severe, although similar, lesions are found in offspring of dams exposed to the virus; this may be due to some degree of immune response (del Cerro et al. 1984).

Lymphocytic choriomeningitis of the newborn rat produces extensive retinitis and retinal dysplasia with minimal uveal involvement and subsequent severe retinal degeneration. This differs from the disease in adult mice, in which there is primarily uveitis with variable involvement of the retina (Silverstein et al. 1976; Ticho et al. 1974a, b). As in the rat, however, the inflammatory changes and concomitant tissue injury follow the distribution of viral antigen (Ticho et al. 1974a). Differences are probably due to the ability of various tissues to support viral replication, in association with the stage of maturation (Silverstein et al. 1976).

◂ **Fig. 93** *(upper left).* Retina from rat on postnatal day 30, infected on the day of birth with lymphocytic choriomeningitis virus. Mononuclear cell (macrophage) infiltration around a retinal vessel *(arrow)* with some similar cells in the vitreous. (From del Cerro et al. 1982) ×200

Fig. 94 *(lower left).* Retinal rosettes *(arrow)* and folds in a rat on postnatal day 15, infected at birth with lymphocytic choriomeningitis virus. Note the focal loss and vacuolization *(arrowhead)* of the retinal pigment epithelium. (From del Cerro et al. 1982) ×200

Fig. 95 *(upper right).* Retina from a 13-month-old rat infected at birth. Total degeneration of the outer nuclear layer and inner and outer segments with the remaining attenuated inner nuclear layer lying on the retinal pigment epithelia. (From del Cerro et al. 1982) ×800

Fig. 96 *(lower right).* Retina from a 65-day-old rat whose dam was infected with lymphocytic choriomeningitis virus. Macrophages with ingested cell debris are in the subretinal space. This congenital infection (del Cerro et al. 1984) has similar lesions to those rats intracerebrally inoculated with LCM virus. (From del Cerro et al. 1984) ×400

Comparison with Other Species

Although lymphocytic choriomeningitis is an interesting experimental model, it has no direct spontaneous counterpart in other species. Some aspects of the response, namely retinal dysplasia and neovascularization, are similar to simian virus 40 induced retinopathy in the neonatal rat (Friedman et al. 1973). Gliosis, atrophy, retinal dysplasia, and perivascular lymphocytic cuffing are also features of the retinopathy induced by intracerebral inoculation of measles virus into suckling Wistar rats (Percy and Coulter-Mackie 1982).

References

del Cerro M, Grover DA, Monjan AA, Pfau CJ, Dematte JE (1982) Chronic retinitis in rats infected as neonates with lymphocytic choriomeningitis virus: a clinical, histopathologic, and electroretinographic study. Invest Ophthalmol Vis Sci 23: 697–714

del Cerro M, Grover D, Monjan AA, Pfau C, Dematte J (1984) Congenital retinitis in the rat following maternal exposure to lymphocytic choriomeningitis virus. Exp Eye Res 38: 313–324

Friedman AH, Bellhorn RW, Henkind P (1973) Simian virus 40-induced retinopathy in the rat. Invest Ophthalmol 12: 591–595

Monjan AA, Hogan RN (1979) Virus-induced retinal dystrophy in the immunologically compromised host. In: Silverstein AM, O'Connor GR (eds) Immunology and immunopathology of the eye. Masson, New York, pp 370–374

Percy DH, Coulter-Mackie M (1982) Measles virus encephalitis and retinopathy in the Wistar rat. Exp Mol Pathol 36: 435–446

Silverstein AM, Ticho U, Monjan AA, Cole GA (1976) Lymphocytic choriomeningitis virus-induced ocular immunopathology. Mod Probl Ophthalmol 16: 208–214

Ticho U, Cole GA, Silverstein AM (1974a) Immunopathologic uveitis in the mouse due to lymphocytic choriomeningitis virus. Invest Ophthalmol 13: 33–38

Ticho U, Silverstein AM, Cole GA (1974b) Immunopathogenesis of LCM virus-induced uveitis: the role of T lymphocytes. Invest Ophthalmol 13: 229–231

Cytomegalovirus Infection, Experimental, Eye, Mouse

Herbert E. Whiteley, Sally S. Atherton, and John A. Shadduck

Synonyms. None.

Gross Appearance

Not described.

Microscopic Features

Intravitreal inoculation of murine cytomegalovirus into mice initiates a neutrophilic inflammatory response within 1 day, involving the ciliary body, iris, and cornea. This progresses within 4 days to a mixed cellular response containing mononuclear cells and neutrophils and the additional involvement of the anterior chamber, optic nerve, and sclera. The inflammation is most severe at the iridocorneal (filtration) angle and in the optic nerve. Fibrosis of the iris with anterior and posterior synechia subsequently develop (Schwartz et al. 1974).

Intranuclear and intracytoplasmic eosinophilic inclusion bodies can be identified by the 2nd day after inoculation in the epithelium of the iris and ciliary body (Fig. 97), corneal endothelium, and retinal pigment epithelium. Degeneration and loss of photoreceptor cell nuclei and inner and outer segments occur in areas overlying retinal pigment epithelial cells that contain viral inclusion bodies. Inflammation is not a feature of this change (Schwartz et al. 1974).

Ultrastructure

Viral particles are found in cells that have histologically identifiable inclusion bodies. Degeneration of photoreceptor cells, characterized by fragmentation and disorganization of outer segments, is found in areas adjacent to viral particles in retinal pigment epithelial cells. Viral particles are not found in any of the retinal cells including ganglion cells, cells of the inner nu-

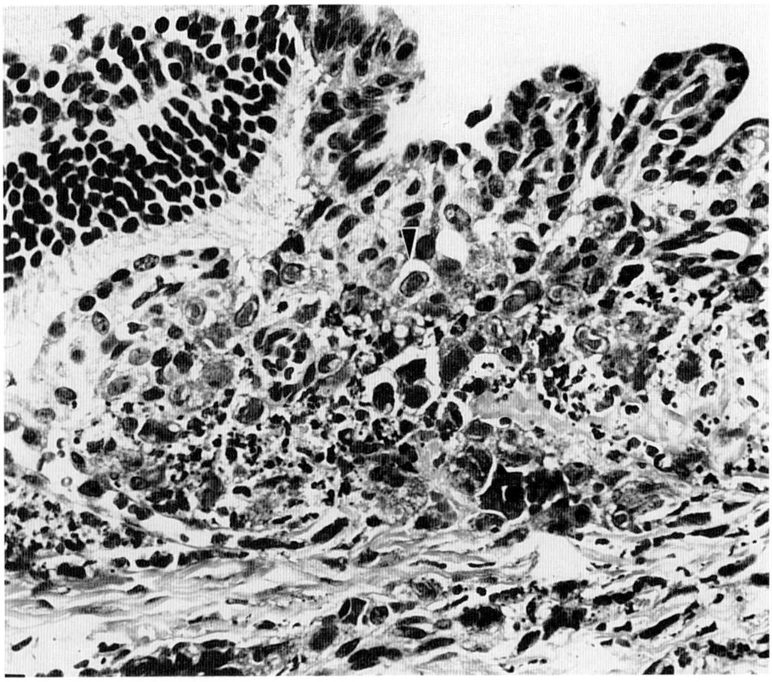

Fig. 97. Anterior uveitis from a mouse injected with the Smith strain of murine cytomegalovirus via the supraciliary route. Note numerous intranuclear inclusion bodies in the ciliary body *(arrowhead)* and suppurative inflammatory infiltrate and necrotic debris. (From Atherton and Cousins 1990) ×400

clear layer, and photoreceptor cells (Schwartz et al. 1974).

Differential Diagnosis

The presence of intranuclear inclusion bodies should distinguish cytomegalovirus infections from spontaneously occurring ophthalmitis.

Biologic Features

The inflammatory lesions in the anterior uveal tract are associated with cell necrosis and release of virus as indicated by a rising titer of recoverable virus (Schwartz et al. 1974). Virus inoculated by the intraperitoneal or intracranial route will often produce a transient mononuclear inflammatory reaction in the anterior uveal tract and persist in a latent stage for at least 90–120 days in intraocular fluid or optic nerve (Bale et al. 1984; Hayashi et al. 1985). Virus reaches its highest titer in intraocular fluid by 20 days after infection. Virus can also persist in extraocular structures including the lacrimal gland and extraocular muscles (Hayashi et al. 1985). The degree of tissue involvement is probably related to virus passage history, mouse strain, and age at time of infection (Hayashi et al. 1985).

Comparison with Other Species

The lesion produced by intravitreal exposure of mice to virus differs from that found in humans in which a severe chronic necrotizing retinitis is often associated with immunosuppression (Schwartz et al. 1974) or congenital infections (Smith et al. 1966).

References

Atherton SS, Cousins SW (1990) A model of focal necrotizing retinitis using murine cytomegalovirus. Invest Ophthalmol Vis Sci [Suppl] 31: 570
Bale JF Jr, O'Neil ME, Hogan RN, Kern ER (1984) Experimental murine cytomegalovirus infection of ocular structures. Arch Ophthalmol 102: 1214–1219
Hayashi K, Kurihara I, Uchida Y (1985) Studies of ocular murine cytomegalovirus infection. Invest Ophthalmol Vis Sci 26: 486–493
Schwartz JN, Daniels CA, Shivers JC, Klintworth GK (1974) Experimental cytomegalovirus ophthalmitis. Am J Pathol 77: 477–492
Smith ME, Zimmerman LE, Harley RD (1966) Ocular involvement in congenital cytomegalic inclusion disease. Arch Ophthalmol 76: 696–699

Scrapie and Other Experimental Infections, Eye, Mouse

Herbert E. Whiteley, Sally S. Atherton, and John A. Shadduck

Synonyms. None.

Gross Features

Gross lesions are not seen.

Microscopic Features

Intracerebral inoculation of the scrapie agent into young mice affects the sensory retina, in which there is loss of photoreceptor inner and outer segments and a marked reduction in the thickness of the outer nucelar layer (Figs. 98, 99). In the most severe cases, there is almost complete loss of the outer nuclear and outer plexiform layer, permitting the inner nuclear layer to rest on the retinal pigment epithelium (Kozlowski et al. 1982). The most severe lesions occur in the central portion of the retina. Although not a major feature of the change, macrophages are occasionally found in the subretinal space (Foster et al. 1986a, b). Acute inflammation or changes in other retinal layers or ocular structures are not a histologic feature of the response.

Ultrastructure

Electron microscopic lesions of murine scrapie have not been described; however, these lesions may be similar to those of the hamster scrapie

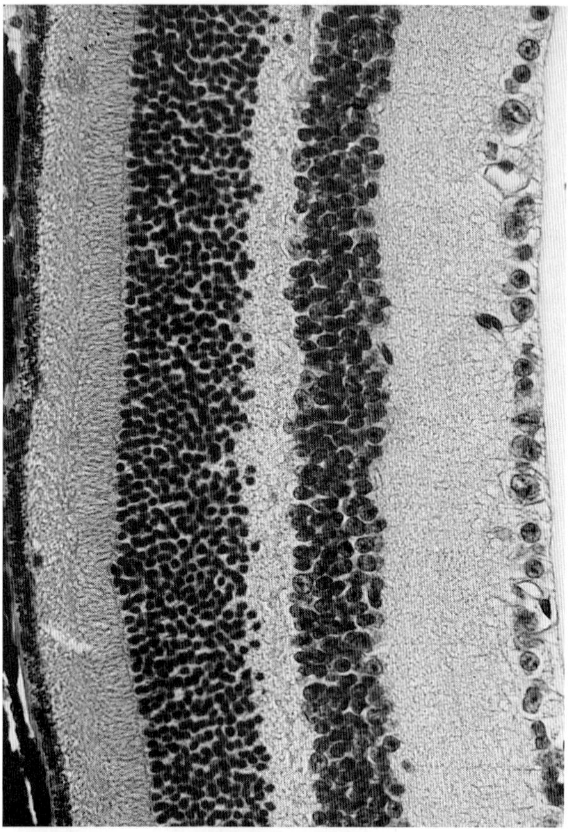

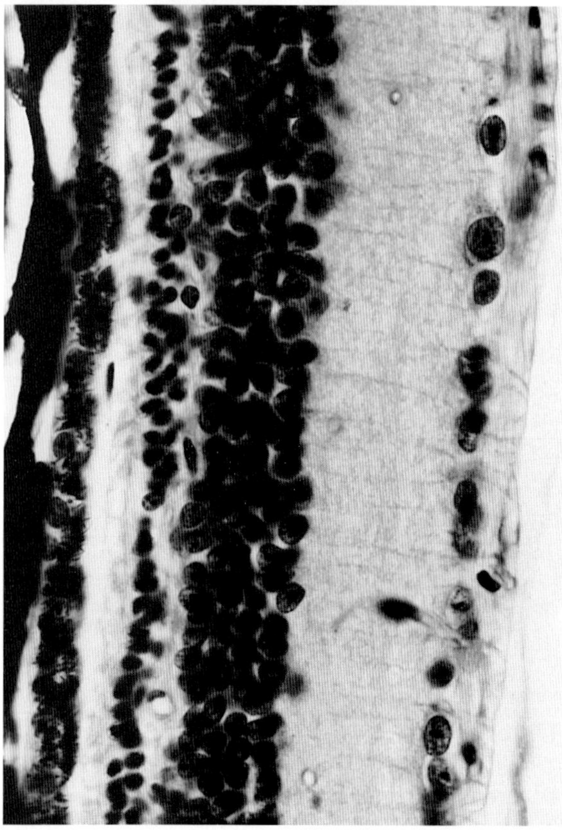

model (Buyukmichi et al. 1982) and to experimental Creutzfeldt-Jakob disease in mice (Hogan et al. 1983). Degenerative changes of the retina initially affect the outer and inner segments of photoreceptor cells. Membranous whorls and cell debris are found in the subretinal space or within macrophages found in this region. Eventually all outer segments are lost and few inner segments remain. Extant photoreceptor cell bodies are often surrounded by Müller cell processes. Retinal pigment epithelial cells are usually unaffected.

Differential Diagnosis

Light-induced retinopathy (see p. 82, this volume) has similar histologic features.

Biologic Features

Scrapie, a naturally occurring spongiform encephalopathy of sheep and goats, is characterized by spongy vacuolar degeneration of gray and sometimes white matter (Fraser 1976) and can be transmitted to laboratory rodents such as mice and hamsters. Retinal degeneration involving the photoreceptor cell layer is found in both naturally occurring (Barnett and Palmer 1971) and experimental disease.

The severity of scrapie-induced retinopathy in mice depends on the interaction between strain of virus and strain of mouse (Foster et al. 1986a). Light-induced retinopathy has a similar histologic appearance to the degenerative changes induced by the scrapie agent. Lesions of scrapie, however, were induced in mice maintained in total darkness (Foster et al. 1986b) and in pigmented mice (Kozlowski et al. 1982), indicating a direct effect of the scrapie agent and not a change secondary to excessive exposure to light.

◂ **Fig. 98** *(above).* Retina, C57BL control mouse. (From Fraser 1976) H & E, ×350

Fig. 99 *(below).* Retina from a 195-day-old C57BL mouse that was inoculated intracerebrally with the 79A strain of scrapie virus as a neonate. Note degeneration and loss of inner and outer segments with a severe loss of cells in the outer nuclear layer. (From Fraser 1976) H & E, ×550

When mice are inoculated intracerebrally with Creutzfeldt-Jakob disease material, they develop a marked retinal degeneration characterized by loss of inner and outer segments and a severe reduction in the thickness of the outer nuclear layer. Macrophages are also found in the outer nuclear layer and subretinal space (Hogan et al. 1983). Vacuolation and slight astrocytosis occur in the optic nerve. Other ocular structures, including retinal pigment epithelium, lens, cornea, vitreous, and choroid are not affected.

Table 10. Ocular lesions of scrapie and Creutzfeldt-Jacob disease in mice and hamsters

	Scrapie[a], mice	Early CJD[b], mice	Terminal scrapie,[c] hamster
Extensive degeneration, ONL, IS, OS	+	+	+
Ganglion cell degeneration	+/–	+/–	+/–
Macrophage infiltration			
Subretinal	+	+	+
ONL	+/–	+	+
INL	–	+/–	–
GCL	–	+/–	–
Spongiform vacuolation			
Retina	–	–	–
Optic nerve	–	+	–

Abbreviations: ONL, outer nuclear layer; IS, inner segment; OS, outer segment; INL, inner nuclear layer; GCL, ganglion cell layer; +, lesion present; +/–, lesion occasionally found; –, lesion usually not found; CJD, Creutzfeldt-Jacob disease.
[a] Kozlowski et al. 1982.
[b] Hogan et al. 1983.
[c] Buyukmichi et al. 1982.

Comparison with Other Species

The lesions of scrapie and Creutzfeldt-Jakob disease in mice are similar to those of experimental scrapie in hamsters (Buyukmichi et al. 1982), although the rapidity with which lesions develop is variable (Table 10). The lesions of these experimental systems are also similar to those thought to occur with spontaneous Creutzfeldt-Jakob disease in man (Lesser et al. 1979; Albert and Weiss 1983).

Other Infections

Several other infectious agents have been demonstrated to cause ocular lesions when experimentally introduced into the eye or nervous system. Some of these are outlined in Table 11.

Table 11. Other experimental viral infections, rat and mouse

Agent	Major lesions	References
Suckling mouse Cataract agent	Cataract formation, panophthalmitis, phthisis bulbi	Olmsted et al. 1966 Clark 1969
St. Louis encephalitis virus	Cataract, micophthalmus	Hanna et al. 1968
Rubella	Cataract, retinopathy	Bohigian et al. 1968
Borna virus	Retinitis	Narayan et al. 1983
Semliki forest virus	Optic nerve demyelination	Tansey et al. 1985
Simian virus 40	Retinal neovascularization, retinal folds, gliosis	Friedman et al. 1973
Measles virus	Retinitis, perivascular cuffing, gliosis, atrophy, dysplasia of retina	Percy and Coulter-Mackie 1982

References

Albert DM, Weiss JS (1983) Experimental Creutzfeldt-Jakob disease: clue to etiology of certain human retinal degenerative diseases (editorial). Lab Invest 49: 633–635

Barnett KC, Palmer AC (1971) Retinopathy in sheep affected with natural scrapie. Res Vet Sci 12: 383–385

Bohigian GM, Fox J, Cotlier E (1968) Immunofluorescent localization of rubella virus in the lens, retina and heart of congenital rubella-infected rats. Am J Ophthalmol 65: 196–201

Buyukmichi N, Goehring-Harmon F, Marsh RF (1982) Retinal degeneration during clinical scrapie encephalopathy in hamsters. J Comp Neurol 205: 153–160

Clark HF (1969) Rat cataract induced by suckling mouse cataract agent. Am J Ophthalmol 68: 304–308

Foster JD, Davies DJ, Fraser H (1986 a) Primary retinopathy in scrapie in mice deprived of light. Neurosci Lett 72: 111–114

Foster JD, Fraser H, Bruce HE (1986 b) Retinopathy in mice with experimental scrapie. Neuropathol Appl Neurobiol 12: 185–196

Fraser H (1976) The pathology of a natural and experimental scrapie. Front Biol 44: 267–305
Friedman AH, Bellhorn RW, Henkind P (1973) Simian virus 40-induced retinopathy in the rat. Invest Ophthalmol 12: 591–595
Hanna C, Jarman RV, Keatts JG, Duffy CE (1968) Virus-induced cataracts – incidence and development in rats after intracerebral inoculation of St. Louis encephalitis virus. Arch Ophthalmol 79: 59–63
Hogan RN, Kingsbury DT, Baringer JR, Prusiner SB (1983) Retinal degeneration in experimental Creutzfeldt-Jakob disease. Lab Invest 49: 708–715
Kozlowski PB, Moretz RC, Carp RI, Wisniewski HM (1982) Retinal damage in scrapie mice. Acta Neuropathol 56: 9–12
Lesser RL, Albert DM, Bobowick AR, O'Brien FH (1979) Creutzfeldt-Jakob disease and optic atrophy. Am J Ophthalmol 87 (3): 317–321
Narayan O, Herzog S, Frese K, Scheefers H, Rott R (1983) Pathogenesis of Borna disease in rats: immune-mediated viral ophthalmoencephalopathy causing blindness and behavioral abnormalities. J Infect Dis 148: 305–315
Olmsted E, Prasad S, Sheffer J, Clark HF, Karzon DT (1966) Ocular lesions induced in C57 mice by the suckling mouse cataract agent (SMCA). Invest Ophthalmol 5: 413–420
Percy DH, Coulter-Mackie M (1982) Measles virus encephalitis and retinopathy in the Wistar rat. Exp Mol Pathol 36: 435–446
Tansey EM, Pessoa VF, Fleming S, Landon DN, Ikeda H (1985) Pattern and extent of demyelination in the optic nerves of mice infected with Semliki Forest virus and the possibility of axonal sprouting. Brain 108 (1): 29–41

Retinoblastoma, Experimental, Rat and Hamster

John A. Shadduck and Jeffrey I. Everitt

Synonyms. None.

Gross Appearance

These lesions occur when human adenovirus type 12 (Huie strain) is administered in high doses intraocularly to CD rats (Kobayashi and Mukai 1973, 1974). They also appear in hamsters inoculated intraocularly as newborns with JC (human papovavirus) (Ohashi et al. 1978). The gross appearance is that of a gray-pink, soft, mottled mass extending into the vitreous. In larger tumors, neoplastic cells invade the anterior chamber producing dislocation or damage of the lens. The tumor may extend extraorbitally into the optic nerve. Necrosis of these cells tends to occur at the posterior edge of the ciliary body.

Microscopic Features

Most experimental retinoblastomas are composed primarily of small, uniform hyperchromatic, undifferentiated cells that form perivascular wreaths. Tumor cells have irregularly shaped, round, or slightly elongated hyperchromatic nuclei and small amounts of poorly defined cytoplasm. The small tumor cells are arrayed in uniform tubular alignment or in columnar patterns suggestive of neuroepithelium. Numerous incomplete rosettes (often referred to as Homer-Wright rosettes) are seen. Mitotic figures are frequent and many tumors undergo hemorrhagic necrosis. The degenerated tumor cells often surround nondegenerated cells adjacent to blood vessels, resulting in a trabecular or papillary appearance. Uniform, neuroblastic cells sometimes form syncytial giant cells. Clusters of bizarre ganglioneuronic tumor cells are common, especially in highly vascularized areas between the more solid portions of the tumor (Kobayashi and Mukai 1974).

A zone of transition sometimes occurs between the tumor proper and the retina. This zone is characterized by dysplastic ganglioneuronic cells that lie within the inner half of the retina adjacent to the tumor. The giant cells in the innermost layer of the otherwise normal-appearing retina are sometimes accompanied by an intense inflammatory response characterized by large numbers of eosinophils. In more advanced cases, tumor cell infiltration into the sclera may be accompanied by episcleral lymphocytic inflammation. Intraocular inflammation characterized by plasma cells and large lymphocytes may occur in the anterior chamber and choroid. Immunofluorescence techniques reveal the presence of adenovirus 12 T antigens in the retinal tumor cells. Ohashi et al. (1978) reported that 11 of 54 hamsters given JC (human papovavirus) intraocularly as newborns developed intraocular neoplasms by 7.5–13 months after inoculation. Eight of the tumors were classified as retinoblastomas based on a morphologic picture characterized by rich cellularity, high mitotic index, Homer-Wright rosettes, cilia with a 9 + 0 tubular pattern, and neuronal processes with microtubules and microfilaments. Other tumors, including neoplasms of the central and peripheral nervous system, also occurred in these animals. Similar tumors were produced in mice following intraocular inoculation of adenovirus 12 (Mukai et al. 1977).

Transformed cells have been induced in vitro by human adenovirus type 12 in retinal cultures derived from weanling hamsters (Albert et al. 1968). Upon intraocular injection of these transformed retinal cells into irradiated hamsters, neoplasms were observed which were composed of layers of dark cells with scant cytoplasm and large dark nuclei. No rosettes or neural elements could be identified (Albert et al. 1974).

Ultrastructure

In rats inoculated with adenovirus 12, the tumor cells that form the incomplete rosettes possess elongated, oval, or slightly indented nuclei and evenly distributed chromatin. The apical processes of the tumor cells form irregularly shaped lumens but there are no terminal bars. Triple-layered nuclear membrane profiles are variably present. Cytoplasmic processes which face the lumen of a rosette contain poorly differentiated intracytoplasmic organelles. Solitary cilia with a 9 + 0 tubular pattern are seen in the apical portion of the rim of cytoplasm where mitochondria appear to converge. Several projecting cilia associated with multiple pairs of centrioles can be seen in the syncytial giant cells (Kobayashi and Mukai 1974; Mukai et al. 1974). Viral particles are not recognizable (Mukai et al. 1980).

Other structures commonly found include intercellular junctions of the zonula adherens type, triple-membrane structures, especially in association with the nuclear envelope, annulate lamellae, coated vesicles, and microtubules (Mukai et al. 1980).

Differential Diagnosis

Ocular neoplasms rarely appear spontaneously in rats or hamsters. No reports of spontaneously occurring retinoblastomas were obtained from the literature nor from a search of the files of the Registry of Comparative Pathology at the Armed Forces Institute of Pathology (Courtesy of George Migaki, DVM, Chief Pathologist).

Biologic Features

Adenovirus 12 induced retinoblastomas occur with various degrees of frequency in rats depending upon the age at which the animals are inoculated and on whether methylnitrosourea is used. Tumors are most easily produced if the experimental animals are inoculated intravitreously within a few hours after birth and the latent period is shorter if methylnitrosourea is used as a pretreatment. The incidence ranges from a low of about 5% to a high of about 45% of inoculated animals, and the latency ranges from approximately 40 to 360 days.

Much more consistent and rapid tumor induction was achieved when human adenovirus 12 transformed cell line of rat origin was transplanted to the vitreous of newborn inbred CDF rats (Kobayaski et al. 1982). All of 39 rats had clinical evidence of tumors within 30 days after implantation. The light and electron microscopic appearance of the tumors was essentially identical to that of the lesions induced in situ by adenovirus 12.

The tumors seem to grow relatively slowly and are observable clinically either as masses behind the lens or because they enlarge and distort the globe or produce exophthalmos by invading beneath the sclera. Tumors produced in rats by intraocular transplantation of adenovirus 12 transformed cells may perforate the eye (Winther 1986).

Comparison with Other Species

Mukai et al. (1980) listed five specific and five nonspecific features of human retinoblastomas. Of the five specific features, the tumors induced in rats with adenovirus 12 displayed two-namely, Homer-Wright rosettes (poorly differentiated rosettes, characteristic of neuroblastic tumors) and cilia with a 9 + 0 doublet microtubular pattern. Missing were Flexner-Wintersteiner rosettes (characteristic of more differentiated retinoblastomas), fleurettes, and photoreceptor differentiation (although ganglioneuronic differentiation was seen). All five of the nonspecific but commonly encountered features of human retinoblastomas were seen in the adenovirus 12 induced rat tumors. These included intercellular junctions, triple-membrane structures, annulate lamellae, coated vesicles, microtubules, and neurofilaments.

Lesions induced in immunosuppressed hamsters given retinal cells transformed in vitro by adenovirus 12 were not compared with human retinoblastomas, but the published description of the hamster lesions (Albert et al. 1968) suggests they are not classical retinoblastomas. Too few morphologic features of the JC virus induced rat tumors (Ohashi et al. 1978) were provided to permit adequate comparisons. Poorly differentiated retinoblastomas were also produced, among several other types of tumors, after intraocular injection of nickel subsulfide in rats (Albert et al. 1982). But these also do not seem to be classical retinoblastomas as seen in man. The available evidence indicates that neither adenovirus 12n nor JC virus is associated with human neuroblastomas (Ueno et al. 1987).

References

Albert DM, Rabson AS, Dalton AJ (1968) In vitro neoplastic transformation of uveal and retinal tissue by oncogenic DNA viruses. Invest Ophthalmol Vis Sci 7: 357–365

Albert DM, Lahav M, Lesser R, Craft J (1974) Recent observations regarding retinoblastoma. I. Ultrastructure, tissue culture growth, incidence, and animal models. Trans Am Ophthalmol Soc 94: 909–928

Albert DM, Gonder JR, Papale J, Craft JL, Dohlman HG, Reid MC, Sunderman FW Jr (1982) Induction of ocular neoplasms in Fischer rats by intraocular injection of nickel subsulfide. Invest Ophthalmol Vis Sci 22: 768–782

Kobayashi S, Mukai N (1973) Retinoblastoma-like tumors induced in rats by human adenovirus. Invest Ophthalmol Vis Sci 12: 853–856

Kobayashi S, Mukai N (1974) Retinoblastoma-like tumors induced by human adenovirus type 12 in rats. Cancer Res 34: 1646–1651

Kobayashi M, Mukai N, Solish SP, Pomeroy ME (1982) A highly predictable animal model of retinoblastoma. Acta Neuropathol (Berl) 57: 203–208

Mukai N, Kobayashi S, Oguri M (1974) Ultrastructural studies of human adenovirus-produced retinoblastoma-like neoplasms in Sprague-Dawley rats. Invest Ophthalmol Vis Sci 13: 593–601

Mukai N, Nakajima T, Freddo T, Jaobson M, Dunn M (1977) Retinoblastoma-like neoplasm induced in C3H/BifB/Ki strain mice by human adenovirus serotype 12. Acta Neuropathol (Berl) 39: 147–155

Mukai N, Nishida T, Nakajima T (1980) A DNA virus-induced model of retinoblastoma. Int Ophthalmol Clin 20: 223–245

Ohashi T, ZuRhein GM, Varakis JN, Padgett BL, Walker DL (1978) Experimental (JC virus-induced) intraocular and extraocular orbital tumors in the Syrian hamster. J Neuropathol Exp Neurol 37: 667

Ueno T, Suzuki N, Kaneko A, Fujinaga K (1987) Analysis of retinoblastoma for human adenovirus and human JC virus genome integration. Jpn J Ophthalmol 31: 274–283

Winther J (1986) In vitro and in vivo growth of an intraocular retinoblastoma-like tumour in F-344 rats. Acta Ophthalmol (Copenh) 64: 657–663

Toxic Retinopathy, Rat, Mouse, and Hamster

Steven R. Frame and William W. Carlton

Synonyms. Chemically induced retinal degeneration.

Gross Appearance

Retinal alterations produced in rodents by toxic compounds are usually not detected grossly except in cases of severe retinal atrophy, retinal detachment, or changes in the pigment content of the retina in the nonalbino rodent. These changes may be detected by careful gross examination (dissecting microscope and indirect illumination) at the time the globes are sectioned, prior to their preparation for histologic sectioning. Also, fundiscopic examination may allow for detection of retinal alterations after administration of toxic compounds.

Table 12. Microscopic alterations produced by some compounds retinotoxic to rodents

Compound	Species	Microscopic alterations	Reference
Urethan	r	Loss of PRC outer segments, decreased melanin granules in RPE, debris in subretinal space → loss of ONL, thinning of INL and focal proliferation of RPE	Bellhorn et al. 1973
Trimethyltin	r	Pyknotic nuclei in ONL and INL, swollen dark staining PRC inner segments	Bouldin et al. 1984
Vigabatrin	r	Disruption of ONL with outward displacement of PRC nuclei	Butler et al. 1987
P-1727	r	Loss of rods and cones, disorganization of ONL and INL	Delahunt et al. 1963
N-Methyl-*N*-nicrosourea	h	Arcades within the ONL, degeneration of RPE → retinal atrophy	Herrold 1967
	m	Retinal thinning and rosette formation in offspring following maternal administration	Smith and Yielding 1986
Cycasin	m, r	Necrosis of the neuroblastic layer of the retina in neonates → retinal rosette formation	Hirono 1972
Carbon disulfide	r	Acute degeneration of retinal ganglion cells	Ide 1958
Fenthione	r	Thinning of central retina, swelling and disorganization of RPE, melanin pigment about vessels	Imai et al. 1983
L-Ornithine hydrochloride	r	Degeneration and focal denuding of RPE → secondary disruption of PRC outer segments	Kuwabara et al. 1981
2-Aminoxy propionic acids	r	Fragmentation of PRC outer segments with outward migration and arcade formation by nuclei of ONL	Lee et al. 1979
Kainic acid	r	Pyknotic cells in inner aspect of INL and edema in the IPL → thinning and increased mitosis in INL	Lessell et al. 1980
Glutamate	m, r	Necrosis and loss of cells in the ganglion cell layer and INL, vacuolation in plexiform layers	Lucas and Newhouse 1957 Sisk and Kuwabara 1985
Doxorubicin	r	Decreased chromatin staining in ganglion cells, swollen axons in NFL → massive loss of ganglion cells	Parhad et al. 1984
L-Cysteine	r	Marked reduction in thickness of the NFL, ganglion cell layer, IPL and ONL	Pedersen and Karlsen 1980
Cytosine arabinoside	r	Retinal dysplasia characterized by rosette formation and retinal disorganization and thinning	Percy and Danylchuk 1977

r, rat; h, hamster; m, mouse; ONL, outer nuclear layer; INL, inner nuclear layer; RPE, retinal pigment epithelium; PRC, photoreceptor cell; NFL, nerve fiber layer; IPL, inner plexiform layer P-1727, *dl*-(*p*-trifluoromethylphenyl) isopropylamine hydrochloride.

Microscopic Features

Drugs and toxins may produce microscopic retinal degeneration with the primary effects on the inner retinal layers, retinal pigment epithelium, or photoreceptor complex. Also, some compounds, such as trimethyltin, may produce lesions in multiple retinal cell types (Santos-Anderson et al. 1984). Microscopic alterations produced by some compounds retinotoxic to rodents are given in Table 12.

Compounds Primarily Affecting the Inner Retinal Layers

Of toxic retinopathies with lesions primarily in the inner layers of the retina, those produced by the acidic amino acids, such as glutamate, are perhaps the best characterized. Within a few hours after the parenteral administration of sodium L-glutamate to 2- to 4-day-old mice, nuclear pyknosis was observed in cells destined to become the inner nuclear layer. By 1 week of age a reduction in the number of ganglion cells was apparent and the inner nuclear layer was one-half its normal thickness. Destruction of the inner retinal layers was complete by 17 days of age (Lucas and Newhouse 1957). Other compounds produce degeneration of the inner retinal layers associated with alteration in cytoplasmic storage of lipids or other materials. Various cationic amphiphilic drugs, such as chloroquine, induce generalized storage of polar lipids and these may be associated with alterations in retinal neurons as well as retinal pigment epithelium (Drenckhahn and Lullmann-Rauch 1978). Chloroquine has induced retinopathy in humans and experimental animals (Grant 1974; Drenckhahn and Lullmann-Rauch 1978; Thompson 1975; Abraham and Hendy 1970). Microscopically, in toluidine blue-stained thick sections, chloroquine retinopathy in rats was characterized by the accumulation of discrete orthochromic granules in the perinuclear cytoplasm of retinal ganglion cells (Thompson 1975).

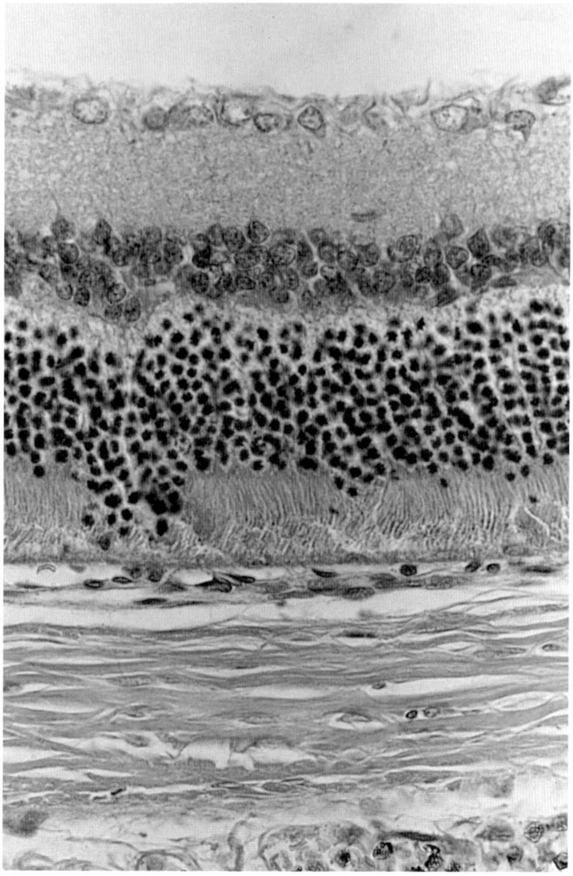

Fig. 100. Retina, rat. Degeneration of photoreceptor inner and outer segments and outward migration of photoreceptor nuclei in the retina of a rat fed a diet containing 1500 ppm methyl 2-(ureidooxy) propionate for 4 weeks. (Courtesy of Dr. K. P. Lee) H & E, ×325

Compounds Primarily Affecting the Retinal Pigment Epithelium

Iodate, which produces lesions in the retinal pigment epithelium, was one of the first compounds identified as producing lesions in a specific retinal layer (Potts 1965). Numerous other compounds including aminophenoxyalkanes, fluoride, napthalene, and aspartate have produced alterations in the retinal pigment epithelium of various animal species (Grant 1974). However, few reports are available on the ocular effects of such compounds in rodents. *N*-Methyl-*N*-nitrosourea, a potent carcinogen in animals, produced pigmentary degeneration in the retina of hamsters when administered intravenously (Herrold 1967). Early alterations in retinal pigment epithelium were cellular swelling and disruption and release of pigment granules. Numerous acute-angled folds or arcades were present in the outer nuclear layer. Lesions progressed to widespread disruption of photoreceptor cells. As previously discussed, amphiphilic cationic drugs, in addition to their effects on the sensory retina, may also produce lipid changes in the retinal pigment epithelium (Drenckhahn and Lullmann-Rauch 1978).

Compounds Primarily Affecting the Photoreceptor Cell

Several compounds have produced retinal degeneration in laboratory rodents with primary lesions in the outer sensory retina. Typical of such compounds is methyl 2-(ureidooxy) propionate (MUP). MUP administered by intragastric intubation to rats for 10 days produced fragmentation and disorganization of the outer limbs of the photoreceptor cells and outward migration of photoreceptor cell nuclei which formed arcades and rosettes (Fig. 100). Phagocytosis by pigment epithelium was secondary to extensive disruption of photoreceptors and loss of the layer of rods and cones (Fig. 101) (Lee et al. 1979). In Long-Evans rats, urethan produced alterations similar to those described for hereditary retinal degeneration when administered as weekly subcutaneous injections beginning at 7 weeks of age (Bellhorn et al. 1973). Alterations were characterized by fragmentation and vacuolation of outer segments of photoreceptor cells and accumulation of debris and macrophages in the subretinal space. In addition to complete loss of photoreceptors, older animals had clumping and depletion of pigment in the retinal pigment epithelium and extension of vascularized tufts of proliferating pigment epithelium into the inner retinal layers.

Compounds Producing Retinal Dysplasia

The retina of the rat at birth is considered to be the equivalent in development to the human retina at 4 or 5 months of gestation (Percy and Danylchuk 1977). Thus, it is not surprising that retinotoxicity manifested as retinal dysplasia has been produced in rodents by certain compounds, such as antimitotic agents. Retinal dysplasia was produced in newborn rats given cytosine arabinoside by subcutaneous injection for 5 consecutive days beginning 1 day after birth. Microscopically, retinal alterations in rats examined at 6 and 60 days of age were retinal rosette formation, abnormal alignment of photoreceptor cells, cellular degeneration, and infiltration of the retina by phagocytic cells (Percy and Danylchuk 1977).

Ultrastructure

Except for some studies with the rat, few reports are available describing chemically induced ultrastructural changes in the retina of rodents. Ultrastructural alterations produced by some compounds retinotoxic to rats are given in Table 13.

Compounds Primarily Affecting the Inner Retina Layers

Ultrastructural alterations produced by compounds affecting the inner retinal layers may reflect the abnormal accumulation of lipid in cells of the inner retina as with the amphiphilic cationic compounds (Drenckhahn and Lullmann-Rauch 1978) (see p.87), or they may result from more direct cellular injury as is seen in the retinopathy produced by monosodium glutamate. Intravitreal injection of sodium glutamate into the eyes of rats produced early ultrastructural alterations of swelling of nucleus, cytoplasmic

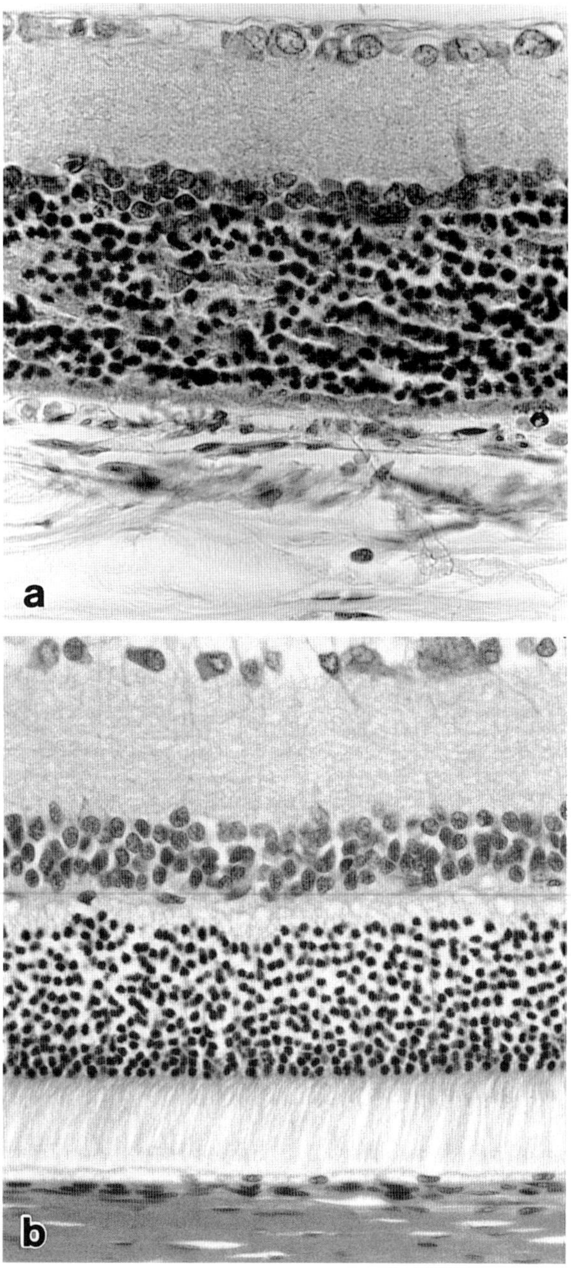

Fig. 101. **a** Retina, rat. Complete loss of rod and cone layer with abutting of photoreceptor nuclei to retinal pigment epithelium in the retina of a rat fed a diet containing 1500 ppm methyl 2-(ureidooxy) propionate for 21 weeks. H & E, ×325 (Courtesy of Dr. K. P. Lee). **b** Retina, rat. Normal retina, control for **a** H & E, ×325 (Courtesy of Dr. K. P. Lee)

Table 13. Ultrastructural alterations produced by some compounds retinotoxic to rats

Compound	Ultrastructural alterations	Reference
Vitamin A	Increased lipid droplets and mitochondrial destruction in RPE, mitochondrial destruction in PRC inner segments	Amemiya 1967
Trimethyltin	Membrane-bound vacuoles and polymorphic dense bodies in PRC inner segments, PRC necrosis, dense-cored visicles and tubules in ganglion cells, intracytoplasmic dense bodies in INL	Bouldin et al. 1984
Amphiphilic cationic drugs	Accumulation of crystalloid or lamellated inclusions in the cytoplasm of RPE or neuroretina; chloroquine only: multilamellated bodies in PRC inner segments	Drenckhahn and Lullmann-Rauch 1978
Fenthione	Loss of PRC outer segments, hypertrophy of RPE, pigment granules in subretinal space and penetrating OLM	Imai et al. 1983
Perhexiline maleate	Lamellar and reticular cytoplasmic inclusions in all retinal cell types, crystalloid inclusions in RPE	Jung et al. 1979
L-ornithine hydrochloride	Marked expansion of cytoplasmic matrix and destruction of organelles in RPE → RPE degeneration/hyperplasia → secondary disruption of PRC outer segments	Kuwabara et al. 1981
2-Aminoxy propionic acid	Disorientation, vacuolation and disruption of PRC outer segments → secondary increase in lysosomal bodies and phagosomes in RPE	Lee et al. 1979
Zinc chelators	Non-membrane-bound, electron opaque, scalloped inclusions in basal cytoplasm of RPE	Leure-duPree 1981
Doxorubicin	Neurofilament accumulation in cell body and proximal axon of ganglion cells	Parhad et al. 1984
Guanidinoethane sulfonate and β-alanine	Disorganization of PRC outer segment membrane disks	Pasantes-Morales et al. 1983
D, L α-Amino-adipic acids	Decreased electron density, cytoplasmic vacuolation and necrosis of Müller cells	Pedersen and Karlsen 1979
Lead	PRC necrosis with electron-dense, shrunken inner and outer segments; necrosis in INL	Santos-Anderson et al. 1984
AY9944	Niemann-Pick disease-like inclusions in various retinal cell types especially ganglion cells	Sakuragawa 1976
Glutamate	Swelling of nucleus, cytoplasm and dendritic processes of ganglion cells; swelling and pyknosis in inner aspect of INL	Sisk and Kuwabara 1985
Hexachlorophene	Vacuolation and tubulovesicular degeneration of PRC outer segment membrane disks	Towfighi et al. 1975

RPE, retinal pigment epithelium; PRC, photoreceptor cell; INL, inner nuclear layer; OLM, outer limiting membrane; Ay9944, *trans*-1,4-bis(2-chlorobenzylaminomethyl) cyclohexane dihydrochloride.

matrix, mitochondria, and dendritic processes of ganglion cells. These changes were followed by loss of cytoplasmic components, nuclear pyknosis and cell shrinkage, and phagocytosis of degenerated dendritic processes by Müller cells. Cellular swelling and nuclear pyknosis were also present in cells of the inner aspect of the inner nuclear layer (Sisk and Kuwabara 1985).

Compounds Primarily Affecting the Retinal Pigment Epithelium

Compounds producing primary lesions in the retinal pigment epithelium may produce cellular hypertrophy and hyperplasia, cellular degeneration, and pigment release, or they may produce cytoplasmic inclusions. Examples of compounds that produce inclusions are the amphiphilic cationic compounds, which are associated with the accumulation of abundant membrane-bound crystalloid or lamellar cytoplasmic inclusion in the retinal pigment epithelium and other retinal cells (Drenckhahn and Lullmann-Rauch 1973), and zinc chelators which produce non-membrane-bound, electron opaque cytoplasmic inclusions in the retinal pigment epithelium (Leure-duPree 1981). Because of the functional relationship between the retinal pigment epithelium and photoreceptor cells, ultrastructural alterations in the outer layers of the sensory retina are frequent sequelae to toxic injury to the retinal pigment epithelium.

Compounds Primarily Affecting the Photoreceptor Cell

Ultrastructural alterations produced by compounds that primarily affect the outer layers of the sensory retina are most frequently found in the outer segment of the photoreceptor cell. In rats, MUP, a 2-aminooxy propionic acid derivative, produced ultrastructural alterations consisting initially of disorganization of the lamellar disks followed by the formation of myelin figures, disruption of the inner segments, and increased membrane-containing phagosomes in the retinal pigment epithelium (Lee et al. 1979). Similarly, hexachlorophene retinopathy in rats was characterized by early vacuolation and disorganization of outer segment disks and destruction of photoreceptor cell bodies (Towfighi et al. 1975).

Compounds Affecting Multiple Retinal Layers

Trimethyltin is an example of a compound producing a retinopathy which, ultrastructurally, has changes in multiple retinal layers, although the degree of severity varies between cell types (Bouldin et al. 1984). The most frequent and severe changes were in the inner segments of photoreceptor cells and consisted of intracytoplasmic, membrane-bound vacuoles and various polymorphic dense bodies. Nerve cell bodies of the ganglion-cell layer neurons had intracytoplasmic clusters of dense-cored vesicles and tubules in addition to membrane-bound vesicles and polymorphic dense bodies. Intracytoplasmic dense bodies were also present in perikaryon of the neurons of the inner nuclear layer, where they occurred more short term than in other retinal layers. Alterations were notably absent in the plexiform layers, retinal pigment epithelium, and Müller cells.

Compounds Producing Retinal Dysplasia

Retinal dysplasia was produced in neonatal rats by multiple subcutaneous injections of cytosine arabinoside (Percy and Danylchuk 1977). Early ultrastructural changes included scattered clefts between the neural retina and the retinal pigment epithelium and abnormal alignment of photoreceptor cells. Rosettes of photoreceptor cells were delineated by terminal bars, and lumens of the rosettes contained cilia and primordial photoreceptor cell processes. Phagocytic cells containing cellular debris were present in the subretinal space.

Differential Diagnosis

Retinal changes may also occur secondary to glaucoma, retinal edema, retinal hemorrhage, and retinal vascular disturbances, including those induced by diabetogenic agents (Grant 1974; Sosula et al. 1973; Heath and Rutter 1966).
Spontaneous lesions may also occur in the retina of laboratory animals, and some of these lesions are similar to those produced by toxic chemicals. Thus it is sometimes difficult to separate chemically induced retinal changes from senile or genetic disorders or light-induced retinopathy. Also, for some compounds, the only manifestation of toxicity may be an increase in the incidence or an earlier age of onset of spontaneous lesions (Taradach and Greaves 1984). Therefore, knowledge of the morphologic characteristics and incidence of such lesions is important in distinguishing compound-related changes from intercurrent spontaneous lesions. In addition, microscopic changes such as postnecrotic atrophy and scarring produced following chronic retinotoxicity are similar regardless of the layer or layers of the retina initially affected. Changes include thinning of the retina with decreased nuclei and loss of the normal-layered architecture.

Biologic Features

Mechanisms of chemically induced retinal degeneration vary with chemical and species. The site and severity of injury within the retina may also vary due to the high degree of subspecialization among neurons of the different retinal layers (Bouldin et al. 1984). However, for most

Table 14. Proposed mechanism of action of some compounds retinotoxic to rodents

Compound	Area affected	Mechanism of action	Reference
Vitamin A	RPE, PRC inner segments	Inhibition of alcohol dehydrogenase system, alteration in mitochondrial membranes	Amemiya 1967
Ferrous sulfate	Rod outer segments	Free radical-induced oxidation of PRC outer segment phospholipid membranes	Anderson et al. 1984
Amphiphilic cationic drugs	RPE, ganglion cells and Müller cells	Formation of poorly catabolized lipid complexes which accumulate in lysosomes	Drenckhahn and Lullmann-Rauch 1978
Fenthione	RPE and sensory retina	Inhibition of esterases and proteases and altered DNA and RNA synthesis	Imai et al. 1983
Kainic acid	Amacrine cells	Stimulation of mitosis via sustained depolarization of neurons	Lessell et al. 1980
Glutamate	Inner retinal layers	Neuronal depolarization → influx of Na^+, Ca^{2+}, and Cl^- → cell swelling and death	Rothmann and Olney 1986
Doxorubicin	Ganglion cells	Inhibition of slow transport → neurofilamentous axonal swelling and cell death	Parhad et al. 1984
Guanidinoethane sulfonate and β-alanine	PRC outer segments	Inhibition of taurine transport	Pasantes-Morales et al. 1983
Ay9944	Various retinal cell types	Inhibition of sphingomyelinase → deposition of lamellar inclusion bodies	Sakuragawa 1976

RPE, retinal pigment epithelium; PRC, photoreceptor cell; Ay9944, *trans*-bis(2-chlorobenzyl aminomethyl) cyclohexane dihydrochloride.

retinotoxic compounds, a pathogenesis is not known. Proposed mechanisms of action for some retinotoxic compounds are given in Table 14.

Determination of the mechanisms involved in chemically induced retinal degeneration may be facilitated by identification of the retinal cell initially affected. However, because of the close interrelationship between the retinal pigment epithelium and photoreceptor cells, it is not always possible to determine morphologically which of those two cell layers is the primary target when retinal degeneration occurs in the outer retina. Also, few clinical electrodiagnostic means are available to detect primary toxic action on the retinal ganglion cells (Grant 1974), and identification of the primary cell type or types affected by a compound may be difficult to determine based on morphology alone.

Comparison with Other Species

Species considerations are especially important in evaluation of compounds which are potentially retinotoxic. For example, ethylenimine and 4,4"-diaminosiphenylmethane caused selective atrophy of rods and cones in the retina of the cat but not in several other laboratory animals species studied; chloroquine produced swelling of ganglion cells in the retina of the pig but the retinal pigment epithelium was affected in humans, the cat, and the rabbit (Grant 1974).

The predictive value of safety evaluations in laboratory rodents with respect to the determination of ocular toxicity in other species, including humans, has been questioned (Heywood 1982). In a survey of the toxicologic profile of 50 compounds, the incidence of ocular toxicity varied considerably between rodent and nonrodent species. In the dog and monkey, 26% and 7%, respectively, of the compounds induced some form of ocular toxicity, whereas in the rodent none of the compounds produced lesions in the eye.

In addition to species considerations, ocular pigmentation may influence retinotoxicity of some compounds in rodents. Thus, in chronic lead retinopathy in rats, pathologic changes in the retina were less severe in pigmented rats than in a nonpigmented strain (Santos-Anderson et al. 1984). Also, vigibatrin, an inhibitor of GABA transaminase, produced retinal degeneration in albino Sprague-Dawley rats, but no retinal changes were produced in pigmented Lister-Hooded rats (Butler et al. 1987). In contrast, retinal degeneration in rats exposed to fenthione was more severe in pigmented rats (Imai et al. 1983).

Age and route of administration of test compounds are also considerations when evaluating potential retinotoxicity. Thus, the severity of alterations produced in the inner layers of the retina in mice by parenteral administration of glutamate increased with age up to the 10th postnatal day, but beyond 10 days of age lesions were difficult to produce even with lethal doses (Olney 1969). However, lesions similar to those produced in neonatal rodents by the parenteral administration of glutamate were produced in mature rats by intravitreal administration of the compound (Sisk and Kuwabara 1985).

References

Abraham R, Hendy RJ (1970) Irreversible lysosomal damage induced by chloroquine in the retina of pigmented and albino rats. Exp Mol Pathol 12: 185–200

Amemiya T (1967) Cytochemical and electron microscopic examination of the retina of rats with hypervitaminosis A. Nippon Ganka Gakkai Zasshi (Acta Soc Ophthalmol Jpn) 71: 2236–2251

Anderson RE, Rapp LM, Wiegand RD (1984) Lipid peroxidation and retinal degeneration. Curr Eye Res 3: 223–227

Bellhorn RW, Bellhorn M, Friedman AH, Henkind P (1973) Urethan-induced retinopathy in pigmented rats. Invest Ophthalmol 12: 65–76

Bouldin TW, Goines ND, Krigman MR (1984) Trimethyltin retinopathy. Relationship of subcellular response to neuronal subspecialization. J Neuropathol Exp Neurol 43: 162–174

Butler WH, Ford GP, Newberne JW (1987) A study of the effects of vigabatrin on the central nervous system and retina of Sprague-Dawley and Lister-Hooded rats. Toxicol Pathol 15: 143–148

Delahunt CS, O'Connor RA, Yeary RA, Kuwabara T (1963) Toxic retinopathy following prolonged treatment with *dl*-(*p*-trifluoromethylphenyl) isopropylamine hydrochloride (P-1727) in experimental animals. Toxicol Appl Pharmacol 5: 298–305

Drenckhahn D, Lullmann-Rauch R (1978) Drug-induced retinal lipidosis: differential susceptibilities of pigment epithelium and neuroretina toward severe amphiphilic cationic drugs. Exp Mol Pathol 28: 360–371

Grant WM (1974) Toxicology of the eye. Thomas, Springfield

Heath H, Rutter AC (1966) Retinal angiopathy in the iminodipropionitrile-treated, alloxan-diabetic rat. Br J Exp Pathol 47: 116–120

Herrold KM (1967) Pigmentary degeneration of the retina induced by *N*-methyl-*N*-nitrosourea. Arch Ophthalmol 78: 650–653

Heywood R (1982) Histopathological and laboratory assessment of visual dysfunction. Environ Health Perspect 44: 35–45

Hirono I (1972) Carcinogenicity and neurotoxicity of cycasin with special reference to species differences. Fed Proc 31: 1493–1497

Ide T (1958) Histopathological studies on retina, optic nerve and arachnoidal membrane of mouse exposed to carbon disulfide poisoning. Nippon Ganka Gakkai Zasshi (Acta Soc Ophthalmol Jpn) 62 A: 85–108

Imai H, Miyata M, Uga S, Ishikawa S (1983) Retinal degeneration in rats exposed to an organophosphate pesticide (fenthion). Environ Res 30: 453–465

Jung HJ, Weisenfreund J, Willson NJ, Suzuki K (1979) Pexid-induced retinal pathology. Acta Neuropathol 47: 33–37

Kuwabara T, Ishikawa Y, Kaiser-Kupfer MI (1981) Experimental gyrate atrophy in animals. Ophthalmology 88: 331–335

Lee KP, Gibson JR, Sherman H (1979) Retinopathic effects of 2-aminooxy propionic acid derivatives in the rat. Toxicol Appl Pharmacol 51: 219–232

Lessell S, Craft JL, Albert DM (1980) Kainic acid induces mitoses in mature retinal neurons in rats. Exp Eye Res 30: 731–738

Leure-duPree AE (1981) Electron-opaque inclusions in the rat retinal pigment epithelium after treatment with chelators of zinc. Invest Ophthalmol Vis Sci 21: 1–9

Lucas DR, Newhouse JP (1957) The toxic effect of sodium L-glutamate on the inner layers of the retina. Arch Ophthalmol 58: 193–201

Olney JW (1969) Glutamate-induced retinal degeneration in neonatal mice. Electromicroscopy of the acutely evolving lesion. J Neuropathol Exp Neurol 28: 455–574

Parhad IM, Giffin JW, Clark AW, Koves JF (1984) Doxorubicin intoxication: neuro-filamentous axonal changes with subacute neuronal death. J Neuropathol Exp Neurol 43: 188–200

Pasantes-Morales H, Quesada O, C'arabez A, Huxtable RJ (1983) Effects of the taurine transport antagonist, guanidinoethane sulfonate, and beta-alanine on the morphology of rat retina. J Neurosci Res 9: 135–143

Pedersen OO, Karlsen RL (1979) Destruction of Müller cells in the adult rat by intravitreal injection of D,L-alpha-aminoadipic acid. An electron microscopic study. Exp Eye Res 28: 569–575

Pedersen OO, Karlsen RL (1980) The toxic effect of L-cysteine on the rat retina: a morphological and biochemical study. Invest Ophthalmol Vis Sci 19: 886–892

Percy DH, Danylchuk KD (1977) Experimental retinal dysplasia due to cytosine arabinoside. Invest Ophthalmol Vis Sci 16: 353–364

Potts AM (1965) Selective action of chemical agents on individual retinal layers. In: Graymore CN (ed) Biochemistry of the retina. Academic, New York, pp 155–162

Rothman SM, Olney JW (1986) Glutamate and the pathophysiology of hypoxic-ischemic brain damage. Ann Neurol 19: 105–111

Sakuragawa M (1976) Niemann-Pick disease-like inclusions caused by a hypocholesteremic agent. Invest Ophthalmol Vis Sci 15: 1022–1027

Santos-Anderson RM, Tso MO, Valdes JJ, Annau Z (1984) Chronic lead administration in neonatal rats: electron microscopy of the retina. J Neuropathol Exp Neurol 43: 175–187

Sisk DR, Kuwabara T (1985) Histological changes in the inner retina of albino rats following intravitreal injection of monosodium L-glutamate. Greafes Arch Clin Exp Ophthalmol 223: 250–258

Smith LB, Yielding KL (1986) Retinal degeneration in the mouse. A model induced transplacentally by methylnitrosourea. Exp Eye Res 43: 791–801

Sosula L, Beaumont P, Hollows FC, Jonso KM (1973) Dilatation and endothelial proliferation of retinal capillaries in steptozotocin-diabetic rats: quantitative electron microscopy. Invest Ophthalmol Vis Sci 11: 926–935

Taradach C, Greaves P (1984) Spontaneous eye lesions in laboratory animals: incidence in relation to age. CRC Crit Rev Toxicol 12: 121–147

Thompson SW (1975) Chloroquine retinopathy in the rat. Vet Pathol 12: 71

Towfighi J, Gonatas NK, McCree L (1975) Hexachlorophene retinopathy in rats. Lab Invest 132: 330–338

Microphthalmia and Anophthalmia, Mouse and Rat

Cynthia S. Cook

Synonyms. Ocular retardation, colobomatous microphthalmia, cystic microphthalmia.

Gross Appearance

The microphthalmic eye appears grossly smaller than normal. The palpebral fissure will usually be proportionally reduced in size (Fig. 102). In addition, the globe may be deeply recessed into the orbit, making examination difficult. Microphthalmia is often accompanied by corneal and/or lens opacities, which may be grossly apparent.

Congenitally, microphthalmic eyes may appear to become progressively smaller as the animal reaches adult size since the abnormal eye does not grow normally as the orbit expands during maturation. A mucoid to mucopurulent discharge may accumulate within the palpebral fissure.

A presumptive diagnosis of apparent anophthalmia is made based upon the absence of a grossly identifiable palpebral fissure. The presence of any palpebral fissure, however small, is evidence that underlying ocular tissue exists.

Microscopic Features

An eye which is small but otherwise normal is described as nanophthalmic and is uncommon. Microphthalmia is nearly always associated with multiple intraocular abnormalities including colobomas of the anterior and/or posterior segment, microphakia (with or without cataract), retinal dysplasia (with or without detachment), persistent hyperplastic primary vitreous, and anterior segment dysgenesis (Figs. 103–105).

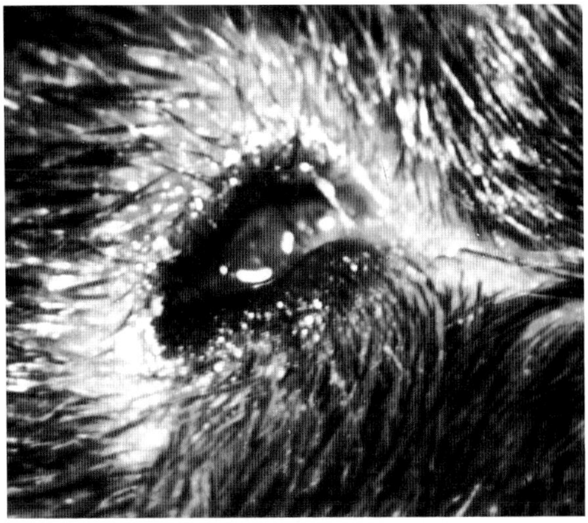

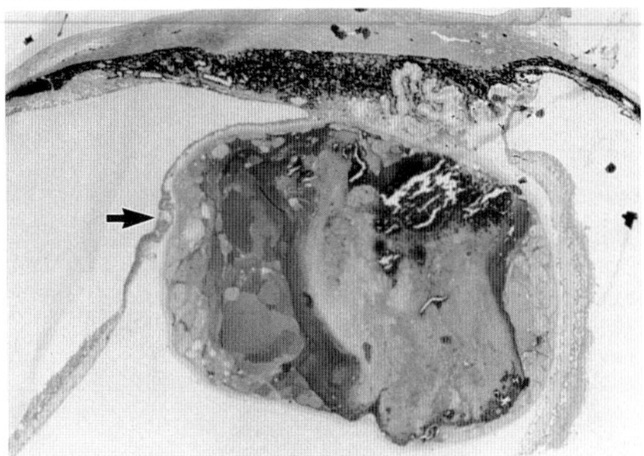

Fig. 102 *(above)*. Microphthalmia in a C57 Black mouse demonstrating a very small palpebral fissure obscuring visualization of the rudimentary globe

Fig. 103 *(below)*. Microphthalmia in a mutant mouse strain with a small, cataractous lens adherent to the dysplastic retina *(arrow)* and ciliary epithelium. Methylene blue/acid fuchsin, ×28.3

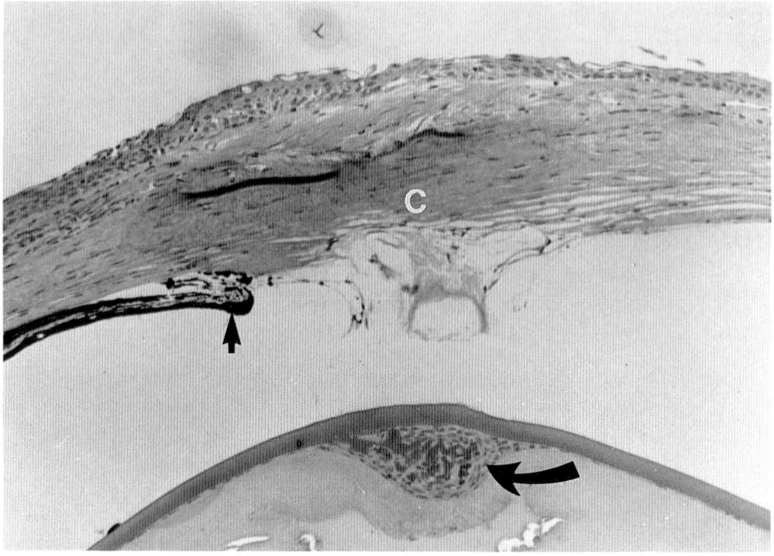

Fig. 104. Anterior segment dysgenesis in a C57 Black mouse characterized by an anterior polar cataract *(curved arrow)* and defects in the posterior corneal *(C)* stroma and endothelium with fibrous attachments to the anterior lens. The iris is hypoplastic and has failed to separate from the cornea (indicated by the *small arrow*). These anomalies are characteristic of Peters' anomaly in man. (Cook and Sulik 1986) PAS, ×142

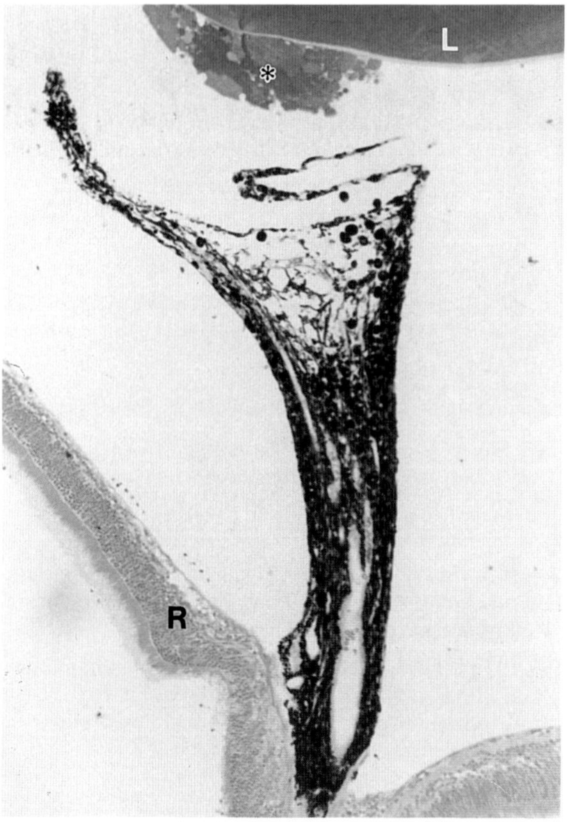

Fig. 105. Persistent hyperplastic primary vitreous associated with microphthalmia in a C57B1/6J mouse. A posterior polar cataract (*) is present. *L*, lens; *R*, retina (artifactually detached). (Cook and Sulik 1986) Methylene blue/acid fuchsin, ×160

Ultrastructure

Embryogenesis

The optic sulci become apparent following gastrulation (formation of the mesodermal germ layer) as bilateral evaginations of the forebrain neural ectoderm during the 8th day of gestation in the mouse. In the C57 Black/6J mouse, microphthalmia occurs secondary to deficiency in the forebrain primordia, resulting in formation of small optic vesicles and correspondingly small optic cup structures. This deficiency may be asymmetric, resulting in a relatively normal optic cup paired with a rudimentary, neural ectoderm-lined cyst (Fig. 106).

A wide spectrum of anomalies accompanies the embryogenesis of microphthalmia. By day 14 of gestation in the mouse, the optic cup is well developed and the lens vesicle has detached from the surface ectoderm; the eyelids have not yet begun to close.

Evaluation at this time using a dissecting microscope reveals a slightly irregular anterior margin of the normal optic cup (the future pupil) (Fig. 107). In contrast, the affected eye in this individual is smaller, with an elliptical pupil, elongated inferiorly due to incomplete closure of the optic (choroid) fissure (Fig. 108). Scanning electron microscopy (SEM) demonstrates deficiency in the size of the palpebral fissure as-

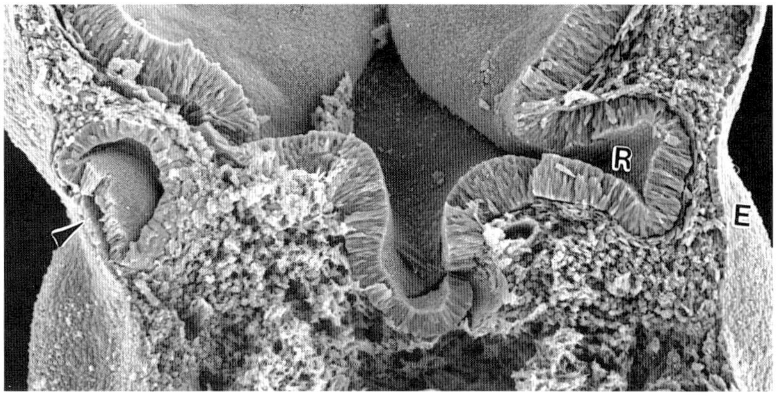

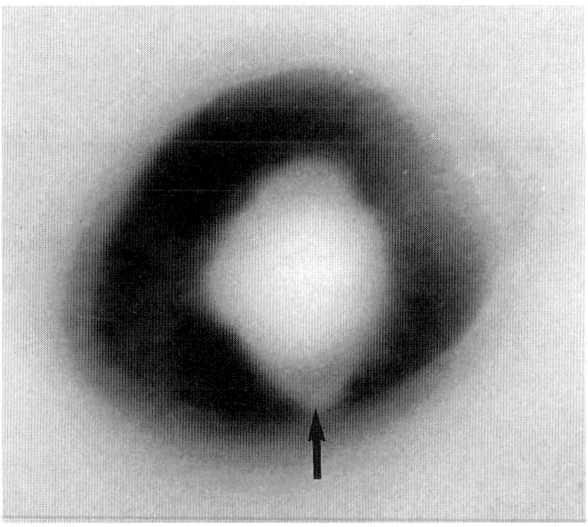

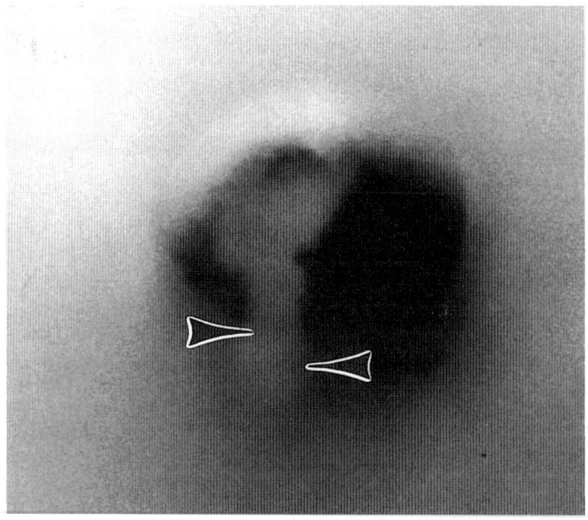

Fig. 106 *(above).* Frontal fracture of a day 10 mouse embryo (34 somite pairs) with marked asymmetry in development of the optic cups. *On the left side,* the optic cup and lens vesicle have invaginated (*arrow* indicates invaginating lens); however, the right optic vesicle *(R)* has failed to reach the surface ectoderm *(E).* The result of this abnormality would be aphakia and severe microphthalmia in the adult. SEM, ×127

Fig. 107 *(lower left).* Normal eye of day 14 mouse embryo as viewed through a dissecting microscope. The outer layer of the optic cup is pigmented and has an irregular anterior margin (the future pupil). A small notch is present inferiorly *(arrow)* indicating the final stages of closure of the choroid fissure, ×74

Fig. 108 *(lower right).* The microphthalmic right eye of the same embryo as in Fig. 107. The palpebral fissure is correspondingly deficient and the choroid fissure has failed to close *(arrowheads).* (Cook and Sulik 1986) ×65

sociated with severe microphthalmia (Figs. 109, 110). Coronal fracture and SEM evaluation of affected embryos on day 14 of gestation in the mouse reveal a small optic cup and lens vesicle surrounded by an apparent excess of hyaloid vasculature compared with normal embryos of the same age (Figs. 111, 112).

Delay or failure of detachment of the lens vesicle from the surface ectoderm (Fig. 113) may be associated with microphthalmia, resulting in anterior segment dysgenesis characterized by cornela opacity, dyscoria, persistent pupillary membranes, and cataract in affected adults (Fig. 104).

Differential Diagnosis

The diagnosis of microphthalmia is usually not difficult. Enophthalmos secondary to ocular pain may present a similar appearance. Identification of a corneal ulcer or other cause for blepharospasm and response to topical anesthesia will aid in the diagnosis of pain-induced enophthalmos. Microphthalmia is often accompanied by a small palpebral fissure; comparison with the fellow eye if asymmetric may be helpful.

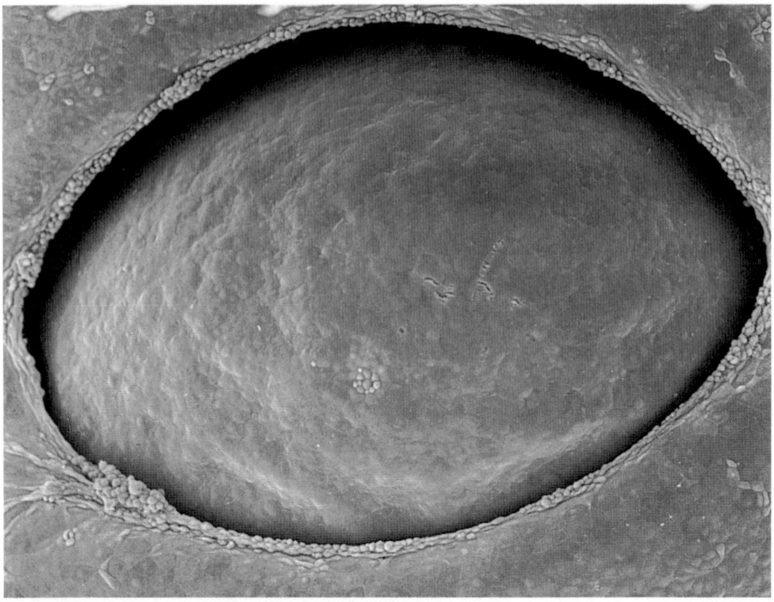

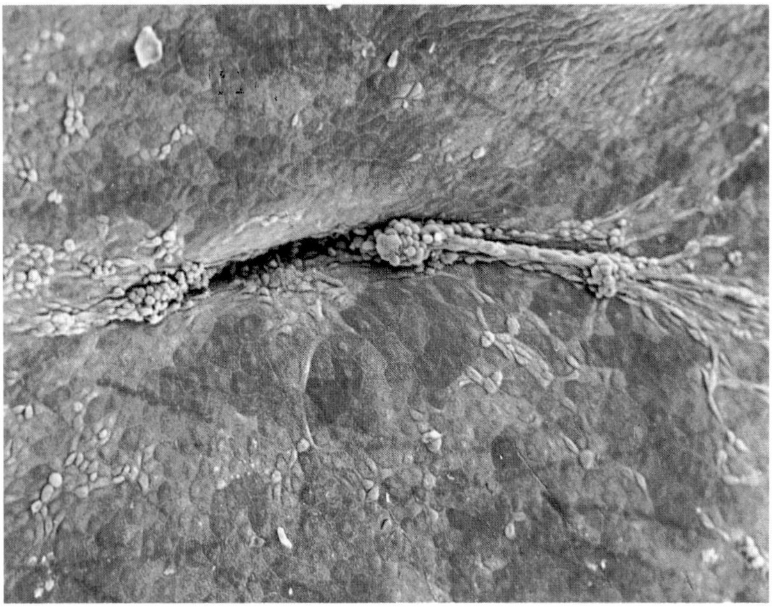

Fig. 109 *(above)*. Normal palpebral fissure of day 14 mouse embryo. The ectodermal margins of the fissure are beginning to close. (Cook and Sulik 1986) SEM, ×114

Fig. 110 *(below)*. Opposite eye of same embryo as in Fig. 109 demonstrating a severely deficient palpebral fissure. (Cook and Sulik 1986) SEM, ×200

Biologic Features

Microphthalmia has been described in a mutant mouse strain (129/Sv-SIJCP) with a recessively inherited gene called ocular retardation *(OR)* (Truslove 1962; Robb et al. 1978). Ocular retardation is accompanied by optic nerve aplasia, early arrest of retinal development, and secondary cataract. Controversy exists regarding the earliest identifiable abnormality in the *OR* mouse.

Truslove (1962) reported that ocular development progressed normally until day 11 of gestation, when the central artery and vein failed to establish their normal pathway in the optic cup; early closure of the optic (choroid) fissure was described. In contrast, Robb et al. (1978) describe normal vascular development in the

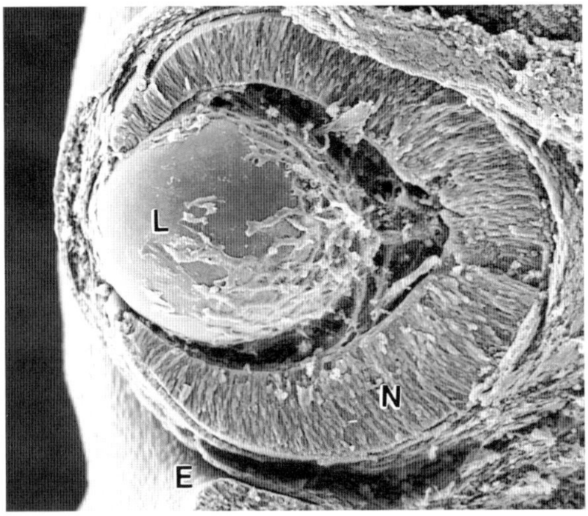

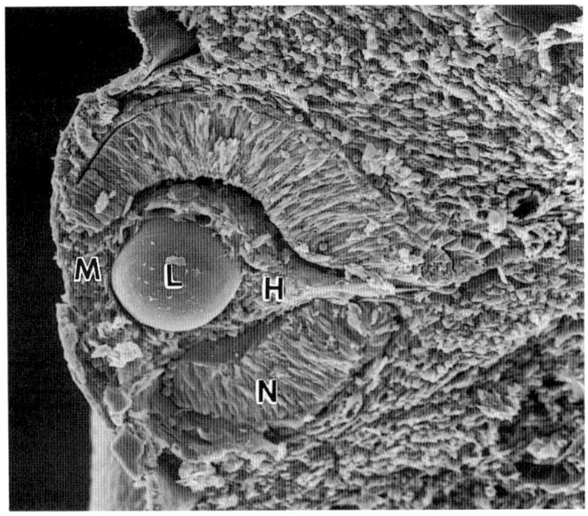

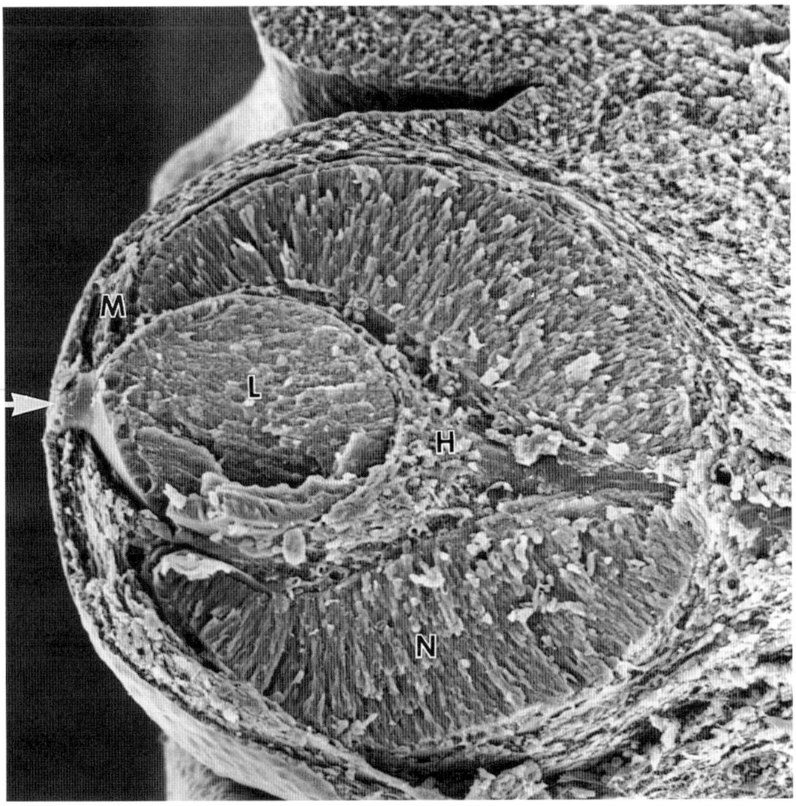

Fig. 111 *(upper left).* Normal eye of day 14 mouse embryo. The lens *(L)* nearly fills the optic cup and is surrounded by hyaloid vasculature. *E,* surface ectoderm covering eyelid margin; *N,* inner layer of optic cup, anlage of neural retina. SEM, ×120

Fig. 112 *(upper right).* Microphthalmic eye of day 14 mouse embryo. The optic cup and lens *(L)* are markedly reduced in size. Note the apparent excess of hyaloid vasculature *(H). M,* neural crest mesenchyme which fills the future anterior chamber; *N,* anlage of the neural retina. (Cook and Sulik 1986) SEM, ×183

Fig. 113 *(below).* Mouse embryo (day 14) with microphthalmia and persistent attachment of the lens vesicle *(L)* to the surface ectoderm *(arrow).* This keratolenticular attachment prevents axial migration of mesenchyme *(M)* of neural crest origin to form the corneal stroma, endothelium, and iridial stroma. In the adult, this malformation would appear similar to Fig. 104. *H,* hyaloid vasculature; *N* anlage of the neural retina. (Cook and Sulik 1986) SEM, ×188

OR mouse and related the occurrence of microphthalmia to the absence of normally occurring cell death in the retinal anlage identified on day 10.5 of gestation.

The ZRDCT mouse strain was originally described by Chase and Chase (1941) as exhibiting bilateral anophthalmia in 90% of individuals and a variable degree of microphthalmia in the remaining 10%. Inhibited growth of the optic vesicle with failure of lens induction was described (Chase and Chase 1941). A different sequence was proposed by Silver and Hughes (1974), who described persistence and proliferation of mesenchyme between the optic vesicle and lens placode displacing the deficient lens vesicle. A variant of this strain was evaluated by Harch et al. (1978), who described normal development of the optic vesicle and apparently normal contact with the surface ectoderm to induce the lens placode. However, following induction, the lens vesicle was smaller than normal and often positioned abnormally within the optic cup. If the deficient lens was not within the boundaries of the optic cup, it was excluded and the optic cup collapsed resulting in anophthalmia. Persistence of a small lens results in microphthalmia. Horch et al. (1978) specifically exclude persistence of mesenchyme between the optic cup and lens placode in the pathogenesis of this condition. Salaun (1982) demonstrated that optic primordia taken from ZRDCT mouse embryos on day 10 of gestation developed more normally in vitro or when grafted onto host tissue of control origin, implicating an environmental mechanism for production of microphthalmia.

Mice homozygous for the fidget gene *(fi/fi)* exhibit microphthalmia due to deficiency in the optic vesicle, associated with a reduction in the mitotic index in the neural ectoderm (Konyukhov and Vakhrusheva 1969). In contrast, Truslove (1956) described microphthalmia as occurring secondary to deficiency in the lens vesicle. Associated findings include keratolenticular dysgenesis with failure of detachment of the lens vesicle from the surface ectoderm. A very similar sequence has been described for the C57B1/6J mouse, where a primary forebrain deficiency is postulated to result in microphthalmia (Cook and Sulik 1986). In this mouse strain, teratogen exposure during gastrulation (day 7 of gestation) has been demonstrated to dramatically increase the incidence and severity of eye malformations (Cook et al. 1987; Cook and Sulik 1988), further demonstrating the induction of microphthalmia very early in gestation. Dickie's small eye is an early lethal mutation when homozygous. Heterozygotes are small and exhibit microphthalmia (Theiler et al. 1978).

Microphthalmia in mice homozygous for the gene *MI* undergoes deficient ocular development attributed to failure of formation of secondary (gel) vitreous secondary to coloboma (Scholtz and Chan 1987). In these mice an unusual dysplasia of the outer layer of the optic cup occurs with aberrant differentiation into neural retina.

Microphthalmia is less frequently described in rats and has been linked to inadequate blood supply through failure in development of the hyaloid vasculature (Browman 1961; Browman and Ramsey 1943). Other descriptions of microphthalmia in rats identify abnormal optic cup formation (Kobayashi and Otani 1981). In these studies, earlier development of the optic vesicle and induction of the lens vesicle were apparently normal. Kobayashi and Otani (1981) describe failure of formation of the proximal (stalk) portion of the optic fissure preventing subsequent access of the optic cup to the primary hyaloid vessel (central artery). These authors believed that failure of closure of the anterior portion of the fissure (retinal fissure) ventrally resulted in failure to establish intraocular pressure and expansion of the optic cup. A similar sequence in the chick was induced experimentally by Coulombre (1956). An earlier initiation of an abnormal sequence has been described in yet another strain of rat exhibiting microphthalmia by Kinney et al. (1982). These authors identified a deficiency in the optic vesicle and postulate that agenesis of the central (hyaloid) artery occurs secondarily in this and other strains with microphthalmia.

Syndromes of microphthalmia/anophthalmia have been described in several species, usually as an inherited abnormality. Most authors agree that anophthalmia represents the most severe manifestation of a spectrum of microphthalmia. Thus, the same etiologic and morphogenetic features apply to both conditions.

Pathogenesis

Silver and Hughes (1973) described the role of morphogenetic cell death during normal ocular morphogenesis, suggesting that cell necrosis may function to inhibit cell movements, thus integrating invaginations which form the optic cup, lens vesicle, and choroid fissure. Inadequate cell death has been postulated by these authors (Silver and Hughes 1974) to be responsible for reductions in the lens and retina primordia.

Although there is controversy regarding the sequence of events leading to microphthalmia in laboratory animals, it is most likely that the initiation of abnormal ocular morphogenesis occurs much earlier than may be readily appreciated. Careful examination of early embryonic stages is challenging because of their small size and the meticulous dissection required to expose the optic primordia. Recent studies utilizing scanning electron microscopy have provided a three-dimensional illustration of the relative tissue relationships involved in normal and abnormal ocular morphogenesis (Cook and Sulik 1986). Investigations of acute teratogen exposure have identified the gastrulation stage as a critical period of sensitivity during ocular development. Ocular malformations were induced by ethanol exposure during a period equivalent to the 3rd week of human gestation. Exposure 24 h later (equivalent to 1 week later in human gestation) did not result in an increased incidence of microphthalmia (Cook et al. 1987). Thus, a narrow, very early, critical period exists for induction of microphthalmia. It is likely that spontaneous, inherited microphthalmia is also initiated during early forebrain differentiation.

Comparison with Other Species

Microphthalmia and anophthalmia occur in many species, including man (O'Keefe et al. 1987). In one survey, the condition was present bilaterally in 2/15 patients, and abnormalities were present in 6/13 cases in the fellow eye. Systemic abnormalities associated with microphthalmia and anophthalmia in humans include facial and CNS malformations which implicate a sequence initiated very early in gestation, prior to formation of the optic sulci.

Studies on the anophthalmic white hamster (Jackson 1981) have described a sequence including incomplete invagination of the optic cup, failure of closure of the choroid fissure, and dysgenesis of the outer layer of the optic vesicle to form apparent neural retina.

Inherited anophthalmos has been described to occur in 82% of progeny from matings between bilaterally affected guinea pigs (Komich 1971). The optic nerves and optic tracts were also absent in affected individuals and the central visual pathways (lateral geniculate and superior colliculi) were hypoplastic.

Syndromes of microphthalmia with multiple ocular anomalies have been described in several breeds of dog, including the Australian shepherd dog (Bertram et al. 1984; Gelatt and McGill 1973), Old English sheepdog (Barrie et al. 1979), Cavalier King Charles spaniel (Narfstrom and Dubielzig 1984), miniature schnauzer (Gelatt and McBill 1973; Gelatt et al. 1983), and Doberman pinscher (Arnbjerg and Jensen 1982; Bergsjo et al. 1984; Peiffer and Fischer 1983). Associated malformations include coloboma, retinal dysplasia, cataract, lenticonus, and aterior segment dysgenesis in a similar spectrum to that described in laboratory rodents.

Anophthalmia and microphthalmia have been described in several breeds of cattle including purebred shorthorn and Jersey as well as crossbred animals (Rupp and Knight 1984; Leipold et al. 1971; Leipold and Huston 1968). The condition occurs spontaneously with a variable incidence; an inherited etiology is possible but not established.

Acknowledgments. The author acknowledges the support of NIH Fellowship # 1 F32 EY05918 and IROI EY 08147 for the original research described in this manuscript.

References

Arnbjerg J, Jensen OA (1982) Spontaneous microphthalmia in two Doberman puppies with anterior chamber cleavage syndrome. J Am Anim Hosp Assoc 18: 481–484

Barrie KP, Peiffer RL, Gelatt KN, Williams LW (1979) Posterior lenticonus, microphthalmia, congenital cataracts, and retinal folds in an Old English sheepdog. J Am Anim Hosp Assoc 15: 715–717

Bergsjø T, Arnesen K, Heim P, Nes N (1984) Congenital blindness with ocular developmental anomalies including retinal dysplasia, in Doberman Pinscher dogs. J Am Vet Med Assoc 184: 1383–1386

Bertram T, Coignoul F, Cheville N (1984) Ocular dysgenesis in Australian shepherd dogs. J Am Anim Hosp Assoc 20: 177–182

Browman LG (1961) Microphthalmia and optic blood supply in the rat. J Morphol 109: 37–55

Browman LG, Ramsey F (1943) Embryology of microphthalmos in *Rattus norvegicus.* Arch Ophthalmol 30: 338–351

Chase HB, Chase EB (1941) Studies on an anophthalmic strain of mice. I. Embryology of the eye region. J Morphol 68: 279–301

Cook CS, Sulik KK (1986) Sequential scanning electron microscopic analyses of normal and spontaneously occurring abnormal ocular development in C57B1/6J mice. Scan Electron Microsc III: 1215–1227

Cook CS, Sulik (1988) Keratolenticular dysgenesis (Peters' anomaly) as a result of acute embryonic insult during gastrulation. J Pediatr Ophthalmol Strabismus 25: 60–66

Cook CS, Nowotny AZ, Sulik KK (1987) Fetal alcohol syndrome: eye malformations in a mouse model. Arch Ophthalmol 105: 1576–1581

Coulombre AJ (1956) The role of intraocular pressure in the development of the chick eye. J Exp Zool 133: 211–225

Gelatt KN, McGill LD (1973) Clinical characteristics of microphthalmia with colobomas of the Australian shepherd dog. J Am Vet Med Assoc 162: 393–396

Gelatt KN, Samuelson DA, Barrie KP, Das ND, Wolf ED, Bauer JE, Andresen TL (1983) Biometry and clinical characteristics of congenital cataracts and microphthalmia in the Miniature Schnauzer. J Am Vet Med Assoc 183: 99–102

Harch C, Chase HB, Gonsalves NI (1978) Studies on an anophthalmic strain of mice. VI. Lens and cup interaction. Dev Biol 63: 352–357

Jackson CG (1981) Prenatal development of the microphthalmic eye in the golden hamster. J Morphol 167: 65–90

Kinney HC, Klintworth GK, Lesiewicz J, Goldsmith LA, Wilkening B (1982) Congenital cystic microphthalmia and consequent anophthalmia in the rat: a study in abnormal ocular morphogenesis. Teratology 26: 203–212

Kobayashi K, Otani K (1981) Morphogenesis of the hereditary microphthalmia in a new strain of rat. J Morphol 167: 265–276

Komich RJ (1971) Anophthalmos: an inherited trait in a new stock of guinea pigs. Am J Vet Res 32: 2099–2105

Konyukhov BV, Vakhrusheva MP (1969) Abnormal development of eyes in mice homozygous for the fidget gene. Teratology 2: 147–157

Leipold HW, Huston K (1968) Congenital syndrome of anophthalmia-microphthalmia with associated defects in cattle. Pathol Vet 5: 407–418

Leipold HW, Gelatt KN, Huston K (1971) Multiple ocular anomalies and hydrocephalus in grade beef shorthorn cattle. Am J Vet Res 32: 1019–1026

Narfstrom K, Dubielzig R (1984) Posterior lenticonus, cataracts and microphthalmia; congenital ocular defects in the Cavalier King Charles Spaniel. J Small Anim Pract 25: 669–677

O'Keefe M, Webb M, Pashby RC, Wagman RD (1987) Clinical anophthalmos. Br J Ophthalmol 71: 635–638

Peiffer RL Jr, Fischer CA (1983) Microphthalmia, retinal dysplasia, and anterior segment dysgenesis in a litter of Doberman Pinschers. J Am Vet Med Assoc 183: 875–878

Robb RM, Silver J, Sullivan RT (1978) Ocular retardation *(or)* in the mouse. Invest Ophthalmol Vis Sci 17: 468–473

Rupp GP, Knight AP (1984) Congenital ocular defects in a crossbred beef herd. J Am Vet Med Assoc 184: 1149–1150

Salaun J (1982) Differentiation of the optic cups from an anophthalmic murine strain, in culture and in intrafoetal grafts. J Embryol Exp Morphol 67: 71–80

Scholtz CL, Chan KK (1987) Complicated colobomatous microphthalmia in the microphthalmic *(mi/mi)* mouse. Development 99: 501–508

Silver J, Hughes AF (1973) The role of cell death during morphogenesis of the mammalian eye. J Morphol 140: 159–170

Silver J, Hughes AF (1974) The relationship between morphogenetic cell death and the development of congenital anophthalmia. J Comp Neurol 157: 281–302

Theiler K, Varnum DS, Stevens LC (1978) Development of Dickie's small eye, a mutation in the house mouse. Anat Embryol (Berl) 155: 81–86

Truslove GM (1956) The anatomy and development of the fidget mouse. J Genet 54: 64–86

Truslove GM (1962) A gene causing ocular retardation in the mosue. J Embryol Exp Morphol 10: 652–660

Adenoma and Adenocarcinoma, Harderian Gland, Mouse, Rat, and Hamster

William W. Carlton and James A. Render

Synonyms. Papillary cystadenoma.

Gross Appearance

Neoplasms of the harderian gland vary in size, shape, and color and some enlarge the gland. The larger neoplasms are often grayish white, fill the orbit, and become obvious by causing protrusion of the eyelid and proptosis of the eyeball. Proptosis prevents closure of the eyelids and results in drying of the cornea and the development of exposure keratitis which may progress to ulceration (Upton et al. 1960). Unilateral keratitis was noted in 7% of BALB/c female mice with harderian gland neoplasms (Sheldon and Greenman 1979).

Microscopic Features

Adenomas of the harderian gland are lobular collections of cuboidal to tall columnar cells much like those found in the normal gland (Fig. 114). The cells have abundant foamy, pale-staining cytoplasm (Figs. 115, 116) (Holland and Fry 1982). The nuclei are round to avoid, basally located, and fairly uniform in size and histologic features. The cells are usually arranged in papillary formations, but areas of some neoplasms are cystic.

Carcinomas of the harderian gland are poorly differentiated solid neoplasms composed of sheets of cells with little adenomatous differentiation and with cellular and nuclear pleomorphism (Figs. 117, 118). These neoplasms infiltrate the orbital contents and periorbital tissues and some metastasize to regional lymph nodes and to the lungs (Fig. 119). The neoplasms are generally nonencapsulated, but capsulation of the neoplasm by fibrous connective tissue is prominent in some animals. Degeneration of the neoplastic cells occurs in some neoplasms, especially in the larger ones.

Ultrastructure

A description of the ultrastructural features of a harderian gland adenoma was not found. In the mouse, the normal harderian gland contains two types of secretory cell. The more numerous (type A) cells are responsible for secretion of the lipid droplets and are probably the cell of origin of the harderian gland neoplasms. The least numerous cells (type B) have dark granules (Woodhouse and Rhodin 1963).

Differential Diagnosis

Harderian gland neoplasms may be confused with those arising in other lacrimal glands. However, neoplasms of the other lacrimal glands in rodent species are extremely rare and occur less frequency than harderian gland neoplasms.

Biologic Features

The harderian gland is present in most laboratory animals with a third eyelid (except the dog). In rodents, the gland lies deep within and occupies most of the orbit medial to the eyeball. In the rat and mouse, it has a horseshoe shape and partially encircles the optic nerve. This tubuloalveolar gland is divided into lobules of alveoli lined by columnar epithelial cells with a round, pale-staining, basally located nucleus. The abundant cytoplasm is vacuolated due to a large amount of lipid. The gland produces a secretion with a high concentration of lipids and a brown pigment containing fluorescent porphyrins (Woodhouse and Rhodin 1963).

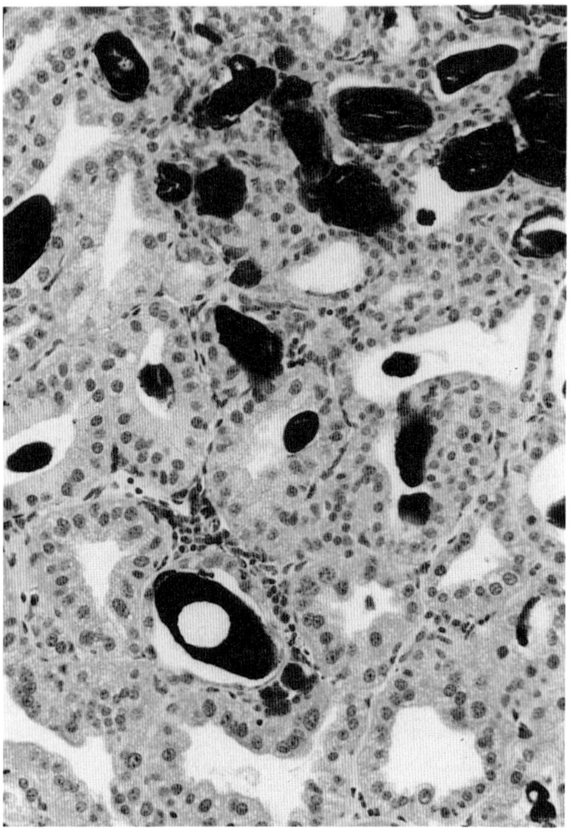

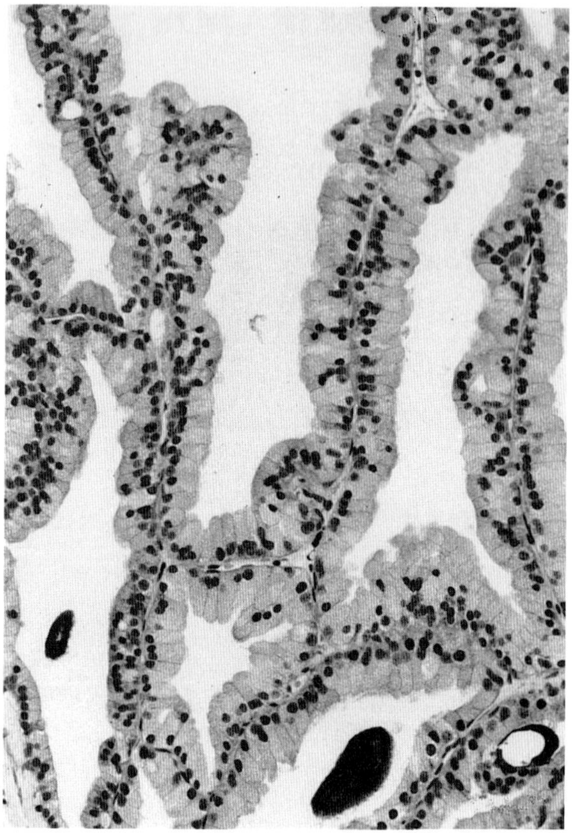

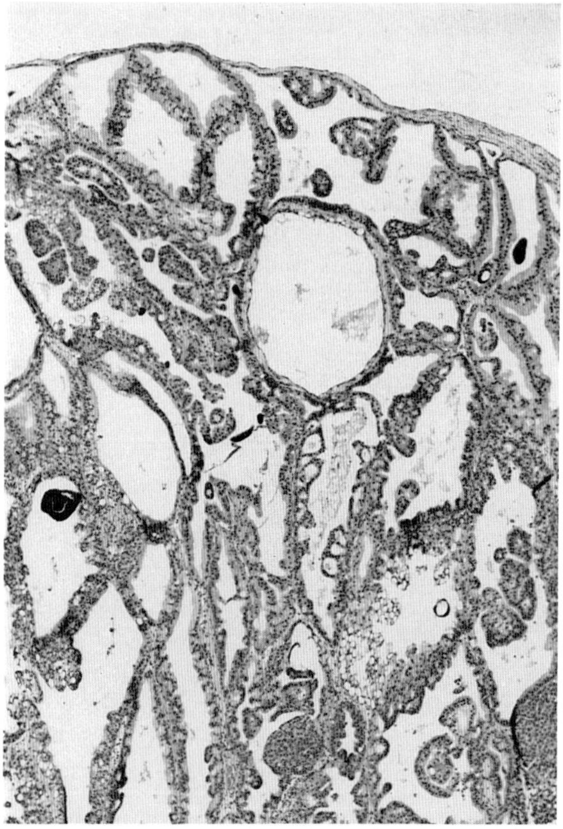

Fig. 114 *(upper left).* Harderian gland of a mouse. Note acini lined by cuboidal to columnar cells with round to oval basally located nuclei and abundant finely vacuolated cytoplasm. Variable-size clumps of dark-brown pigment fill some of the lumens. (Tissue provided by Dr. G. Long, Eli Lilly Co., Greenfield, IN, USA) H & E, ×192

Fig. 115 *(lower left).* Adenoma of harderian gland, mouse. Alveoli are often cystic and lined by a variable number of rows of cuboidal to columnar epithelium. Papillary structures are present in some alveoli. (Tissue provided by Dr. G. Long, Eli Lilly Co., Greenfield, IN, USA) H & E, ×48

Fig. 116 *(upper right).* Adenoma of harderian gland, mouse. The alveoli are lined by columnar epithelial cells with round to oval nuclei and abundant finely vacuolated cytoplasm. Note that most nuclei are at the base of the cells, and some are at different levels in the lining epithelium. (Tissue provided by Dr. G. Long, Eli Lilly Co., Greenfield, IN, USA) H & E, ×192

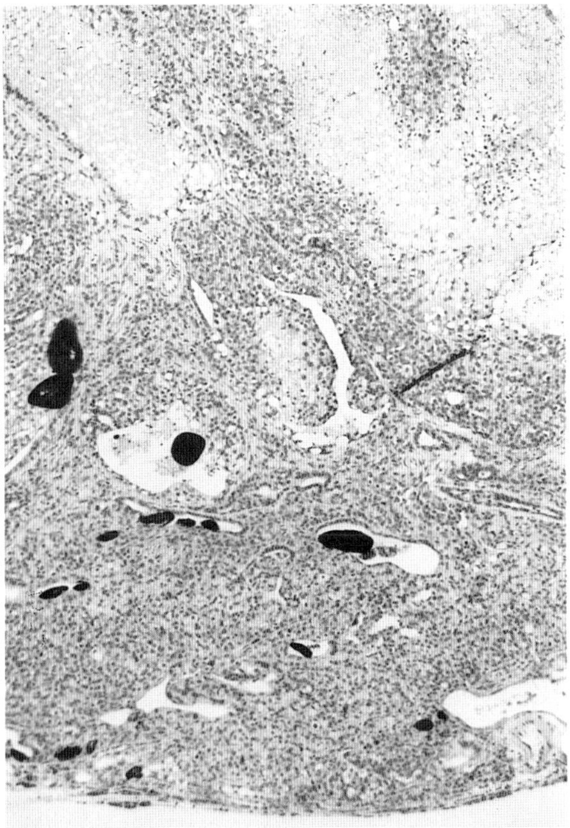

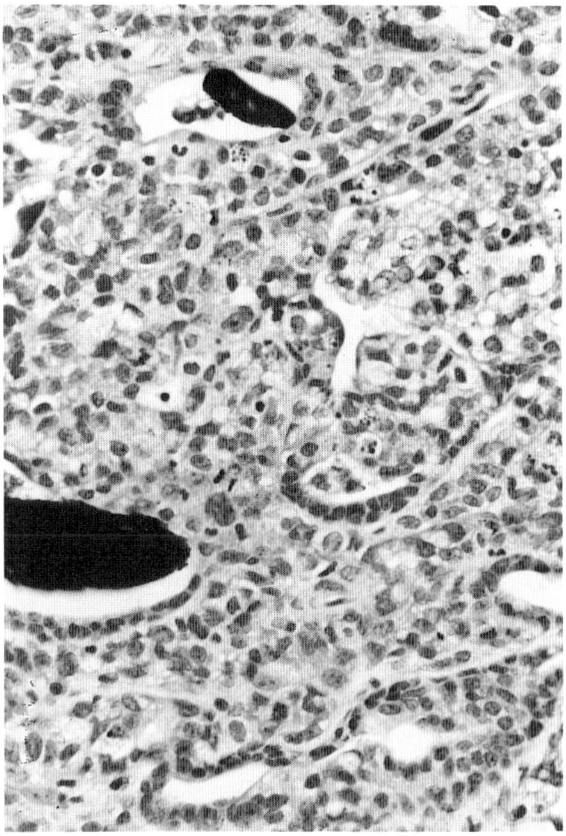

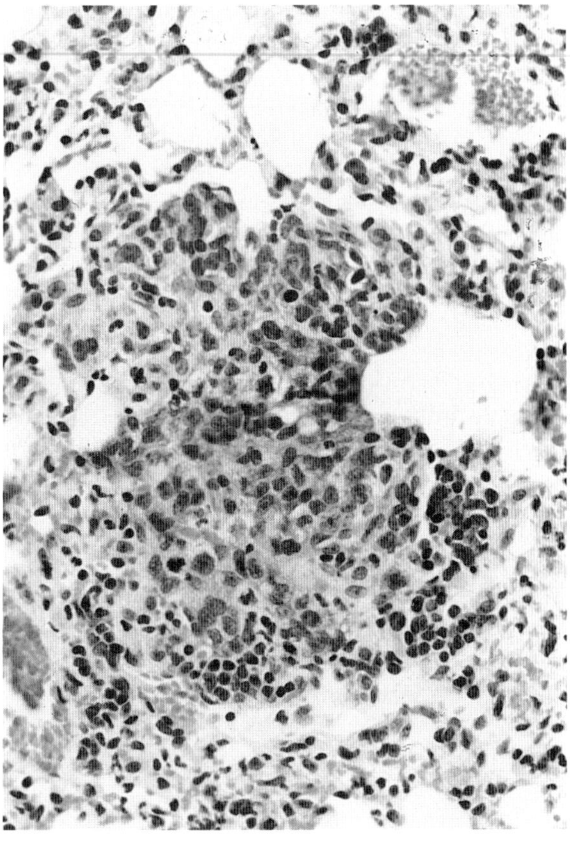

Fig. 117 *(upper left).* Adenocarcinoma of harderian gland, mouse. Note multiple foci of necrosis *(top)*. Most of the neoplasm consists of a solid sheet of epithelial cells with a few alveoli. (Tissue provided by Dr. G. Long, Eli Lilly Co., Greenfield, IN, USA) H & E, ×76

Fig. 118 *(upper right).* Adenocarcinoma of harderian gland, mouse. Neoplasm is composed mostly of a sheet of epithelial cells with nuclear pleomorphism and foamy, vacuolated cytoplasm. Some epithelium is organized into alveoli, two containing pigment. (Tissue provided by Dr. G. Long, Eli Lilly Co., Greenfield, IN, USA) H & E, ×300

Fig. 119 *(lower right).* Adenocarcinoma of harderian gland, mouse. Metastatic focus in the lung. Note the nuclear pleomorphism of the neoplastic cells which fill alveoli. (Tissue provided by Dr. G. Long, Eli Lilly Co., Greenfield, IN, USA) H & E, ×300

Neoplasms of the harderian gland occur primarily in certain strains of mice and rarely in the rat. One adenocarcinoma was found in 1945 Osborne-Mendel rats and one adenoma and one adenocarcinoma were recorded in 3548 aging Fisher 344 rats (Goodman et al. 1979, 1980). The neoplasm has been observed in several strains of mice and the incidence has varied with strain. The incidence was 1.2% in a sample of over 4000 RFM/Un female mice (Ullrich and Storer 1979a), 0.8% in male and 0.5% in female B6C3FI mice (Ward et al. 1979), and 11% in C3Hf/He female mice (Holland et al. 1978). The incidence of harderian gland adenoma was about 2.0% in the Eppley colony of hamsters (Pour et al. 1979) and about 1% in the Hannover colony (Pour et al. 1976). Sheldon et al. (1983) described primary harderian gland neoplasms (574) in 3123 male and 9024 female experimental mice of various ages and of 6 inbred strains and substrains and 3 hybrid stocks. The incidence was about 2.75% in the males and about 5.07% in the females. The BALB/c strain accounted for about 80% of the neoplasms.

Naturally occurring harderian gland neoplasms in mice are found most commonly in aged mice and are slow growing. In the mouse, the glands of the right and left orbit appear affected with equal frequency. Bilateral neoplasms may be both benign and malignant. Most of the neoplasms are benign, and carcinomas with metastases are rare. The carcinoma is poorly differentiated and is considered highly malignant as some metastasize to the lungs (Holland and Fry 1982; Tucker and Baker 1967; Sheldon and Greenman 1979).

The incidence of harderian gland neoplasms has been increased in the mouse by various experimental procedures such as exposure to gamma-radiation (Furth et al. 1960; Ullrich and Storer 1979a, b) X-irradiation (Vesselinovitch et al. 1971a), neutron irradiation (Upton et al. 1954, and treatment with certain chemical carcinogens. The incidence of harderian gland neoplasms has been increased by treatment with such chemicals as urethan (Della Porta et al. 1963; Deringer 1965; Tannenbaum and Silverstone 1958; Vesselinovitch et al. 1970, 1971b), benzidine (Vesselinovitch et al. 1975), ethylnitrosourea (Vesselinovitch et al. 1974), nitrogen mustard nitrous oxide (Matsuyama et al. 1968), and rifampicin (Della Porta et al. 1978). In mice, the harderian glands were more responsive to carcinogenesis when exposed to the carcinogen after opening of the eyelids and functional development of the glands.

Harderian gland neoplasms have also been increased in rats by chemical carcinogens. Harderian gland neoplasms were observed in MRC rats repeatedly injected with 10% urethan (Vesselinovitch and Mihailovich 1968) and in rats fed from weaning a low-fat diet containing 0.03% 2-acetylaminofluorene (Engel and Copeland 1951).

Harderian gland neoplasms that develop in mice treated with carcinogenic chemicals and after exposure to irradiation occur earlier, grow more rapidly, and appear more malignant than naturally occurring neoplasms (Upton et al. 1960). Some of these neoplasms grow invasively and some metastasize to local lymph nodes and to the lungs.

Comparison with Other Species

The harderian gland is not present in humans. Adenomas and carcinomas are observed in the lacrimal and nictitans gland of the dog, but are considered rare. Neoplasms of the nictitans glands (gland of the third eyelid) in the dog have been mistakenly identified as a harderian gland neoplasm. In fact, the dog has no harderian gland. Neoplasms of the harderian gland in domestic animals species are either undescribed or rare.

References

Della Porta G, Capitano J, Montipo W, Parmi L (1963) A study of the carcinogenic action of urethan in mice (in Italian). Tumori 49: 413–428

Della Porta G, Cabral JR, Rossi L (1978) Carcinogenicity study of rifampicin in mice and rats. Toxicol Appl Pharmacol 43: 293–302

Deringer MK (1965) Response of strain DBA/2eBDe mice to treatment with urethan. JNCI 34: 841–847

Engel RW, Copeland DH (1951) Influence of diet on the relative incidence of eye, mammary, ear-duct and liver tumors in rats fed 2-acetylaminofluorene. Cancer Res 11: 180–183

Furth J, Buffett RF, Haran-Ghera N (1960) Pathogenesis and character of radiation-induced pituitary tumors. Acta Unio Int Contra Cancrum 16: 138–142

Goodman DG, Ward JM, Squire RA, Chu KC, Linhart MS (1979) Neoplastic and nonneoplastic lesions in aging F344 rats. Toxicol Appl Pharmacol 48: 237–248

Goodman DG, Ward JM, Spuire RA, Paxton MB, Reichardt WD, Chu KC, Linhart MS (1980) Neoplastic and nonneoplastic lesions in aging Osborne-Mendel rats. Toxicol Appl Pharmacol 55: 433–447

Holland JM, Fry RJM (1982) Neoplasms of the integumentary system and Harderian gland. In: Foster HL, Small JD, Fox JG (eds) The mouse in biomedical research, vol IV. Academic, London, pp 513–528
Holland JM, Mitchell TJ, Gipson LC, Whitaker MS (1978) Survival and cause of death in aging germfree athymic nude and normal inbred C3Hf/He mice. JNCI 61: 1357–1361
Matsuyama M, Suzuki H, Nakamura T (1968) Carcinogenesis in *dd/I* mice injected during suckling period with urethane, nitrogen mustard *N*-oxide and nitroseurethane. Br J Cancer 23: 167–171
Pour P, Mohr U, Althoff J, Cardesa A, Kmoch N (1976) Spontaneous tumors and common diseases in two colonies of Syrian hamsters. IV. Vascular and lymphatic systems and lesions of other sites. JNCI 56: 963–974
Pour P, Althoff J, Salmasi SZ, Stepan K (1979) Spontaneous tumors and common diseases in three types of hamsters. JNCI 63: 797–811
Sheldon WG, Greenman DL (1979) Spontaneous lesions in control BALB/c female mice. J Environ Pathol Toxicol 3: 155–167
Sheldon WG, Curtis MB, Kodell RL, Weed L (1983) Primary Harderian gland neoplasms in mice. JNCI 71: 61
Tannenbaum A, Silverstone H (1958) Urethan (ethyl carbamate) as a multipotential carcinogen. Cancer Res 18: 1225–1231
Tucker MJ, Baker SB (1967) Diseases of specific pathogen-free mice. In: Cotchin E, Roe FJC (eds) Pathology of laboratory rats and mice. Blackwell, Oxford, pp 787–824
Ullrich RL, Storer JB (1979a) Influence of gamma irradiation on the development of neoplastic disease. II. Solid tumors. Radiat Res 80: 317–324
Ullrich RL, Storer JB (1979b) Influence of gamma irradiation on the development of neoplastic disease. III. Dose rate effects. Radiat Res 80: 325–342
Upton AC, Furth J, Christenberry KW (1954) Late effects of thermal neutron irradiation in mice. Cancer Res 14: 682–690
Upton AC, Kimball AW, Furth J, Christenberry KW, Benedict WH (1960) Some delayed effects of atom bomb-radiations in mice. Cancer Res 20 (2): 1–60
Vesselinovitch SD, Mihailovich N (1968) The development of neurogenic neoplasms, embryonal kidney tumors, Harderian gland adenomas, Anitschkow cell sarcomas of the heart, and other neoplasms in urethan-treated newborn rats. Cancer Res 28: 888–897
Vesselinovitch SD, Mihailovich N, Itze L (1970) Comparative studies on the kinetics of the neoplastic competence in mice. Cancer Res 30: 2548–2551
Vesselinovitch SD, Simmons EL, Mikailovich N, Rao KVN, Lombard LS (1971a) The effect of age fractionation and dose on radiation carcinogenesis in various tissues of mice. Cancer Res 31: 2133–2142
Vesselinovitch SD, Mihailovich N, Rao KVN, Itze L (1971b) Perinatal carcinogenesis by urethan. Cancer Res 31: 2143–2147
Vesselinovitch SD, Rao KVN, Mihailovich N, Rice JM, Lombard LS (1974) Development of broad spectrum of tumors by ethylnitrosourea in mice and the modifying role of age, sex and strain. Cancer Res 34: 2530–2538
Vesselinovitch SD, Rao KVN, Mihailovich N (1975) Factors modulating benzidine carcinogenicity bioassay. Cancer Res 35: 2814–2819
Ward JM, Goodman DG, Squire RA, Chu KC, Linhart MS (1979) Neoplastic and nonneoplastic lesions in aging (C57BL/6N X C3H/HeN) F_1 ($B6C3F_1$) mice. JNCI 63: 849–854
Woodhouse MA, Rhodin JA (1963) The ultrastructure of the Harderian gland of the mouse with particular reference to the formation of its secretory product. J Ultrastruct Res 9: 76–98

Atrophy and Sclerosis, Harderian Gland, Rat

Georg J. Krinke

Synonyms. Porphyrin granuloma, spontaneous granulomatous dacryoadenitis.

Gross Appearance

Patchy dark discoloration at the surface of the harderian gland indicates the presence of porphyrin accretions.

Microscopic Features

Atrophy and sclerosis characteristically involve the superficial lobules of the harderian gland (Fig. 120) although they may affect deeper located areas as well; the left and right glands are generally damaged to a similar extent. Porphyrin-containing secretory material forms solid accretions distending the acinar lumina. Parenchymal cells lining the acinar walls undergo atrophy and, in more severe lesions, are replaced by reactive cells such as macrophages

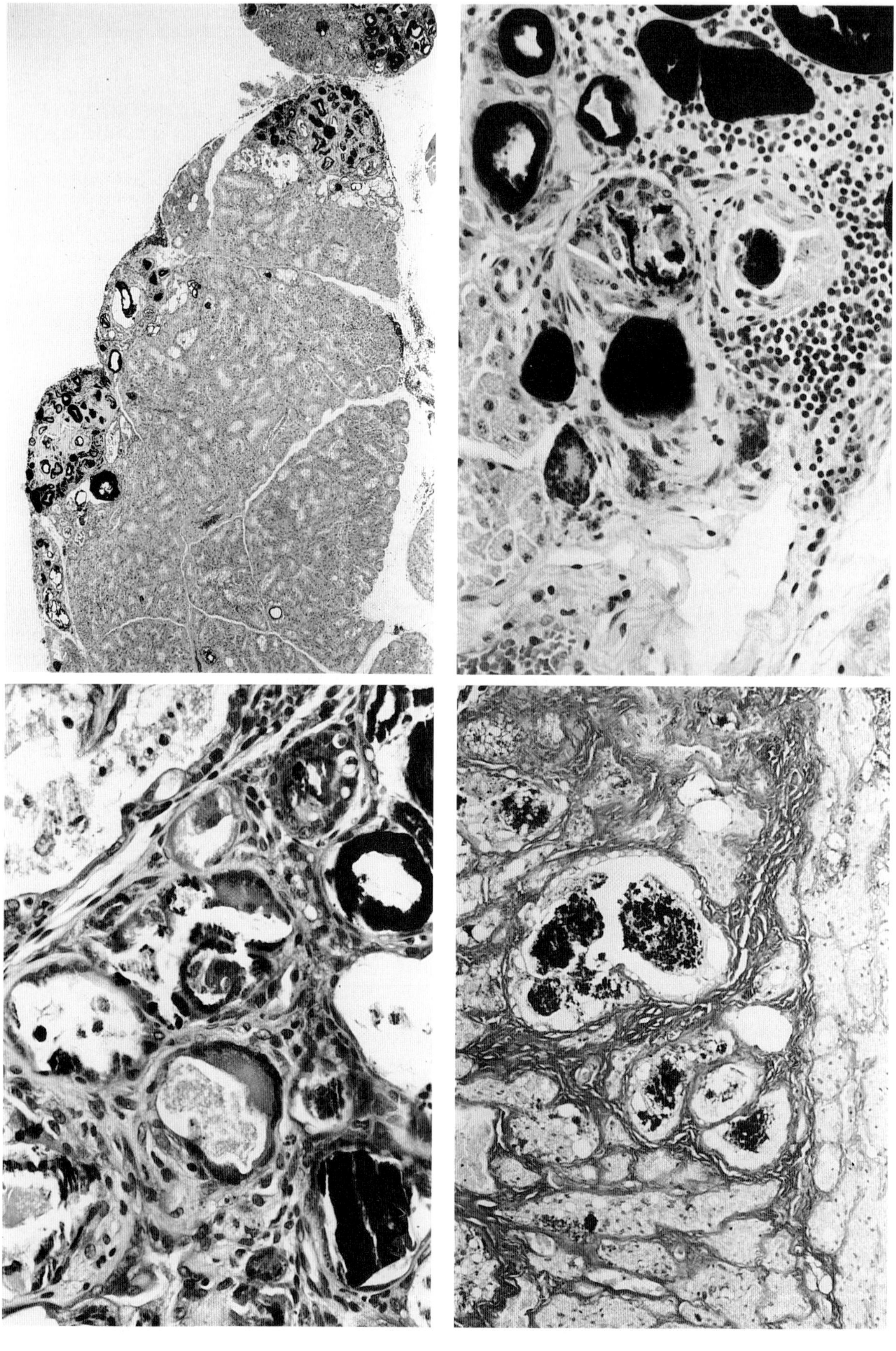

and multinucleate giant cells of foreign body type (Fig. 121). The cytoplasm of macrophages occurring in both the lumina and the interstitium is loaded with porphyrin material, while the presence of epithelioid cells gives the affected area a hyaline appearance. Occasional lymphocytic infiltration may be encountered in the interstitium (Fig. 122).

In advanced lesions, focal sclerosis of the harderian gland is produced by the formation of connective tissue around the acinar units, which retain their function, as well as replacing those which have been destroyed (Fig. 123).

Differential Diagnosis

Localized necrosis and inflammation of the harderian gland may result from trauma following collection of blood from the orbit (McGee and Maronpot 1979). However, in contrast to spontaneous atrophy and sclerosis, the posttraumatic lesion is not accompanied by the presence of porphyrin accretions. Since spontaneous atrophy and sclerosis occur about as frequently in rats subjected to orbital blood collection as in those from which no blood has been withdrawn (Krinke et al. 1988), those changes are considered to occur independently of the procedure.

Although infectious sialodacryoadenitis of rats is characterized by hypersecretion of porphyrin-stained, red tears (chromodacryorrhea), the formation of porphyrin accretions is not observed. The disease produces multilobular inflammatory lesions with variable degrees of squamous metaplasia of the acinar epithelium; moreover the lacrimal and salivary glands may be involved as well (Doi et al. 1980; Eisenbrandt et al. 1982). Some features of experimental autoimmune harderian dacryoadenitis are comparable to those occurring in spontaneous atrophy and sclerosis, but the sequence of events is reversed: spontaneous atrophy and sclerosis are preceded by the formation of porphyrin accretions, but the autoimmune reaction begins as a multifocal, interstitial infiltration of lymphocytes and macrophages, with granulomatous lesions developing later; porphyrin pigment only appears in the advanced stages (Liu et al. 1987).

◀ **Fig. 120** *(upper left)*. Harderian gland, male Sprague-Dawley rat, 25 months old. Accumulation of porphyrin-containing secretory material with a granulomatous reaction within superficial lobules. H & E, ×8.5

Fig. 121 *(lower left)*. Harderian gland, female Sprague-Dawley rat, 26 months old. Multinucleate giant cells of foreign body type adjacent to fragments of porphyrin material. H & E, ×85

Fig. 122 *(upper right)*. Harderian gland, male Sprague-Dawley rat, 25 months old. Large accretions, a focal lymphocytic infiltration *(top)*, and a focal accumulation of macrophages containing scavenged secretory material *(bottom)*. H & E, ×85

Fig. 123 *(lower right)*. Harderian gland, male Wistar rat, 21 months old. Abundant connective tissue fibers are present in the damaged area. Van Gieson, ×35

Biologic Features

Natural History

The harderian gland is considered to be a specialized derivative of an ancestral lacrimal gland, occurring in various vertebrates including some mammalian species. In mammals its function probably varies among species, e.g., in aquatic animals its secretion is thought to protect the eye from sea water. In rodents the gland often contains porphyrin, but its significance is uncertain; it may function as a sebaceous gland, or it may be involved in phermonal (odoripherous, behavior-related) mechanisms (Sakai 1981). The presence of light-absorbing porphyrin may provide photoprotection in those species adapted to a dark environment (Hugo et al. 1987). The porphyrin content of the rat harderian gland increases with age, the male gland invariably containing higher concentrations than that of the female (Rohonyi and Kelenyi 1962).

In neonatal rats, the harderian gland may influence pineal function by acting as an extraretinal photoreceptor (Wetterberg et al. 1970). Its secretory pattern depends on diurnal lighting conditions; sexual dimorphism is evident in that in the female neonatal gland a higher proportion of acini contain secretory material in comparison with the male (Feria-Velasco et al. 1983).

Ovarian function appears to be essential for the maintenance of porphyrin synthesis; in adult female rats ovariectomy decreases the porphyrin content, which may be restored to control values by the administration of oestradiol plus progesterone. In addition, constant light or constant darkness decrease the porphyrin content in comparison with diurnal lighting (Ulrich et al. 1974).

Pathogenesis and Etiology

The superficial localization of the lesions indicates predominant involvement of the terminal portions of selected glandular units. The early changes consist of the formation of porphyrin accretions, possibly due to the accumulation of redundant secretory material (Krinke and Krinke 1987).

The increased frequency of the lesions in aging rats as well as the presence of sex differences may reflect a hormonal influence on the secretory activity of the harderian gland. In female hamsters, ovariectomy brings about the formation of accretions surrounded by foreign body giant cells and macrophages (Spike et al. 1985). In view of the sensitivity of the harderian gland to light, illumination probably plays a role.

The reactive changes have features compatible with the findings in foreign body granulomas. The propensity of the rat harderian gland to produce granulomatous lesions with a significant epithelioid cell component has been demonstrated in experimental autoimmune dacryoadenitis, and tentatively attributed to the sebaceous character of its secretory product (Liu et al. 1987).

Frequency

Spontaneous atrophy and sclerosis of the rat harderian gland are related to advancing age. In Sprague-Dawley rats, changes at 1 year are mild and affect about 34% of the animals, while in the 2nd and 3rd year of life they are more severe and occur in 80%–91%. Females appear to be more susceptible than males of a comparable age (Krinke and Krinke 1987; Krinke et al. 1988); a recent examination of control groups from a long-term study on Wistar rats, however, detected more frequent lesions in male than in female animals (unpublished).

Comparison with Other Species

In aging mice, porphyrin accretions form in the harderian gland, which undergoes atrophy of acinar cells and foci of macrophages and lymphocytes. In comparison with the rat, neither the superficial distribution of the lesion nor the prominent sclerotic change are so obvious in the mouse harderian gland. Interestingly, some of the tumors which occur characteristically in the mouse harderian gland appear to be devoid of redundant porphyrin secretory material, even if the unaffected glandular tissue contains accretions. Atrophy of gland epithelium, the formation of porphyrin accretions, and infiltration by phagocytes and other inflammatory cells have been reported in the harderian gland of aging hamsters (Payne et al. 1985).

References

Doi K, Yasoshima A, Kojima A, Okawa H, Kurabe S, Okaniwa A (1980) Pathological observations on natural cases of sialodacryoadenitis of rats. Exp Anim 29: 419–426

Eisenbrandt DL, Hubbard GB, Schmidt RE (1982) A subclinical epizootic of sialodacryoadenitis in rats. Lab Anim Sci 32: 655–659

Feria-Velasco A, Melendez C, Jaramillo J (1983) Sex differences in secretion pattern of neonatal rat Harderian gland under various environmental lighting conditions. Comp Biochem Physiol [B] 74: 709–714

Hugo J, Krijt J, Vokurka M, Janousek V (1987) Secretory response to light in rat harderian gland: possible photoprotective role of harderian porphyrin. Gen Physiol Biophys 6: 401–404

Krinke AL, Krinke G (1987) Sex-related difference in changes with age of the rat Harderian gland. Verh Anat Ges 81: 665–667

Krinke A, Froehlich E, Kobel W, Krinke G (1988) Does the repeated orbital sinus puncture alter the occurrence of changes with age in the retina, the lens, or the Harderian gland of laboratory rats? Z Versuchstierkd 31: 111–119

Liu SH, Sakai F, Prendergast RA, Silverstein AM (1987) Experimental autoimmune dacryoadenitis II. Harderian gland disease in the rat. Invest Ophthalmol Vis Sci 28: 276–280

McGee MA, Maronpot RR (1979) Harderian gland dacryoadenitis in rats resulting from orbital bleeding. Lab Animal Sci 29: 639–641

Payne AP, McGadey J, Johnston HS (1985) Interstitial porphyrins and tubule degeneration in the hamster Harderian gland. J Anat 140 (Part 1): 25–36

Rohonyi B, Kelenyi G (1962) Porphyrin content of the Harderian gland of the rat. Acta Biol Hung 13: 241–245

Sakai T (1981) The mammalian Harderian gland: morphology, biochemistry, function and phylogeny. Arch Histol Jpn 44: 299–333

Spike RC, Johnston HS, McGadey J, Moore MR, Thompson GG, Payne (1985) Quantitative studies on the effects of hormones on structure and porphyrin biosynthesis in the Harderian gland of the female golden hamster. 1. The effects of ovariectomy and androgen administration. J Anat 142: 59–72

Ulrich R, Yuwiler A, Geller E, Wetterberg L (1974) Effects of sex hormones and environmental lighting on rat Harderian gland porphyrin. J Endocrinol 63: 99–102

Wetterberg L, Geller E, Yuwiler A (1970) Harderian gland: an extraretinal photoreceptor influencing the pineal gland in neonatal rats? Science 167: 884–885

The Ear

Adenoma of the Auditory Sebaceous Glands, Rat

John C. Seely

Synonyms. Sebaceous adenoma, squamous cell papilloma, adenoma or papilloma of Zymbal's gland, papillary adenoma, Zymbal's gland.

Gross Appearance

Most adenomas of the auditory sebaceous glands are not grossly apparent. Usually they are discovered during routine microscopic examination of the glands. Rarely, they may be observed as papillomatous growths within the ear canal or as subcutaneous nodules, lying anterioventral to the ear.

Microscopic Features

Spontaneous auditory sebaceous gland adenomas are usually solitary neoplasms which may be observed within the lumen of the ear canal, immediately below the epithelium of the distal portion of the ear canal or within the portion of the large Zymbal's gland which lies beneath the ear canal. These neoplasms tend to be expansive growths characterized either by a solid proliferation of sebaceous cells (Fig. 124) or by complex patterns of sebaceous cells and papillary growths (Fig. 125) covered predominantly by keratinized, squamous cell epithelium. These latter neoplasms tend to arise within the sebaceous glands underlying the epithelium of the ear canal and proliferate into the ear canal (Fig. 126). Most adenomas are usually well circumscribed, are larger than one individual lobule, and lack significant encapsulation. Cystic spaces or dilated channels are often present in adenomas and, depending upon their size, may be lined by stratified squamous epithelium. These spaces or channels contain varying amounts of eosinophilic secretory material, desquamated necrotic cells, and inflammatory cells. Adenomas are composed of cells which generally resemble sebaceous cells. Disruption of the normal cell maturation process and disorganized lobular architecture further characterize adenomas. Adenomas also contain varying populations of basal cells and intermediate cells. Diffuse enlargement of all glands and intact lobular architecture are characteristic of hyperplasia. An adenoma is seen as an expanding mass involving only part of the sebaceous glands.

Ultrastructure

Zymbal's gland adenomas do not appear to have been studied with the electron microscope. It may be assumed that these neoplasms have the same features observed as other sebaceous gland adenomas. However, this assumption needs to be established by appropriate studies.

Differential Diagnosis

Adenomas of the auditory sebaceous glands must be differentiated from sebaceous gland adenomas arising in the skin in the vicinity of the base of the ear. This differential diagnosis, however, can be established by a careful gross examination to determine its precise location. Squamous papillomas of the ear canal could arise from the squamous epithelium lining the ear canal. A papilloma near the base of the ear canal is more likely to be of Zymbal's gland origin especially if it contains sebaceous cells.

Biologic Features

Benign neoplasms of Zymbal's gland appear to represent a progression from hyperplasia since known carcinogens also cause hyperplasia early in the process (Copeland-Haines and Eustis 1990). Adenomas may or may not progress into carcinomas. Neoplastic features such as size, dysplasia, and cellular atypia (Copeland-Haines and Eustis 1990) are usually insufficient to predict the ultimate behavior.

Etiology and Frequency

Adenomas of the auditory sebaceous glands are uncommon neoplasms. Malignant tumors seem to be reported more frequently than adenomas. Available data from several different rat strains would suggest that the frequency of adenomas

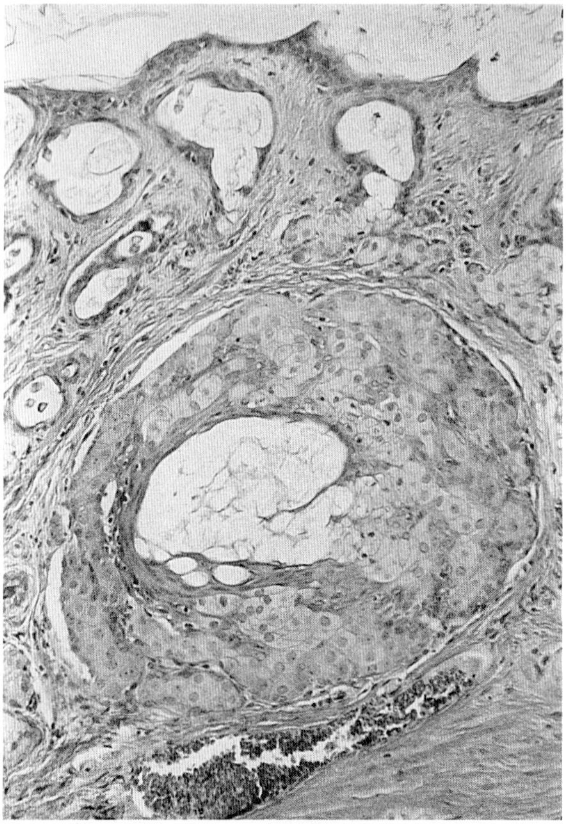

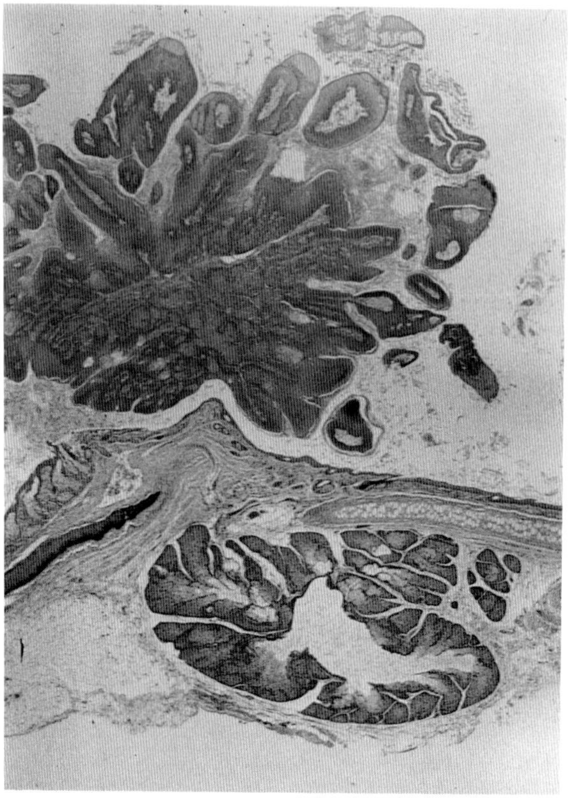

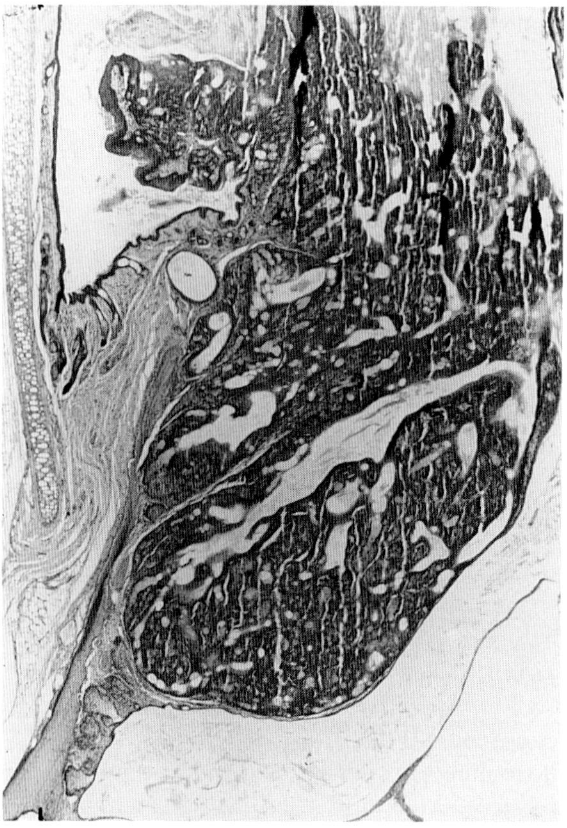

Fig. 124 *(upper left).* Adenoma, Zymbal's gland, rat. A well-circumscribed expanded nodule between the epithelium of the ear canal *(top)* and the aural cartilage *(bottom).* H & E, × 160

Fig. 125 *(lower left).* Adenoma, Zymbal's gland, rat. The mass protrudes into the ear canal and is composed primarily of sebaceous cells and stratified squamous epithelium. (From Seely 1986 with permission of *Lab Animal*) H & E, × 25

Fig. 126 *(upper right).* Adenoma, papillary, Zymbal's gland, rat, within the ear canal. Although the neoplasm is covered by papillomatous stratified squamous epithelium, the central portion (outside the aural cartilage) is made up of sebaceous cells. H & E, × 25 and carcinomas is less than 1% (Deerberg and Rehm 1981; Goodman et al. 1979; Pliss 1973; Schardein et al. 1968; Snell 1965). Since benign neoplasms are rarely observed grossly and routine sections of Zymbal's glands may not be prepared, the reported incidence of spontaneous adenomas may be understated. Neoplasms of the auditory sebaceous glands have been induced by a variety of carcinogens (Pliss 1973; Pohl and Fouts 1983; Seely 1986). However, most of these chemicals induce malignant neoplasms and, therefore, the discussion of induced tumors will be covered under the topic of carcinomas.

Comparison with Other Species

Spontaneous neoplasms of Zymbal's glands appear to occur exclusively in the rat. Zymbal's gland adenomas in other species are either rare or have not been reported. Ceruminous gland tumors in the cat and dog may be compared to Zymbal's gland neoplasms since they tend to be found in the deeper portion of the ear canal and tend to have either glandular or papillary patterns (Carpenter et al. 1987). Morphologically similar neoplasms in man are not known since humans do not have auditory sebaceous glands.

References

Carpenter JL, Andrews LK, Holzworth J (1987) Tumors and tumor-like lesions. Adenocarcinoma of ceruminous glands. In: Holzworth J (ed) Diseases of the cat: medicine and surgery. Saunders, Philadelphia, pp 567–568

Copeland-Haines DC, Eustis SL (1990) Specialized sebaceous glands. In: Boorman GA, Eustis SL, Elwell MR, Montgomery CA, MacKenzie WF (eds) Pathology of the Fischer rat. Academic, San Diego, pp 279–292

Deerberg F, Rehm S (1981) Tumours of the external auditory canal and the auditory sebaceous glands in Han: Wist rats. Z Versuchstierkd 23: 134–137

Goodman DG, Ward JM, Squire RA, Chu KC, Linhart MS (1979) Neoplastic and non-neoplastic lesions in aging F–344 rats. Toxicol Appl Pharmacol 48: 237–248

Pliss GB (1973) Tumours of the auditory sebaceous glands. In: Turusov VS (ed) Pathology of tumours in laboratory animals. IARC Sci Publ 1 (1): 22–30

Pohl RJ, Fouts JR (1983) Cytochrome P-450-dependent xenobiotic metabolizing activity in Zymbal's gland, a specialized sebaceous gland of rodents. Cancer Res 43: 3660–3662

Schardein JL, Fitzgerald JE, Kaump DH (1968) Spontaneous tumors in Holtzman-source rats of various ages. Pathol Vet 5: 238–252

Seely JC (1986) Zymbal glands in the rat. Lab Anim 15: 25–31

Snell KC (1965) Spontaneous lesions of the rat. In: Ribelin WE, McCoy JR (eds) The pathology of laboratory animals. Thomas, Springfield, pp 241–302

Carcinoma of the Auditory Sebaceous Glands, Rat

John C. Seely

Synonyms. Sebaceous adenocarcinoma, squamous cell carcinoma, ceruminous carcinoma, adenosquamous carcinoma, basal-cell carcinoma, carcinosarcoma, Zymbal's gland carcinoma.

Gross Appearance

Carcinomas of the auditory sebaceous glands usually arise as firm, subcutaneous nodules just below the ear canal. Occasionally, they may be apparent as papillary growths within the ear canal. Subcutaneous tumors tend to grow rapidly, ulcerate, and involve the entire side of the face and neck. On cut surface, they usually have a gritty texture. Local invasion into adjacent soft tissue or bone is not uncommon. Pulmonary or regional lymph node metastases may be present.

Microscopic Features

Auditory sebaceous gland carcinomas, like adenomas, are usually solitary neoplasms but are less well circumscribed than adenomas. Because of their large size, it may not always be possible to determine in what portion of the Zymbal's glands the neoplasm originated. Carcinomas may consist of irregular acini or solid sheets of cells and frequently contain cystic cavities filled with cellular and keratinous debris

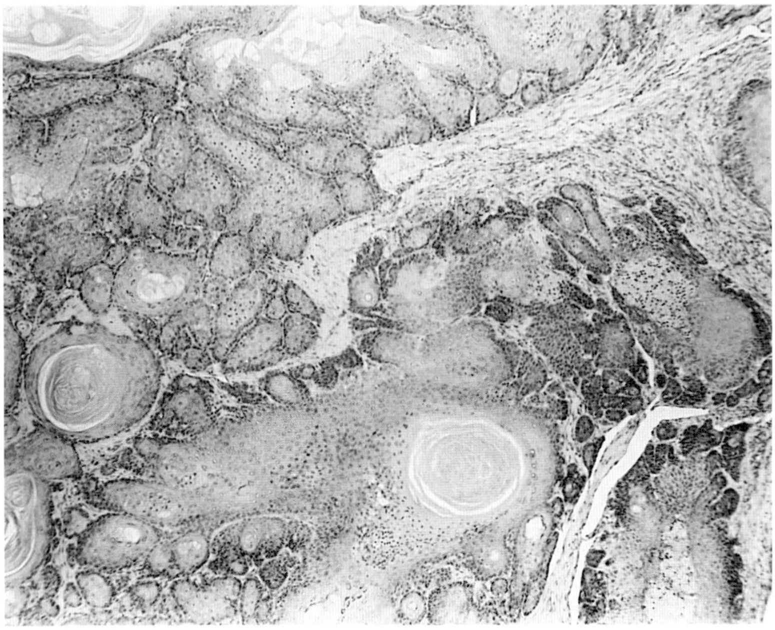

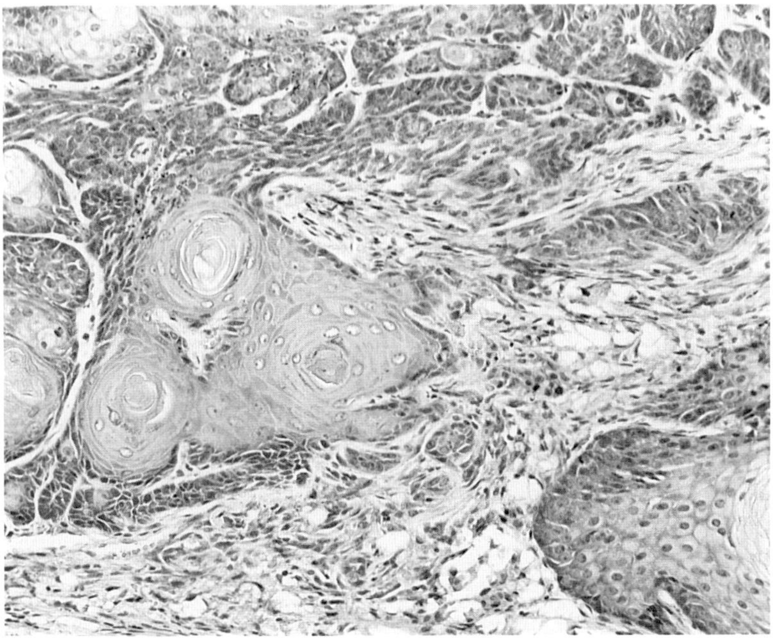

Fig. 127 *(above)*. Carcinoma, auditory sebaceous gland (Zymbal's gland), rat. A well-differentiated, keratinized, infiltrative carcinoma. H & E, ×63

Fig. 128 *(below)*. Carcinoma, auditory sebaceous gland (Zymbal's gland), rat. Higher magnification of the carcinoma in Fig. 127 illustrating tumor cell invasion through the basement membrane. H & E, ×160

(Copeland-Haines and Eustis 1990). Papillary projections covered by squamous epithelium may be observed in the larger cystic spaces. Carcinomas may be well differentiated containing neoplastic sebaceous cells and squamous epithelium with keratin (Fig. 127). Most carcinomas, however, tend to be highly pleomorphic and anaplastic neoplasms. These tumors lose much of their Zymbal's gland appearance and are characterized by local invasion into adjacent soft tissue and/or bone (Fig. 128). These neoplasms are often accompanied by a stromal proliferation or scirrhous reaction. Within some tumors, it may be difficult to distinguish between the nonneoplastic stroma and neoplastic cells which have become fusiform in appearance (Fig. 129).

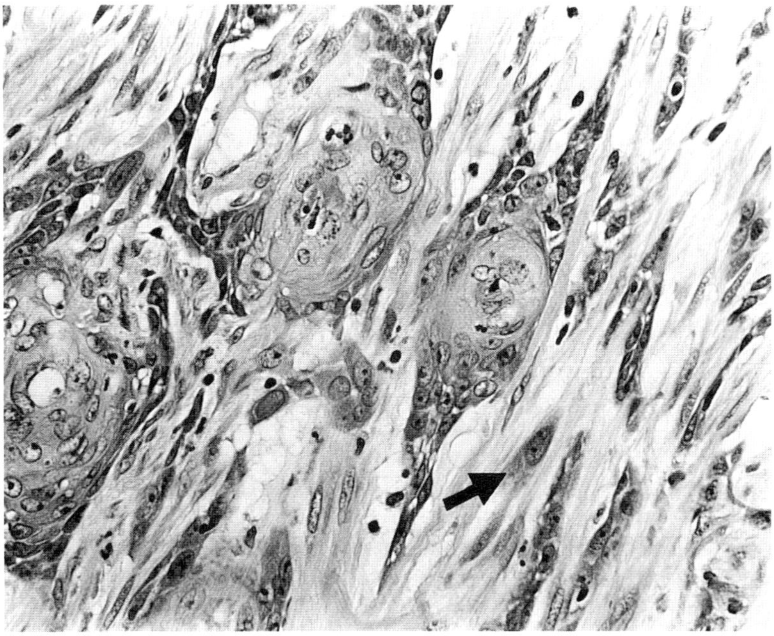

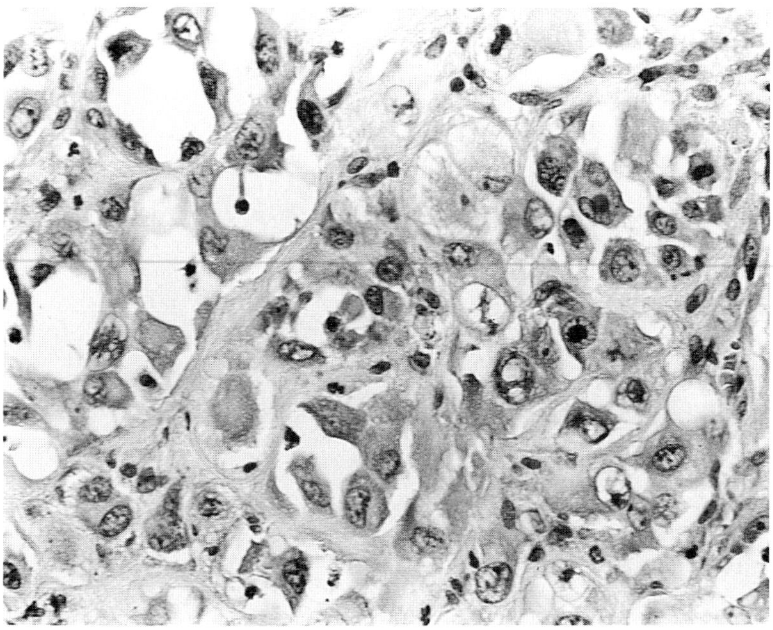

Fig. 129 *(above)*. Carcinoma, auditory sebaceous gland (Zymbal's gland), rat. Islands of poorly differentiated carcinoma cells surrounded by a connective tissue stroma. Fusiform carcinoma cells *(arrow)* admixed with spindle-shaped connective tissue cells are also present. H & E, ×400

Fig. 130 *(below)*. Carcinoma, auditory sebaceous gland (Zymbal's gland), rat. Highly anaplastic neoplasm. H & E, ×400

Occasionally, large proportions of the tumor may contain solid growths of fusiform cells which appear malignant, leading some to diagnose these as carcionsarcomas (Copeland-Haines and Eustis 1990). However, in these neoplasms, it is not clear if this sarcomatous component is derived from the stroma or from anaplastic epithelium. Highly anaplastic neoplasms may contain considerable cellular atypia (Fig. 130) consisting of cells with large nuclei, variable amounts of cytoplasm, and increased numbers of mitotic figures. Metastatic sites may contain one or more of the neoplastic cell types found in the primary tumor.

Ultrastructure

As with adenomas, carcinomas do not appear to have been studied with the electron microscope. It may be assumed that these neoplasms have the same features observed as other sebaceous gland carcinomas. However, this assumption needs to be established by appropriate studies.

Differential Diagnosis

Carcinomas of the auditory sebaceous glands must be differentiated primarily from squamous cell carcinomas arising from the skin in the vicinity of the base of the ear or from the squamous epithelium lining the ear canal. Reports have described tumors as squamous cell carcinomas of skin origin around the ears that most likely were carcinomas of Zymbal's gland (Seely 1986). Zymbal's gland carcinomas would also have to be differentiated from other highly malignant glandular neoplasms which could theoretically arise near the ear. These tumors could represent either sebaceous carcinomas of the skin or salivary gland neoplasms. In any event, a careful and thorough gross examination should always be performed in these cases.

Biologic Features

Malignant neoplasms of the Zymbal's glands appear to represent an "end stage" in the biologic continuum from adenoma or papilloma to carcinoma. Histologic subclassification of carcinomas into primary sebaceous, squamous, or other cell types does not seem warranted in routine carcinogenicity studies.

Etiology and Frequency

Carcinomas of the auditory sebaceous glands are reported more frequently than adenomas. This may be due, in part, to the fact that in some carcinogenic studies routine sections of the Zymbal's glands are not performed and only grossly observed Zymbal's gland masses are selected for histologic examination. Published data from several different rat strains would suggest that their frequency (carcinomas and adenomas) is less than 1% (Deerberg and Rehm 1981; Goodman et al. 1979; Haseman et al. 1985; Pliss 1973; Schardein et al. 1968; Snell 1965). Malignant neoplasms of the auditory sebaceous glands have been induced by a variety of chemical carcinogens (Huff et al. 1988; Laws et al. 1955; Schardein and Kaump 1966; Takayama et al. 1984; Tannenbaum et al. 1962). Nine chemicals which were identified as causing Zymbal's gland neoplasms in rats from a survey of 222 chemicals evaluated for carcinogenicity by NCI/NTP were also mutagenic for *Salmonella typhimurium* (Ashby and Tennant 1988). Many of these chemicals additionally caused preputial/clitoral neoplasms which are also modified sebaceous glands. In addition, reactive metabolites of chemical carcinogens may be formed in Zymbal's gland since homogenates of the gland contain cytochrome P-450-dependent enzyme activity (Pohl and Fouts 1983).

Comparison with Other Species

Spontaneous Zymbal's gland carcinomas in other species are either rare or have not been reported. Malignant neoplasms of the mouse Zymbal's glands have been induced by ingestion of benzene (Maltoni et al 1988). The relative infrequency of the carcinogenic response in mouse Zymbal's glands has been postulated to be due to a lower cytochrome P-450 activity, a lower cellular turnover than that found in the rat, and fewer fully differentiated cells per unit area (Pohl and Fouts 1983). Morphologically similar neoplasms in man are not known since humans do not have the same type of auditory sebaceous glands.

References

Ashby J, Tennant RW (1988) Chemical structure, *Salmonella* mutagenicity and extent of carcinogenicity as indicators of genotoxic carcinogenesis among 222 chemicals tested in rodents by the U. S. NCI/NTP. Mutat Res 204: 17–115

Copeland-Haines DC, Eustis SL (1990) Specialized sebaceous glands. In: Boorman GA, Eustis SL, Elwell MR, Montgomery CA, MacKenzie WF (eds) Pathology of the Fischer rat. Academic, San Diego, pp 279–292

Deerberg F, Rehm S (1981) Tumours of the external auditory canal and the auditory sebaceous glands in Han: Wist rats. Short Communication. Z Versuchstierkd 23: 134–137

Goodman DG, Ward JM, Squire RA, Chu KC, Linhart MS (1979) Neoplastic and non-neoplastic lesions in aging F-344 rats. Toxicol Appl Pharmacol 48: 237–248

Haseman JK, Huff JE, Rao GN, Arnold JE, Boorman GA, McConnell EE (1985) Neoplasms observed in

untreated and corn oil gavage control groups of F344/N rats and (C57 BL/6N X C3H/HeN) F 1 (B6C3F1) mice. JNCI 75: 975–984
Huff JE, Eastin W, Roycroft J, Eustis SL, Haseman JK (1988) Carcinogenesis studies of benzene, methyl benzene, and dimethyl benzenes. Ann NY Acad Sci 534: 427–441
Laws JO, Rudali G, Royer R, Mabrille P (1955) The early changes produced in the auditory sebaceous gland (Zymbal's gland) of the rat by 2-acetylaminofluorine. Cancer Res 15: 139–142
Maltoni C, Conti B, Perino G, DiMaio V (1988) Further evidence of benzene carcinogenicity. Results on Wistar rats and Swiss mice treated by ingestion. Ann NY Acad Sci 534: 412–426
Pliss GB (1973) Tumours of the auditory sebaceous glands. In: Turusov VS (ed) Pathology of tumours in laboratory animals. IARC Sci Publ 1 (1): 23–30
Pohl RJ, Fouts JR (1983) Cytochrome P-450-dependent xenobiotic metabolizing activity in Zymbal's gland, a specialized sebaceous gland of rodents. Cancer Res 43: 3660–3662
Schardein JL, Kaump DH (1966) Auditory canal structures in rats as altered by aging and by the administration of tris (*p*-aminophenyl) carbonium pamoate. Cancer Res 26: 1625–1632
Schardein JL, Fitzgerald JE, Kaump DH (1968) Spontaneous tumors in Holtzman-source rats of various ages. Pathol Vet 5: 238–252
Seely JC (1986) Zymbal glands in the rat. Lab Anim 15: 25–31
Snell KC (1965) Spontaneous lesions of the rat. In: Ribelin WE, McCoy JR (eds) The pathology of laboratory animals. Thomas, Springfield, pp 1–60
Takayama S, Masuda M, Mogami M, Ohgaki H, Sato S, Sugimura T (1984) Induction of cancers in the intestine, liver, and various other organs of rats by feeding mutagens from glutamic acid pyrolysate. Gann 75: 207–213
Tannenbaum A, Vesselinovitch SD, Maltoni C, Mitchell DS (1962) Multipotential carcinogenicity of urethan in the Sprague-Dawley rat. Cancer Res 22: 1362–1371

Auricular Chondritis, Rat

Taisan Chiu

Synonyms. Chondritis, external ear; auricular cartilage, inflammation.

Gross Appearance

The gross appearance of experimentally induced lesions resembles that of naturally occurring ones. The lesions are seen in both ears. In the early stages of the natural disease the affected ears show no clinically detectable abnormality. Slight focal nodular or diffuse swelling and thickening, with or without erythema, develops as the lesions progress. These signs may partially or completely disappear. Nodule size and thickening increase up to a certain point and then stop without further change. The thickness of the ears ranges up to many times normal (Fig. 131). Subsequently, the ears become irregularly thickened (Fig. 132), white, firm, nodular, and droopy (Fig. 133) or remarkably deformed and misshapen (Fig. 134), resembling "cauliflower" or "wrestler" ears in man. Generally, there is no apparent change on the surface of the skin of the affected pinnae but, in some rats, the skin may be scaly, alopercic, or ulcerated.

Microscopic Features

The histologic features of both naturally occurring and experimentally induced lesions are similar. Depending upon the stage of the disease process, the lesions invariably consist of granulomatous inflammation; fibrovascular, fibrochondrous, chondrous, or chondroosseous tissues; or a mixture of these. The lesions are focal or multifocal, which are later coalesced. In the very early stages of the disease, the characteristic histologic change is an active granulomatous inflammation involving the auricular cartilage, which is otherwise normal (Fig. 135). The inflammatory cells involved are mainly neutrophils and histiocytes, and some lymphoid cells and multinucleated giant cells; occasionally, eosinophils may be present. As the disease progresses, the normal cartilage plate is gradually destroyed by inflammation, and fibrovascular tissue develops at the edge of the lesion. This proliferative fibrovascular tissue is then trans-

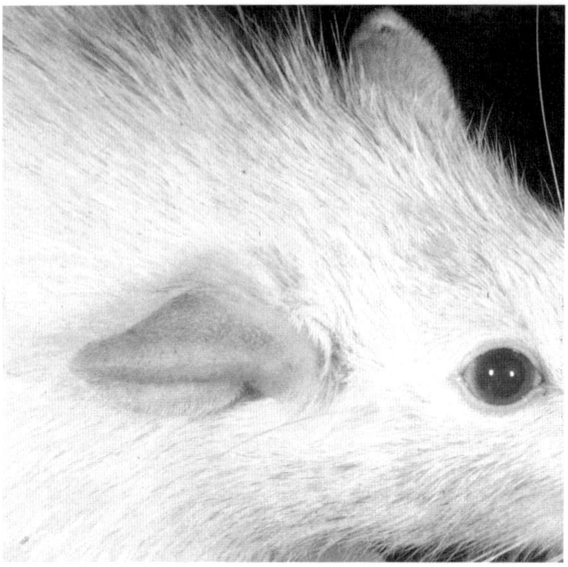

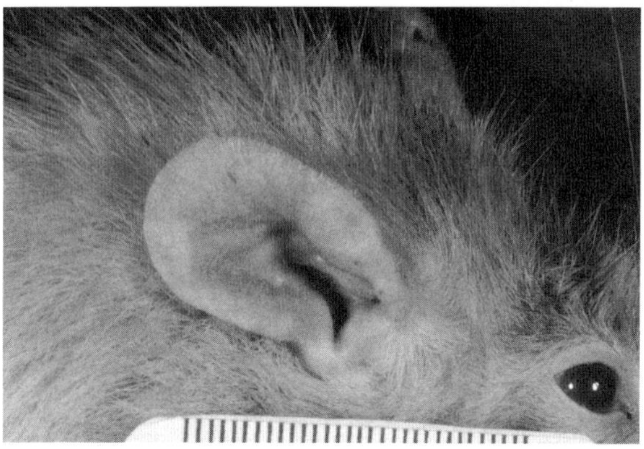

Fig. 131 *(above).* Auricular chondritis, rat. Puffy, evenly thickened external ears. The ears are slightly erythematous

Fig. 132 *(below).* Auricular chondritis, rat. The ears of the same rat as shown in Fig. 131, taken 2 months later. Note a somewhat decreased swelling and an uneven surface with a nodular appearance

formed into nodular masses of proliferating fibrochondrous and chondrous tissue followed by osseous metaplasia (Fig. 136). Some of the osseous tissue contains marrow tissue with hemopoietic activity. The inflammatory reaction may become less active and gradually subside but usually not until the entire cartilage plate has been involved. In rats with chronic disease, the entire central core of the thin cartilage may be replaced by irregularly thickened, newly formed nodular masses of fibrovascular, fibrochondrous, chondrous, and/or chondroosseous tissues (Figs. 137, 138). In the fibrovascular areas between the nodular masses of fibrochondrous and chondrous tissues, there are focal mononuclear cell infiltrates, mainly lymphocytes and plasma cells (Fig. 139). The dermis and epidermis overlying the lesion usually have no significant microscopic alteration. However, dermal edema and inflammatory infiltrates and epidermal acanthosis and ulceration may be present.

Ultrastructure

The ultrastructural changes of the naturally occurring lesions have not been reported. In experimentally induced lesions, electron-dense deposits that are irregular in shape and size have been observed around the chondrocytes in the clinically normal area (Cremer et al. 1981).

Differential Diagnosis

Nodular masses of fibrochondrous or chondrous tissue in chronic auricular chondritis should be distinguished from fibrochondroma, chondroma, or chondrosarcoma. In auricular chondritis, the irregular nodular masses of fibrovascular, fibrochondrous, chondrous, and/or chondroosseous tissues may partially or entirely replace the central core of the pinnae where the normal cartilage plate was once present. The presence of focal mononuclear inflammatory infiltrates in the fibrovascular tissue is also helpful in making a distinction. In addition, there is frequent osseous metaplasia. In neoplasms, the lesions are localized proliferating tissues which only partially replace the central core of the pinna and are not usually accompanied by granulomatous inflammation.

Advanced lesions of auricular chondritis can be difficult to distinguish grossly and histologically from chronic lesions found in an auricular cartilage disease that develops from a unique and distinctive noninflammatory process – chondrolysis (Chiu and Lee 1984; Enomoto et al. 1983). The damaged and split cartilage caused by chondrolysis may be followed by a regeneration of fibrochondrous, chondrous, and chondroosseous tissues identical to auricular chondritis. The diagnosis becomes even more difficult when both inflammatory and noninflammatory disease processes occur separately in the same ear and coalesce later (Chiu and Lee 1984).

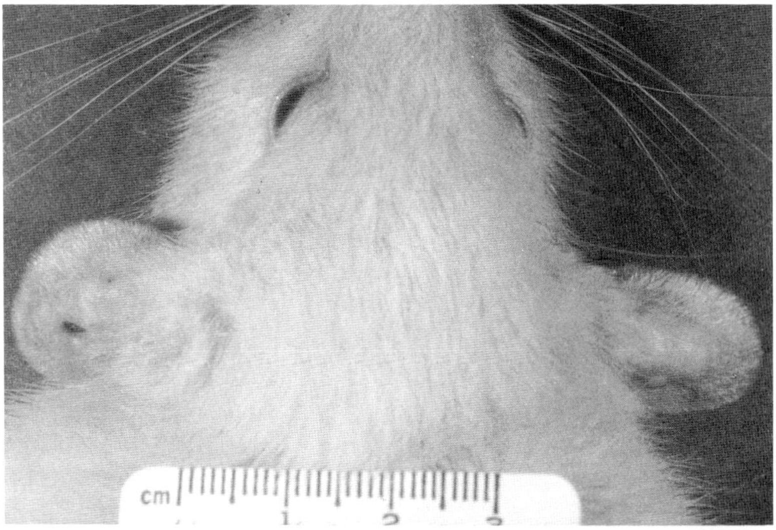

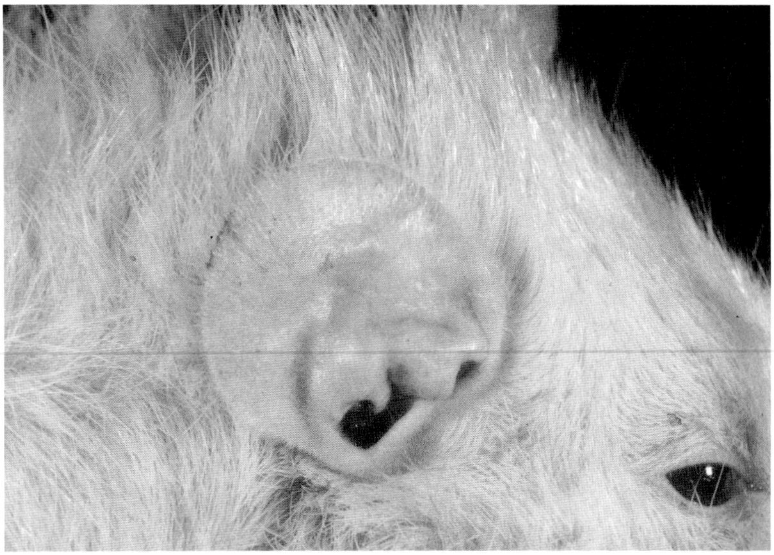

Fig. 133 *(above)*. Chronic auricular chondritis, rat. Both pinnae are thickened, white, nodular, and droopy

Fig. 134 *(below)*. Advanced auricular chondritis, rat. A remarkably misshapen ear

Biologic Features

Auricular chondritis in rats occurs naturally and can also be induced experimentally. There are only a handful of reports of natural or experimental auricular chondritis in rats. The natural diesease has been reported in male and female Sprague-Dawley (S–D) (Chiu and Lee 1984), fawn-hooded (F–H), and F–H x NBR rats (Prieur et al. 1984). The lesions in these rats are identical in their gross, histologic, and biologic features. Auricular chondritis was produced in female rats (males not tested) of the S–D and Wistar but not Wistar-Lewis (W–L) strains by intradermal injection of type II collagen to the back, hind footpad, and tail (Cremer et al. 1981; McCune et al. 1982). However, arthritis was induced in all of these strains of rats and few rats developed only ear lesions without arthritis. In addition to gross and histologic appearances, some biologic features of the experimentally induced ear diseases resemble those of the naturally occurring ones. Both pinnae are affected in most rats. The precise age of onset of the naturally occuring disease is not known; however, a gross ear change was observed in rats approximately 6 months old and older (Chiu and Lee 1984; Prieur et al. 1984). The natural incidence of gross ear deformity in outbred S–D rats which were obtained from Charles River Breeding La-

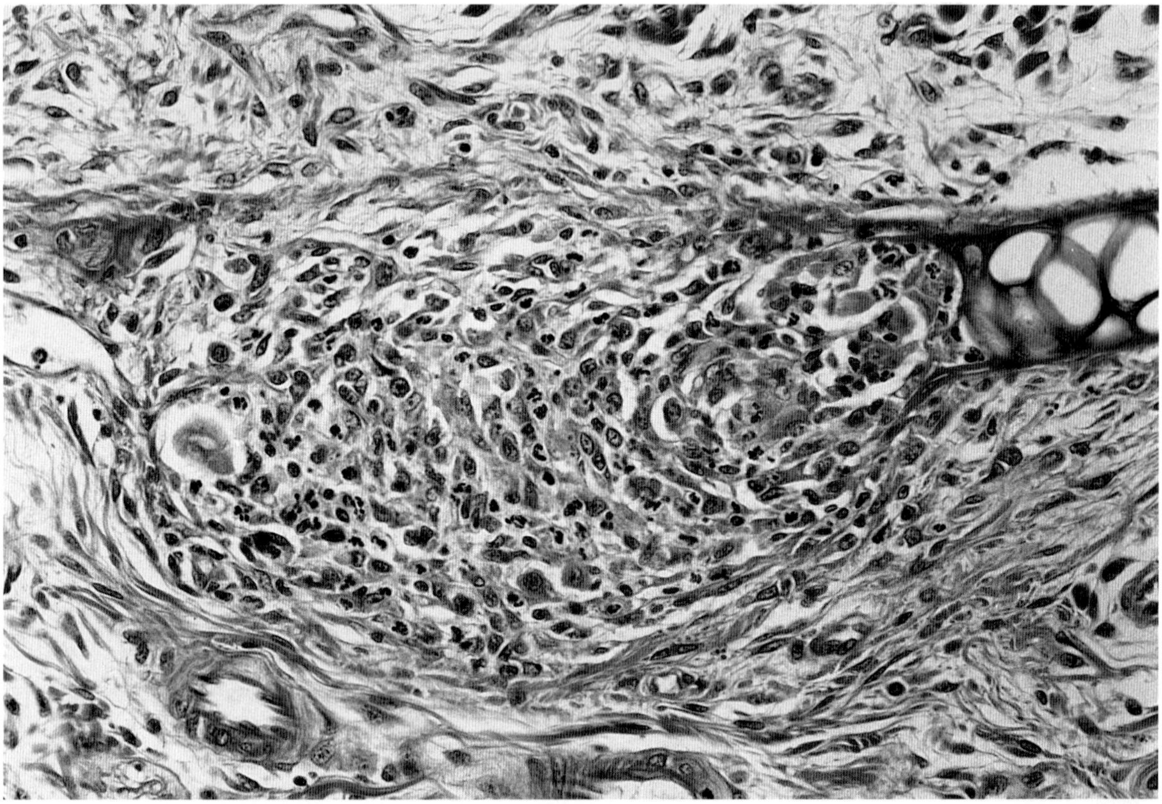

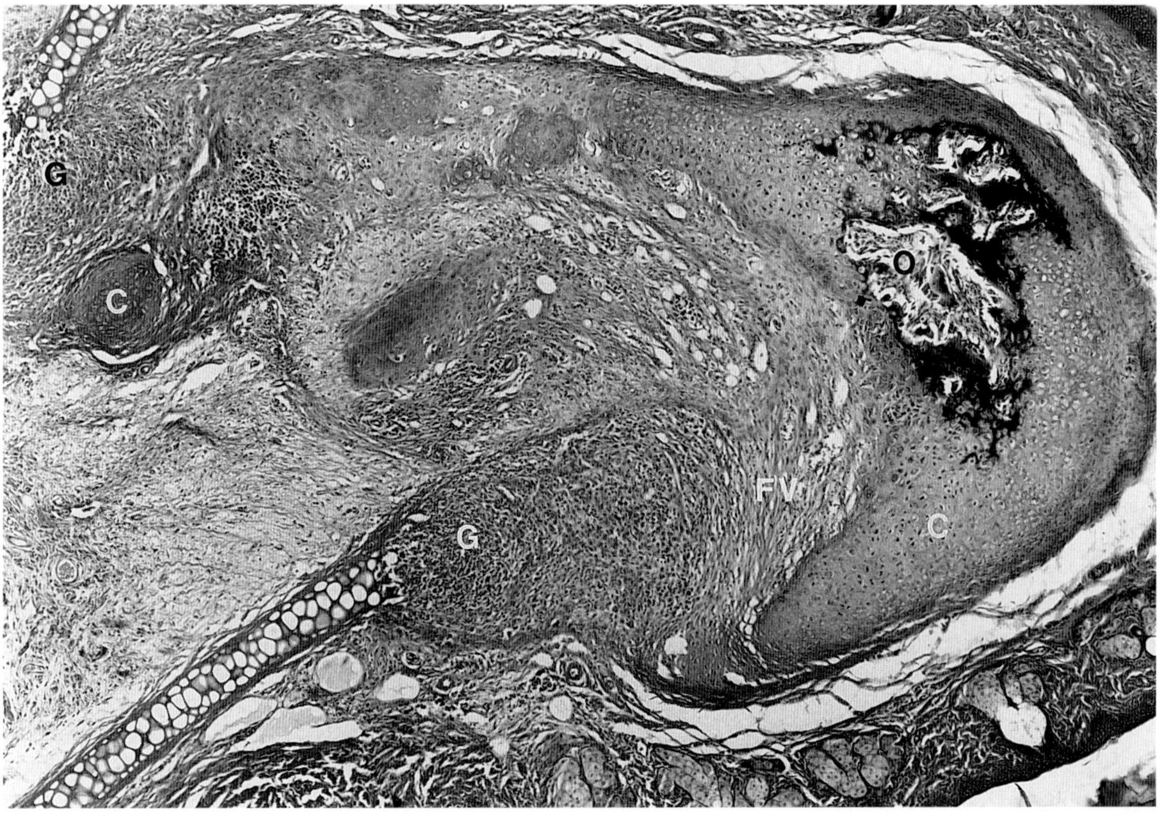

Fig. 135 *(above).* An early lesion of auricular chondritis, rat. Focal granulomatous inflammation involves an otherwise normal cartilage plate. No significant change is present in the surrounding tissues. H & E, ×400

Fig. 136 *(below).* An advanced lesion of auricular chondritis, rat. Note the sequential formation of various regenerative tissues – fibrovascular *(FV)*, chondrous *(C)*, and osseous tissues *(O)* – next to granulomatous *(G)* inflammation. H & E, ×66

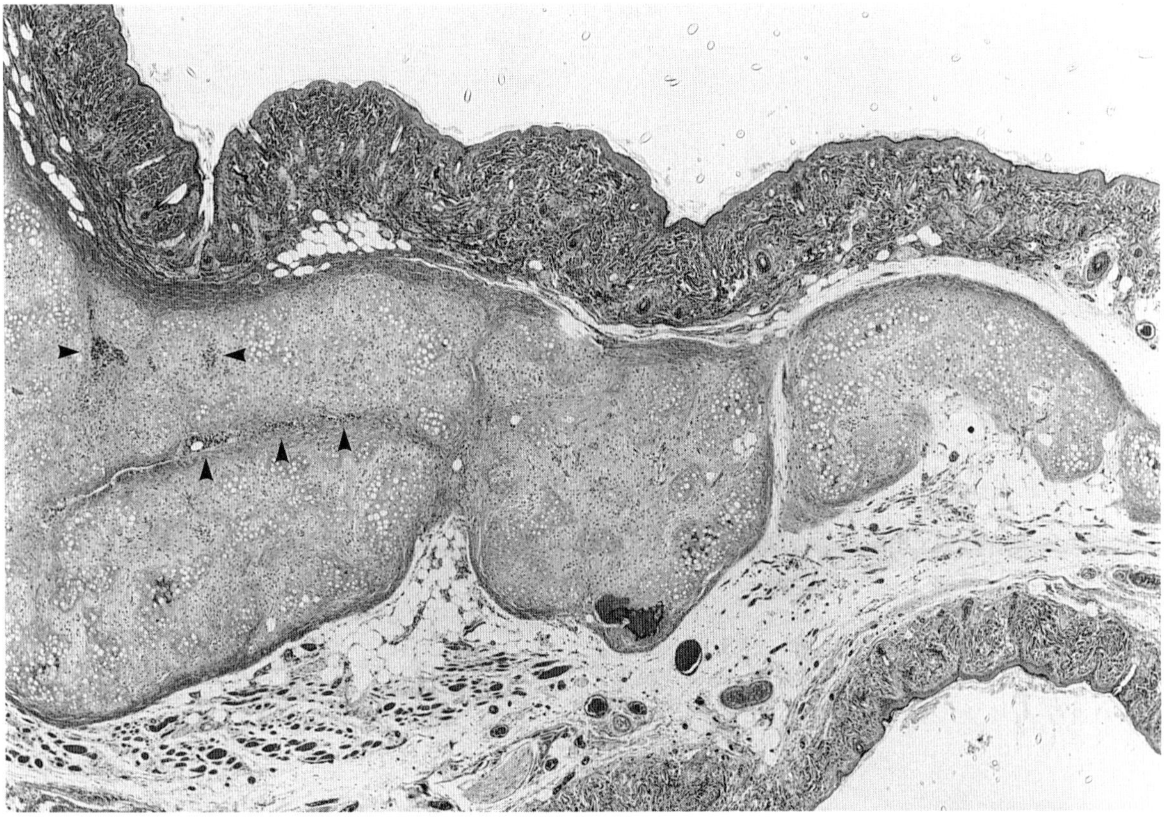

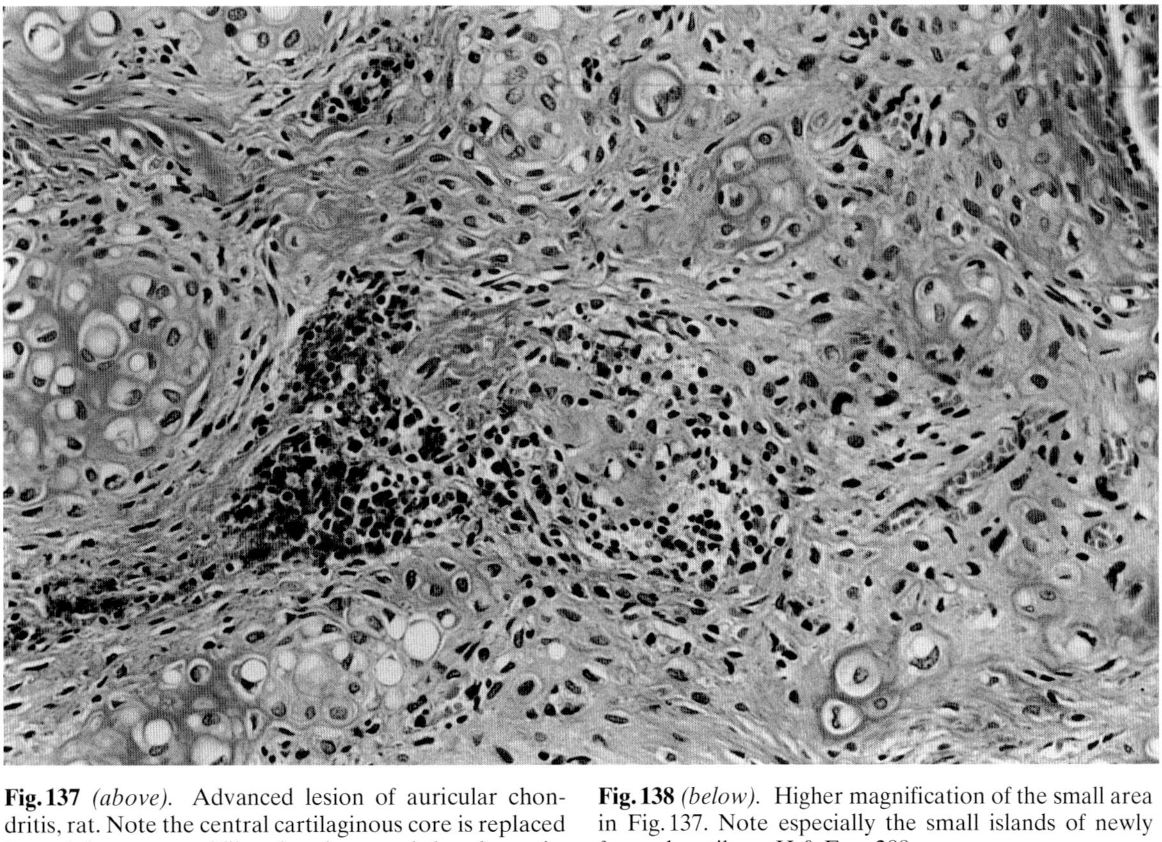

Fig. 137 *(above).* Advanced lesion of auricular chondritis, rat. Note the central cartilaginous core is replaced by nodular masses of fibrochondrous and chondrous tissues. Focal mononuclear cell infiltrates *(arrowheads)* are scattered in the mass. H & E, ×40

Fig. 138 *(below).* Higher magnification of the small area in Fig. 137. Note especially the small islands of newly formed cartilage. H & E, ×288

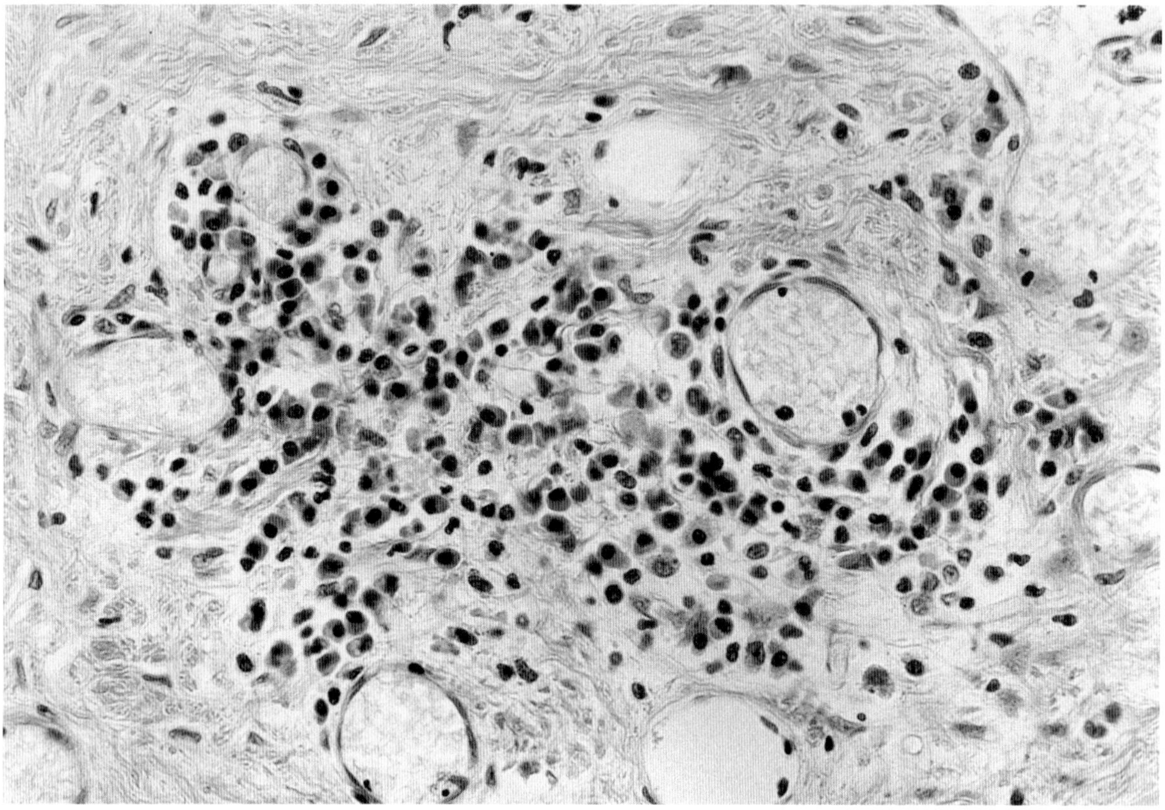

Fig. 139. Advanced auricular chondritis, rat. Higher magnification of a small area of lesion in Fig. 137. Note distended capillaries and mononuclear cell infiltrate, mostly plasma cells. H & E, ×500

boratories, Wilmington, Massachusetts, was reported to be 98 of 2733 (3.6%) males and 82 of 2148 (3.8%) females (Chiu and Lee 1984). However, outbred S–D rats, obtained in recent years from the Kingston, New York, branch of the Charles River Breeding Laboratories for use in long-term studies, had a significantly lower spontaneous incidence of similar gross auricular lesions: 8 of 2035 (0.4%) males and 15 of 2143 (0.7%) females (T-Chiu, unpublished data). Prieur et al. (1984) reported that the incidence was 4 of about 50 male and 22 of about 200 female inbred F–H rats, and 3 of about 200 female F–H x NBR rats. No cases of auricular chondritis were reported in about 700 rats of NBR, S–D, BD-IV, and BD–IX strains.

Experimentally induced auricular chondritis was generally noted between 27 and 106 days after injection of type II collagen (Cremer et al. 1981; McCune et al. 1982). The incidence was 12 of 88 (13.4%) in female outbred Wistar rats and 7 of 78 (9.0%) in female outbred S–D rats.

The unique and characteristic feature of the natural disease in rats is the selective involvement and destruction of the auricular cartilage by granulomatous inflammation.

The other cartilaginous tissues such as trachea, nasal turbinates, joints, and ribs are not affected by this inflammatory process, nor are the tissues surrounding the auricular cartilage significantly altered. The early lesions of the disease may regress since the swelling and erythema in some rats subsided and the ears appeared clinically normal for the remaining observation period in a 2-year study. A subsequent microscopic examination of the ear tissues revealed no lesions (T-Chiu, unpublished observations). In ears with chronic progressive change, microscopic lesions develop in a sequence of temporally distinct morphologic features. Focal or multifocal inflammatory lesions arise at the perichondrium of otherwise normal auricular cartilage. A continuous destruction of the cartilage tissue by the inflammatory process leads to a subsequent formation of regenerative tissues (see "Microscopic Features"), which results in a nodular and thickened appearance of the ears. The periphery of the cartilage plate is usually less severely affected.

A recurrence of the inflammatory reaction has not been reported in rats. Despite variable erythematous swelling of the affected pinnae, the lesions do not appear to be warm, painful, or pruritic; nor does the disease appear to affect the general condition or life of the animals. The etiology of the naturally occurring disease is unknown. It is unrelated to whether animals are used in feeding or inhalation studies, trauma from ear marking, or infectious agents (Chiu and Lee 1984). The disease has been regarded as an autoimmune disorder since ear lesions developed in rats experimentally immunized with type II collagen. There was a positive immunofluorescence reaction using antibodies to fibrinogen, IgG, and C3 in the inflammatory infiltrate (McCune et al. 1982) and in the cartilaginous matrix near the perichondrium adjacent to the chondrocytes from the clinically normal areas, except antifibrinogen (Cremer et al. 1981). The location of these positive reactions corresponded to the areas of electron-dense deposits observed ultrastructurally. Similar immunologic studies in the natural disease have not been reported.

Since the disease occurs naturally and is induced experimentally in certain strains of rats and the incidence of the natural disease varies with the source of animals, genetic factors may play a role in the development of the disease. Furthermore, since the disease involves only the auricular cartilage and is only seen in young adult and older rats, the biochemical nature of auricular cartilage and the age of animals may also be contributory factors in the pathogenesis of the lesion.

Comparison with Other Species

This auricular disease has not been described in other animal species although inflammation may involve the auricular cartilage as an extension of dermatitis. Auricular chondritis in rats has some resemblance to that in man in clinical, biologic, and microscopic features but there are differences. This uncommon human external ear disease has been recognized for many years and is frequently associates with relapsing polychondritis (see Michet et al. 1986). The ear lesions are bilateral and occur without a sexual predisposition in adults and, rarely, children. In the acute phase of the disease, the affected external ears are swollen, red to violaceous, tendcr, warm, and severely painful. The acute episode is recurrent. In the chronic phase, the ears are misshapen. The etiology of this disease in humans is still unknown but a collagen autoimmune disease has been considered for many years (see Homma et al. 1984 and Stuart et al. 1982). A defect of perichondrial cells (Linck et al. 1981) has been suggested to be the initial cause of the inflammatory reaction.

Acknowledgment. The author wishes to thank Dr. William C. Krauss for his kind comments on the manuscript.

Addendum. Since the submission of this manuscript, a report of spontaneous disease in Wistar rats has been published (McEwen and Barsoum 1990).

References

Chiu T, Lee KP (1984) Auricular chondropathy in aging rats. Vet Pathol 21: 500–504

Cremer MA, Pitcock JA, Stuart JM, Kang AH, Townes AS (1981) Auricular Chondritis in rats. An experimental model of relapsing polychondritis induced with type II collagen. J Exp Med 154: 535–540

Enomoto A, Harada T, Maita K, Shirasu Y (1983) Auricular cystic lesions of the external ear in Sprague-Dawley rats. Jpn J Vet Sci 45: 695–698

Homma S, Matusmoto T, Abe H, Fukuda Y, Nagano M, Suzuki M (1984) Relapsing polychondritis. Pathological and immunological findings in an autopsy case. Acta Pathol Jpn 34: 1137–1146

Michet CJ Jr., McKenna CH, Luthra HS, O'Fallon WM (1986) Relapsing polychondritis. Survival and predictive role of early manifestations. Ann Intern Med 104: 74–78

Linck G, Porte A, Mantz JM, Tempe JD, Jaeger A, Hauber C, Batzenschlager A (1981) Light and electron microscopic study of ear cartilage in a case of relapsing polychondritis evolving under corticoid treatment. Virchows Arch [Pathol Anat] 391: 301–308

McCune WJ, Schiller AL, Dynesius-Trentham RA, Trebtham DE (1982) Type II collagen-induced auricular chondritis. Arthritis Rheum 25: 266–273

McEwen BJ, Barsoum NJ (1990) Auricular chondritis in Wistar rats. Lab Anim 24: 280–283

Prieur DJ, Young DM, Counts DF (1984) Auricular chondritis in fawn hooded rats. A spontaneous disorder resembling that induced by immunization with type II collagen. Am J Pathol 116: 69–76

Stuart JM, Townes AS, Kang AH (1982) The role of collagen autoimmunity in animal models and human diseases. J Invest Dermatol 79 [Suppl 1]: 121S–127 S

Cholesteatoma, Aural, Gerbil

G.H. Hottendorf

Synonyms. Aural keratoma, epidermoid cholesteatoma.

Gross Appearance

A firm nodule may protrude from the external ear canal. The tympanic bulla may be thickened and filled with a gray, dry material (Schiffer et al. 1986).

Microscopic Features

Cholesteatoma is a term introduced in 1829 to describe "pearly tumors" (O'Donogbue 1986). Cholesteatoma is keratinizing stratified squamous epithelium on a layer of connective tissue; these two tissues comprise the "matrix" (Schechter 1969). No pilosebaceous units are present in the subepidermal tissue but distinct basal and prickle cells as well as rete pegs can be seen in the epidermis. Because of the continuing production of keratin within the confines of the middle ear, a mass composed primarily of accumulated keratin results (Fig. 140), which may erode bone of the ear canal and labyrinth. Microscopically, cholesteatomas resemble epidermal inclusion cysts (Balogh 1988).

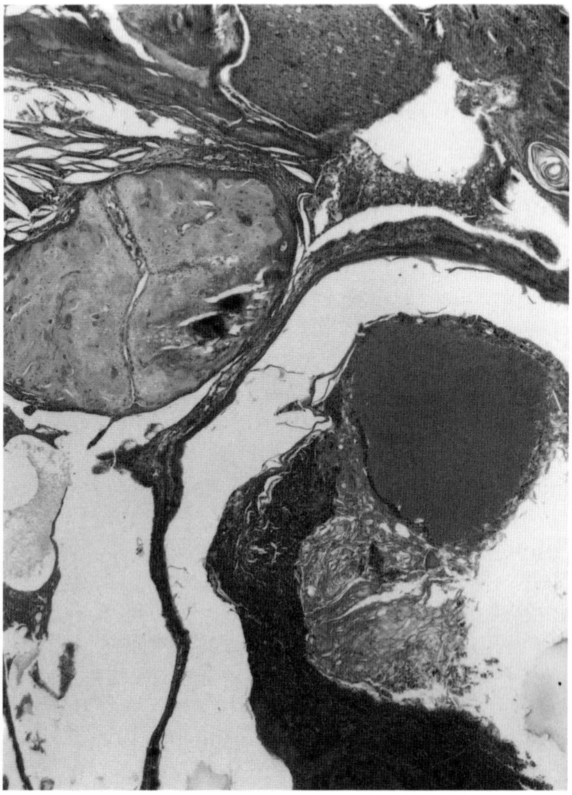

Fig. 140. A predominantly keratin mass in the external meatus *(lower right)* protrudes into the middle ear preceded by the tympanic membrane. The head of the malleus reveals erosion at the interface with the tympanic membrane. The middle ear contains inflammatory debris and cholesterol clefts. A small "microcholesteatoma" is present in the *upper right*

Ultrastructure

The ultrastructural morphology basically represents the observations made with the light microscope with the following exceptions. There are transitional cells of unknown origin at the junction between the migrating squamous epidermis of the cholesteatoma and the normal mucosal cells of the middle ear (Jackson and Lim 1978). The epidermis of human cholesteatomas contains Langerhans' cells and T lymphocytes, which are not present in normal tympanic membrane epidermis. This observation suggests that an immunologic mechanism may be involved in the pathogenesis of this common lesion of human ears (Van Dijk et al. 1986).

Differential Diagnosis

Grossly, the masses protruding in the external ear canal could be confuses with squamous cell carcinomas reported in aged *Meriones libycus* (Rowe et al. 1974). Microscopically, however, the differentiation of the lesions should be more obvious. Granulation tissue and cholesterol clefts may occur in associated sites of chronic inflammation and hemorrhage at various locations.

Biologic Features

The neoplastic nature of this lesion is under debate. In a recently published human pathology text, for example, cholesteatomas are discussed with the inflammatory lesions and not with tumors of the ear (Balogh 1988). The keratinizing squamous epithelium that characterizes the aural lesion does grow, migrate, and expand in order to form a cholesteatoma. This growth may be primarily a response to inflammation, however (Jackson and Lim 1978). A cholesterol-containing lesion in the choroid plexus of horses has been called cholesteatoma but preferably should be designated a cholesterinic granuloma (Jones et Hunt 1983). Cholesteatomas arise spontaneously and can be experimentally induced in gerbils (McGinn et al. 1982; Henry et al. 1983) Cholesteatomas are often associated with tilting of the head to the affectes side in this species (Schiffer et al. 1986). The spontaneous gerbilline cholesteatomas are age related (Fig. 14) and the presence of these masses may be indicated by an increase in the peripheral auditory evoked potential threshold, a parameter of auditory dysfunction (Henry et al. 1983). The lesion can be experimentally induced in Mongolian gerbils *(Meriones unguiculatus)* by surgical ligation of the external auditory canal (McGinn et al. 1982) and these experimentally induced lesions are identical with spontaneous gerbilline cholesteatomas (McGinn et al. 1984). The pathogenesis of spontaneous aural cholesteatomas in gerbils and man involves the expansion of hyperplastic squamous epithelium in a confined space, the middle ear, with subsequent erosion of the ear canal and labyrinth (McGinn et al. 1984). In man, three main, pathogenic theories have been proposed (O'Donoghue 1986). The congenital theory invokes embryonic cell rests as the source of primary (congenital) cholesteatomas. Congenital cholesteatoma can be defined as a collection of squamous epithelium found behind an intact tympanic membrane in the absence of previous infection or perforation of the tympanic membrane. This entrapped epithelium may be present for years before producing symptoms (Lipkin et al. 1986). The metaplastic theory proposes squamous metaplasia of middle ear mucosa as the origin of secondary (acquired) cholesteatomas. The invasive or migration theories of secondary cholesteatoma formation invoke migration of squamous epithelium from the external canal through the tympanic membrane.

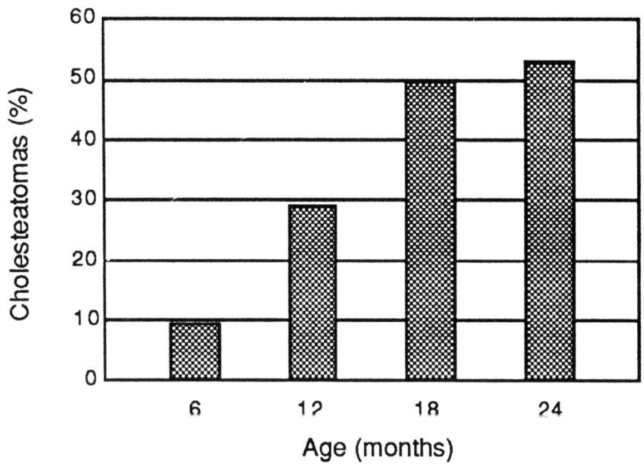

Fig. 141. Age-related frequency of aural cholesteatomas in Mongolian gerbils. (Henry et al. 1983)

Whichever, if any, of these theories might apply to gerbils is unknown. The mechanism of aural cholesteatoma formation in the gerbil apparently involves the failure of clearance of keratin from the squamous epithelium on the tympanic membrane and in the external auditory canal (Henry et al. 1983). Various formation stages of spontaneous aural cholesteatoma in gerbils have been described (McGinn et al. 1984). Stage I represents the accumulation of keratin debris on the outside surface of the tympanic membrane. Stage II results from the continued accumulation of keratin which displaces the tympanic membrane medially into the middle ear; bone resorption in the bony portion of the external auditory canal may begin at this stage. Contact of the expanding cholesteatoma with the prominence of the cochlea occurs in stage III. Stage IV represents the filling of the bulla by the predominantly keratin mass and stage V involves the intracranial extension of the cholesteatoma.

Comparison with Other Species

Aural cholesteatoma is a common lesion of the middle ear of man associated with subsequent hearing loss, recurrent infections, and intracranial complications (Schiffer et al. 1986). The morphologic and biologic characteristics of the gerbilline cholesteatoma closely mimic human cholesteatoma (Jackson and Lim 1978; Henry et al. 1983; McGinn et al. 1982). Although the Mongolian gerbil has been alleged to be the only nonhuman animal to spontaneously develop aural cholesteatomas (Henry et al. 1983; Schiffer et al. 1986), spontaneous cholesteatomas have been reported in rabbits and guinea pigs (Kelemen 1978). When placed in the ear, various irritants will produce cholesteatoma in several species (Steinbach and Grüninger 1980). Mere surgical ligation of the external auditory canal will produce aural cholesteatomas in gerbils and rabbits, but not in cats, guinea pigs, hamsters, mice, and rats (McGinn et al. 1984).

References

Balogh K (1988) The head and neck. In: Rubin E. Farber JL (eds) Pathology. Lippincott, Philadelphia, pp 1297–1299

Henry KR, Chole RA, McGinn MD (1983) Age-related increase of spontaneous aural cholesteatoma in the Mongolian gerbil. Arch Otolaryngol 109: 19–21

Jackson DG, Lim DJ (1978) Fine morphology of the advancing front of cholesteatoma – experimental and human. Acta Otolaryngol 86: 71–88

Jones TC, Hunt RD (1983) Veterinary pathology, 5th edn. Lea and Febiger, Philadelphia, p 1682

Kelemen G (1978) Diseases of the ear. In: Benirschke K, Garner FM, Jones TC (eds) Pathology of laboratory animals, vol I. Springer, Berlin Heidelberg New York, pp 628–629

Lipkin AF, Coker NJ, Jenkins HA (1986) Hereditary congenital cholesteatoma. A variant of broncho-oto dysplasia. Arch Otolaryngol Head Neck Surg 112: 1097–1100

McGinn MD, Chole RA, Henry KD (1982) Cholesteatoma, experimental induction in the Mongolian gerbil, *Meriones unguiculatus*. Acta Otolaryngol 93: 61–67

McGinn MD, Chole RA, Henry KR (1984) Cholesteatoma induction. Consequences of external auditory canal ligation in gerbils, cats, hamsters, guinea pigs, mice and rats. Acta Otolaryngol 97: 297–304

O'Donoghue GM (1986) The migration theory of cholesteatoma formation. Some experimental observations. J Laryngol Otol 100: 395–398

Rowe SE, Simmons JL, Ringler DH, Lay DM (1974) Spontaneous neoplasms in aging gerbillinae. A summary of forty-four neoplasms. Vet Pathol 11: 38–51

Schechter G (1969) A review of cholesteatoma pathology. Laryngoscope 79: 1907–1920

Schiffer SP, Lukas VS, Chrisp CE (1986) Diagnostic exercise: head tilt in a gerbil. Lab Anim Sci 36: 176–177

Steinbach E, Grüninger G (1980) Experimental production of cholesteatoma in rabbits by using non-irritants (skin tolerants). J. Laryngol Otol 94: 269–279

Van Dijk CM, Visser CE, Veldman JE (1986) Spatial distribution of Langerhans' cells and T-lymphocyte subpopulations in human tympanic membrane and aural cholesteatoma. Virchows Arch [B] 52: 143–152

Subject Index*

---

* Page numbers in **boldface** indicate the principal discussion; Figures are designated by the letter "f" following the page number; Tables are found on page numbers followed by the letter "t".